To ·Tish
Dec. 1968

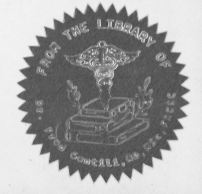

BLOOD FLOW IN ARTERIES

MONOGRAPHS OF THE PHYSIOLOGICAL SOCIETY

Number 7

Editors: H. Barcroft, A. L. Hodgkin, W. D. M. Paton

BLOOD FLOW IN ARTERIES

by

DONALD A. McDONALD

M.A., D.M.(Oxon.), D.Sc.(Lond.)

Reader in Physiology in the University of London
at the Medical College of St. Bartholomew's Hospital, London

LONDON

EDWARD ARNOLD (PUBLISHERS) LTD.

PRINTED IN GREAT BRITAIN
BY W. & J. MACKAY & CO. LTD., CHATHAM

To the memory of my friend

JOHN RONALD WOMERSLEY

(Born June 20, 1907; died in Columbus, Ohio
March 7, 1958)

ACKNOWLEDGMENTS

The goddess of Chance is rarely thanked on occasions such as this. I am sure that this is not so much due to the ingratitude of scientists as to the fact that she plays some part in starting almost any research. In my case her interventions have been so helpful and so perfectly timed that I feel I must pay her homage. For, although this book appears under my name alone, it could never have been written—for there would have been little of any value to write about—without the immense help I have had from my principal collaborators, John Womersley and Michael Taylor.

My interest in the present subject arose from the chance observation of streamline flow in the basilar artery of the rabbit (Fig. 4.2). This was in the course of a severely "practical" research, with Dr. (now Mr.) J. M. Potter, into some problems arising from cerebral radioangiography. This led to the use of high-speed cinematography as the only method we could think of to measure the flow velocity in the basilar artery. I then thought it would be interesting to exploit the technique in a study of pulsatile flow in other systemic arteries—sliding, as it were, into circulatory physiology down the vertebral arteries.

In 1949, and again in 1951, I had the honour to work with Prof. W. R. Hess in Zürich (on neurophysiological problems) and although his own great contributions to circulatory physics were made many years ago he gave me most stimulating help in this field, for which, and for his continuing encouragement, I am most grateful.

The collection of records of pulsatile flow velocity in arteries was interesting but proved unsatisfying because their interpretation was difficult in the absence of a quantitative method of analysis. Progress was only achieved when I had the great good fortune to arouse the interest and enthusiasm of that distinguished mathematician, the late J. R. Womersley, in these problems.

Womersley's career has been so well described by Sir Charles Darwin in his Obituary notice (*Nature*, 3 May 1958) that I need say little of it, except that he had a wide experience in many fields of applied mathematics and so was thoroughly familiar with the experimental approach so necessary in this type of work. Quite apart from the most valuable analyses he did, and the stimulation of his personality as a friend, the three years over which we collaborated were a most valuable experience in the problems of working with someone trained in a different scientific discipline. Long periods of discussion during the first eighteen months of our collaboration (during which Womersley only had his leisure hours to devote to it) were necessary before I could formulate the physiological problems in a way that would make physical sense. Equally it was a long time before he knew enough about the physiology of the circulation to tackle it in a realistic way. Once the main objectives were clearly seen, advance was very rapid, especially as he was able to spend a whole year in this department (June 1954–55) supported by a personal grant from the Medical Research Council. I feel that unless colleagues from the physical sciences are prepared to spend a comparable amount of time in learning some physiology, then the value of such collaboration will always be limited. This field is littered with abstract analyses of the circulation by talented mathematicians which are of slight use because they have little contact with physiological reality. If only brief consultations are available, then my own experience indicates that we, as physiologists, must first get the problem into a mathematical form and use, as it were, our colleague as a translator, skilled in a language we cannot handle with any fluency. For no mathematical treatment is ever better than the primary assumptions on which it is based.

Womersley went to the U.S.A. in 1955 but good luck was still with me for, six months earlier, Dr. Michael Taylor had one day arrived on the doorstep (unannounced from Adelaide), asking if he could work at Bart's for a year during the tenure of a C. J. Martin Research Fellowship. He was thus able to spend a few months in collaboration with John Womersley before the latter's departure. While he remained in England my problems of collaborating with expert mathematicians were over. Taylor, with a training in medicine and physiological research has also a passion for mathematics such that he is technically the equal of many professionals in this field. If I do not here sufficiently express my admiration and gratitude for his contribution to this work it is only because, while we are exhorted to speak only good of the dead, it is deemed fulsome (or at least un-English) to speak too well of the living—especially one's close friends. Let it suffice to say that the organization of the ideas on wave reflection and arterial input impedance (the chapters in the latter part of this book) are almost entirely due to discussions with him. In addition the whole text has been subjected to his critical scrutiny—but I should also apologize to him for not always acceding to his demands for more rigour (in the mathematical sense); any inaccuracies that physicists may find will almost certainly be due to my omissions, for the sake of simplicity, of this kind.

To Professor K. J. Franklin F.R.S. I owe a debt of gratitude for over twenty years of teaching and encouragement. I am also very grateful to John Potter, Peter Helps and John Hale who in the past ten years have severally been most helpful colleagues, and to Derek Bergel who is here at present. Thanks are also freely offered to Miss Mary Morse for typing so painstakingly the many versions of the text, and to Mr. D. C. Moore for lettering and photographing the figures.

All the high-speed cinematography was done by Mr. John Hadland and his expert team, and financed by a grant over several years from the Medical Research Council (who also purchased essential apparatus); the most superficial perusal will show how fundamental this support was for this investigation. Photographic apparatus was also generously provided by the Central Research Fund of the University of London, and the counter-chronometer by the Research Fund of this Medical College.

An important part in the clarification of my ideas (however relative that term may appear) was due to the innumerable discussions I had with my American friends during a visit to the States in the later part of 1956. This tour was due to a most generous travelling Fellowship from the Rockefeller Foundation and to them, and especially to Dr. Pomerat, I offer very grateful thanks. To mention all the physiologists, and physicians, who helped me at that time, whether by providing additional data, or merely by vigorous dispute, would be impossibly long. I must, however, thank Dr. Sam Talbot, of Johns Hopkins, for reading the whole of the first draft of this book so carefully in October–November 1956, and for the advice he gave me. It was particularly stimulating in the U.S.A. to find that this work aroused interest in Departments of Medicine quite as often as in Departments of Biophysics, or of Physiology, in spite of the theoretical or "pure" nature of the research.

I am also very grateful for most helpful suggestions about the final draft from Dr. D. S. Parsons, Dr. L. E. Bayliss and Prof. H. Barcroft.

I am also grateful to the Editors of the *Journal of Physiology* and of *Physics in Medicine and Biology* for permission to use blocks from their publications.

Finally, may I thank all those who have allowed me to use their data either in the text, or as figures (with permission often belatedly sought). In the case of figures their names are given in the relevant legends—where there is no attribution figures are from original graphs of my own.

February 1960.

CONTENTS

CHAPTER I

INTRODUCTION

The most obvious feature of the "blood flow in arteries" is that it is pulsatile. Therefore the field of survey is the character of pulsatile flow and the physical laws governing it. This means that it will also comprehend the form of the pressure-wave of the pulse, both in relation to the flow and the means by which the pulse-wave (of flow as well as pressure) is propagated over the arterial system.

In trying to elucidate the fundamental physical properties of pulsatile flow I offer as justification the fact that circulatory physiology is turning to the measurement of pulsatile flow rather as the pioneers of a previous generation, such as Otto Frank and Carl Wiggers, embarked on the problem of measuring the pulsatile pressure changes in the cardiovascular system. There can be no question of the immense contribution to our understanding of the physiology of the circulation that the clarification of the theory and design of manometers has made. It is my belief that the study of the corresponding flow patterns can make as great, if not greater, contributions. The creation of a flow of blood and its transport to and from the tissues is, after all, the purpose of the cardiovascular system. The accompanying pressure changes, although intimately related to the flow, are essentially of secondary interest.

To interpret the discoveries made by the invention of manometers with adequate recording characteristics, Frank developed the concept of the arterial tree as a compression chamber and its mathematical and physical development, which is universally known in tribute to its German origin as the Windkessel theory, is a monument to the genius of Frank and the outstanding group of physiologists which were trained in his laboratory and others of that period. I do not intend here, however, to review the large field of literature that has been concerned with testing the original theory and its numerous modifications. This has already been done at great length by others, and reference should be made to Wezler and Böger (1939), Gomez (1941), Sinn (1956) and Wetterer (1954, 1956), while many textbooks—notably that by Wiggers (1949)—give short accounts of it.

The Windkessel theory was originated as a means of interpreting the pressure changes in the arterial system. Little was known of pulsatile flow at that time and the theoretical development of the theory since has never concerned itself to any extent with pressure-flow relationships in the arterial tree. This in itself would be no bar if it had been built on a sound physical basis, but many of its primary assumptions are so restrictive and many that have been added to it seem so directly contradictory that I feel it has outgrown its usefulness. Some of these misgivings as to the theoretical assumptions of the Windkessel have been discussed more fully by McDonald and Taylor (1959).

This book will attempt to outline in a simple way the analysis of the circulation as a system in a steady-state oscillation, based on standard principles of hydrodynamics. This requires very few initial assumptions; and approximations that are introduced can always be assessed as to their magnitude. Whether it is an improvement on the Windkessel theory time, and the consensus of opinion, will tell. Thus far it has proved very satisfactory, especially in dealing with the analysis of the relations between pressure and flow, which I consider to be of fundamental importance.

Some mathematics is necessary for the expression of these principles, but this has been kept to a minimum because I am aware that the training of the average physiologist, among whom I include myself, does not include any extensive mathematical course. For the derivation of the mathematical equations used the reader is referred to the original papers. Womersley (1958a) has collected all his personal contributions to the subject, and McDonald and Taylor (1959) have reviewed many of the topics discussed in this book with greater emphasis on the mathematical and physical aspects. The mathematics that are used in discussion are nowhere more advanced than for the syllabus of the Advanced level of the General Certificate of Education in use in English schools, principally in the use of complex numbers. These are quite adequately discussed in a popular best-seller by Hogben (1937), and Smith (1954) is also recommended as a good exposition of the subject for the non-specialist.

THE SCOPE OF THE PRESENT WORK

Described in its simplest form the circulation consists of a pump, the heart, which forces blood periodically into a branching system of elastic tubes. The pulsations generated travel centrifugally and are damped out by the time they reach the smallest branches, the capillaries, which are in intimate contact with the cells of the tissues. The blood then returns in a more or less steady stream to the heart. However, secondary pulsations are imposed on it as it approaches the heart, both from that organ itself and also from the intrathoracic changes in pressure due to respiration.

As already stated, the problems that are the main theme of this book are those concerned with pulsatile flow and the pulsatile pressure changes associated with it. Thus it is mainly concerned with flow in arteries; but where the fundamental physical laws governing this type of flow have been determined they will be equally applicable to pulsatile, that is non-steady or oscillating, flow in veins, and with little modification can be applied to the oscillatory flow of air in the trachea. The physical interpretation of the function of the cardiac pump is not, however, being attempted here. It will be seen that although we start, as it were, at the aortic valves and do not consider in any detail the smallest vessels, the hydrodynamics to be discussed are those concerned throughout the whole peripheral circulation.

Oscillatory, or pulsatile, flow of liquids has received little attention from physicists compared with the tremendous volume of work on steady flow. Circulatory physiology can thus, to a certain extent, congratulate itself on initiating interest in this field. But quite apart from the far from easy solution of the characteristics of oscillatory flow in elastic pipes the circulation in the animal adds other problems. To recapitulate some of these: the blood has anomalous viscous properties owing to the fact that it is a suspension of particles in a colloid solution. The flow-ejection pattern of the heart is complex and the elastic properties of the arteries are non-linear; furthermore the geometry of the branching arterial tree lacks any simple pattern. To analyse such a system it is necessary to simplify. This simplification either can take the form of an analogue model to represent the behaviour of the whole circulation or analyse individual sections of the circulation and attempt to build up a synthesis of the whole from component parts. Of the analogues the "Windkessel" has completely dominated the field.

The alternative approach of building from the investigation of single regions began, in my own case, experimentally with the measurement of phasic flow in arteries at the beginning of the present decade (Potter and McDonald, 1950, McDonald, 1952*a*), but only developed physical and mathematical direction with the collaboration of J. R. Womersley in 1953 (Womersley, 1954; Helps and McDonald, 1954*b*). The first step was the analysis of the pulsatile pressure-flow relationship in the femoral artery, hence in the vascular bed of one limb. For this analysis no model analogies were made but it was treated as a problem in hydrodynamics. The simplifications introduced were effected by making approximations. In this case the first approximation was to neglect the pulsatile variation in arterial diameter. Further investigations were then carried out to show that this dilatation was in fact small and the mathematical analysis was extended to take this into account. This and subsequent work (see Ch. 9) has in fact shown that this first-order approximation is satisfactory until techniques of flow recording are greatly improved in accuracy (Ch. 6). It was also assumed that the flow was laminar throughout the cardiac cycle. There was definite experimental evidence for this in the femoral artery but it remains a questionable point in large arteries (Ch. 3).

The most important innovation made in Womersley's analysis was in the use of the Fourier series to give a numerical description of the pulse wave. This has proved so valuable that it may be regarded as the keystone of the system of physical analysis of the circulation that we have been building. While this is a very widely used method of analysing periodic phenomena in the physical sciences it appears to be relatively unfamiliar to many physiologists. As constant reference will be made to Fourier analysis in the later chapters of this book it needs to be discussed at further length.

FLOW AND PRESSURE PULSATIONS AS "STEADY-STATE" PHENOMENA

In any attempt to apply mathematical techniques to the circulation it is obvious that we must be able to describe the phenomena we are studying in such a way that we can attach numerical values to them. In the case of the pressure wave generated by the heart this appears to be a difficult problem, and no agreement has been reached as to how it should be done. Indeed in the very extensive literature on the subject most authors have contented themselves with describing the shape of the pulse wave in purely literary descriptive terms such as the "foot", the "peak", "anacrotic wave", "dicrotic notch", etc. This is clearly unsatisfactory from the analytical point of view, however familiar it may be in conveying information from one worker to another.

In terms of physical and mathematical practice a wave is either regarded as an isolated phenomenon or as a repetitive one. That is, it is a transient response, or it is a periodic oscillation. As the mathematical description of a periodic oscillation is simpler than that of a transient it would be reasonable to suppose that it was the preferred approach, provided that it is valid. Now the regularity of the heart beat is one of its most characteristic features, and, in terms of the length of an individual pulse, this regularity is normally maintained for a very long time. This is a condition of "steady-state" oscillation. Under these circumstances any wave that is repeated regularly can be represented by a Fourier series, that is, the shape can be described as the sum of a set of sinusoidal waves whose frequencies are all integral multiples of the frequency of repetition of the wave.

The *Fourier series* and the method of performing a Fourier analysis is described more precisely in Appendix 1. It is familiar to most people in terms of the harmonic analysis of musical sounds, a connection that is emphasized by the use of phrases such as "harmonic components" or "overtones". In physiology it is generally accepted as a basis for determining the frequency response of manometers used for recording arterial pressure pulses (see Ch. 11). It is, therefore, logical to extend its use to the flow pulse and the physical relation between pulsatile pressure and flow. It has the advantage of dealing with simple harmonic motion which, mathematically, is the most tractable form of oscillatory motion and the synthesized curve is a simple sum of the component harmonic terms.

This property of summation of its component terms is one reason for its outstanding usefulness in describing curves. From this derives the important practical property of the series that the curve described by a certain number of terms is the best approximation possible for that number of terms. Computing further terms will only improve the fit where it is faulty, and does not require any alteration in the dimensions of the lower harmonics. In applying it to the circulation certain approximations have to be made. In the first place there are irregularities in the pulse frequency. As it is a required condition for the Fourier series that the system should be in a "steady-state" any alteration in frequency must be allowed to settle down, just as the conditions due to starting up in a system must have disappeared before a steady-state is attained. The rapidity with which a steady-state is attained depends largely on the damping in the system which is being driven (see Appendix 2) and in the arterial system of a dog we have evidence (Fig. 12.2) that it is attained within 1 second, and probably in 0·5 sec, i.e. once the pulse has been regular for 2–3 beats at most. A more complex difficulty arises over the question of non-linearity. The circulation is not a linear system so that, although a Fourier series may represent a pressure pulse, or a flow pulse, accurately one cannot, strictly speaking, say that one harmonic term of the pressure is only related to the corresponding harmonic term of the flow. The harmonic components interact with one another. This non-linear effect has been calculated by Womersley (1958a) in respect of the motion of the blood and found to be small enough to be regarded as negligible in a first-order approximation.

The physical reality of the Fourier representation of impulses of complex shape has often been debated. The apparent artificiality of the statement that the only frequencies represented are integral multiples of the fundamental frequency suggests to the sceptic that this is merely a mathematical device. Yet it can easily be seen that if frequencies other than integral multiples were present they would not repeat at the fundamental interval and so successive waves would not be of the same form, which denies the condition for applying the analysis. Put in another way, this means that the cyclical period to be analysed must be one in which the whole pattern is exactly repeated, and this may not, in the circulation, be the cardiac cycle but may, for instance, in venous flow patterns, be the respiratory cycle. Provided that such reservations are made, the validity of Fourier analysis in problems such as pulsatile flow is amply established by its experimental value in such diverse fields as electrical engineering and acoustical physics.

THE PULSE AS A "TRANSIENT" PHENOMENON

It was stated above that a description of the pulse, alternative to that of the steady-state oscillation, could be in terms of an isolated, transient phenomenon. That is to say the arterial system can be regarded as coming to rest by the end of diastole so that the next heart beat excites the system entirely anew. This approach has been taken by the great majority of workers investigating the behaviour of the pulse wave. Unfortunately no one has applied the full mathematical analysis of transient impulses to the pulse form so that it is impossible, at present, to assess the potentialities of the method. The form of analysis corresponding to the Fourier series for the periodic oscillation is that of the Fourier integral. Whereas in the series we deal only with components at discrete frequencies, for a single impulse we have to consider a continuous range of frequencies from zero to infinity and integrate them.

The Fourier integral is used in transient analysis in other branches of physics and there seems no fundamental reason why it should not be used in describing transients in the circulation except that it is rather intractable for computation. It is described fully in mathematical books to which the reader should refer (Goldmann, 1949).

Attempts have been made to describe the pulse as a transient in a somewhat simpler form. Taylor and Womersley (unpublished) devised a method whereby a curve such as that of the pulse wave could be described as a set of exponential curves. The values of the exponential terms were extracted as the roots of a difference equation. A satisfactory fit was not, however, achieved and Taylor (1956) has suggested that this is due to the discontinuity inherent in the curve, owing to the fact that the pressure wave is generated by an impulse (ventricular systole) that only lasts for part of the cycle. Apart from this investigation I know of no other detailed attempt to describe the actual form of the pulse wave mathematically in transient terms, although Frank (1927) discussed the applicability of the Fourier integral and series. It would be of great value to have contributions by mathematicians and physicists with especial experience in this field.

This type of circulatory analysis requires that a hypothetical "model" should be set up. As mentioned above, the one that has, in one form or another, virtually monopolized the field is that of the "Windkessel" or arterial compression chamber. Originally the idea was due to Stephen Hales (1677–1761) who first pointed out in his book *Haemostaticks* that the expansion of the arteries in systole and their elastic recoil in diastole played an important part in determining the arterial blood-pressure. The anonymous author of the first German translation added an explanatory footnote comparing this effect with the air-compression chamber (windkessel) in the pumping apparatus of a fire engine. From a descriptive and picturesque analogy the concept was made into a mathematical model by Otto Frank and his pupils in a long series of papers in the first three decades of this century. In its simplest form the arterial tree was arbitrarily divided into an expansile elastic portion, the windkessel, and the peripheral arteries which acted simply as conduits. The windkessel was treated as a single chamber, that is a lumped system, and wave-transmission along it was neglected in the sense that it was regarded as infinitely fast. Much of the experimental work of this school has been devoted to determining the length of the windkessel, that is the arteries that should be included in it. This has been reviewed by Wezler and Böger (1939) who concluded that, at rest, it included the whole of the aorta and terminated posteriorly about the middle of the iliac arteries. This estimate is derived from the wave-length of the secondary waves in the pulse which are, ex-hypothesi, due to incompletely damped oscillations of the windkessel. The definition of the length of the windkessel as a fraction of the wave-length of the resonant oscillation seems a contradiction of the first assumption that the wave travels over the system infinitely fast. As a result the length of the windkessel varies greatly with changes in vasomotor activity. For example, under the influence of adrenaline it lengthens a great deal, and it is difficult to understand how an elastic chamber can expand and contract in this way under the influence of drugs. The mathematical model has been modified by many workers to make it more realistic. Apéria (1940) has reviewed all these in detail and improved the theory by introducing a consideration of wave-transmission (his "undulatory" theory). His monograph is the most comprehensive one there is in English, although its accuracy has been questioned by Broemser *et al.* (1943). This is, unfortunately, far too wide a field to discuss here. Some reference to it is made in Chapter 10 which is concerned with the interpretation of wave-reflection.

The analysis of the pulse in transient terms has been made in a more practical way by Peterson (1952, 1954) by studying the effects on the arterial pulse of an injected pulse of known volume and velocity. The lack of precise knowledge as to the form of the systolic ejection of blood is one of the principal difficulties in making a full physical interpretation of pressure changes in the arterial system. The technique of using an artificial injection of known parameters is clearly an important advance, but difficulties in interpreting Peterson's results emphasize the difficulties inherent in the analysis of transients. Peterson (1954) and Peterson and Sheppard (1955) have also built models of "windkessels" and criticized the errors inherent in this concept. Interesting results have also been obtained by Starr (technical description— Starr *et al.*, 1953; Starr 1957) in which he simulates one cardiac ejection in a cadaver by a blow from a heavy pendulum on to the plunger of a syringe placed in the aorta.

THE PLAN OF THE SURVEY

The circulatory problems that are discussed in the following chapters fall under three main headings. (1) The nature of the flow in blood-vessels and the questions as to where this may be laminar or if there are any regions where the flow is wholly turbulent (Chs. 2, 3 and 4). These problems are not only of interest in relation to methods of measuring blood flow and the production of heart sounds and murmurs, but form an important starting-point in evaluating the pressure-flow relationships in the blood-vessels. This forms section (2) and is considered especially in Ch. 5. The technical investigation of this in the circulation is bound up with the problems of flow meter design (Ch. 6) and is followed by a survey of present knowledge as to pulsatile flow patterns (Ch. 7). Section (3) is primarily concerned with wave-propagation in the arterial system (Chs. 8, 9, 10 and 11). The elastic properties of the arterial wall are reviewed and then a consideration is made of the properties of wave-propagation in an elastic tube filled with a viscous liquid. This problem (Ch. 9) is almost impossible to investigate in the circulation because of the presence of reflected waves, but nevertheless it is necessary to consider the theoretical analysis and the results of experiments on simple hydraulic models in order to sift out the more complex findings that we do, in fact, record in the arterial tree. The need for theoretical analysis is, in any case, well illustrated by the fact that even such a simple relation as that of Poiseuille's law can only be fully interpreted, e.g. in terms of viscosity, in the form derived mathematically (Ch. 2). The effects of wave-reflection are considered in Ch. 10 and are shown to be borne out by the experimental findings in the arterial system. These may appear to be rather unfamiliar in terms of the usual discussion of reflected waves because here we are dealing throughout with a consistent application of the concept of a steady-state oscillation. Much of the obscurity of the literature on this subject has been due to the introduction of terms, such as "standing waves" which are peculiar to a steady-state oscillation into analyses which are *a priori* based on the assumption that the pulse is a transient phenomenon. This latter assumption in some cases may well be reasonably accurate, e.g. when the pulse-frequency is low. It cannot, however, be profitably analysed in purely qualitative terms and its quantitative analysis is, as pointed out above, difficult. As the aim of the present work is to advance our methods of objective quantitative analysis of arterial pressure and flow the steady-state analysis has been chosen in the belief that it is the most realistic, and the knowledge that it is the simplest. Like all good theories it also forms a clear basis for further experimental work. Although the experimental results are, as yet, far fewer than is desirable I feel that, in this type of work, care in analysis of a small number of experiments is more valuable than the accumulation of a large mass of data. Because it is hoped that the present analysis will be applied to experimental and clinical investigations the pursuit of many small details has been undertaken, not only for their intrinsic interest, but in the hope that they may be proved to be negligible in analyses taken to a reasonable degree of accuracy.

The final chapters deal with a review of available manometer types in relation to the performance required of them (Ch. 11); then follows an interpretation of the changes in the form of the pressure pulse as it travels peripherally (Ch. 12) in the light of the analysis of wave-transmission and reflection set out in previous chapters. Lastly, there is a brief discussion of the way in which the analysis of pressure waves may form a basis for calculating the cardiac output (Ch. 13) and a summary of conclusions (Ch. 14). In spite of the general opinion that the hydrodynamics of the circulation is so complex as to defy analysis it is found that the final picture proves to be reasonably simple in terms of the technical precision of measurements that can, at present, be made in the living animal.

CHAPTER II

THE NATURE OF FLOW IN A LIQUID

In considering the circulation we are naturally concerned with the laws governing the flow of liquids in cylindrical pipes. The simplest example is that of a long straight tube with a constant rate of flow (steady flow) along it. To maintain such a steady flow there must be a constant pressure applied to the liquid because of its viscosity or "internal friction". The law governing such flow in a cylindrical tube is the well-known Poiseuille law which states that the head of pressure is directly proportional to the length of the pipe, to the rate of flow and to the viscosity and is inversely proportional to the fourth power of the radius. If dye is injected into liquid flowing under these conditions it is seen that the liquid in the axis of the tube is moving much faster than that near the wall and the front of the dye assumes a parabolic shape. The explanation for this is that the particles of liquid are flowing in a series of laminae parallel to the sides of the tube and the fluid actually in contact with the wall is stationary and each successive lamina is slipping against the viscous friction of the lamina outside it. When flow occurs in such parallel laminae it is called "laminar". If two tubes join to form a trunk and dye has only been injected into one of them it will be found that there is no mixing transversely across the tube; the streams remain distinct and may be seen to flow side by side in the main trunk. This phenomenon is called streamlining. Hence laminar flow is often called "streamline" flow. Alternatively it may be called "Poiseuille-type" flow because it obeys the Poiseuille law. .

If the rate of flow through a tube is continuously increased there comes a point when the resistance to flow increases quite sharply and Poiseuille's law is no longer applicable. Dye injected at this stage into the stream shows that the fluid is mixing across the tube and that the particles of dye and hence of the liquid are no longer moving regularly in the line of flow but are following more or less random paths across the tube in addition to their main movement along the tube. The flow is then said to be "turbulent". The laws governing the pressure-flow relationships of turbulent flow are

11

not predictable with precision, so that for this reason alone it is important to know whether any flow being studied is laminar or turbulent. It should be emphasized, however, that this classical distinction of types of flow is only correctly defined for steady flow in rigid tubes and there are intermediate stages of instability in the liquid which become of importance in the irregular flow systems of the living animal and which will be considered in the next chapter.

Laminar flow in viscous liquids

The concept of viscosity is quite inseparable from the consideration of the way that liquids flow. Stated in its most general way we can say that if a force is applied to a portion of a mass of liquid it will begin to flow but that if the force is removed the movement will be brought to rest. On the other hand, if a similar portion of a body of liquid is kept moving, the movement will be communicated to the rest of the fluid. This property is clearly analogous to that of friction between solid bodies and hence was termed "internal friction" by the earlier workers on the subject. Hatschek (1928) gives an interesting account of the development of these concepts from which the following account is derived.

The first theoretical consideration of the subject was made by Newton in the *Principia Mathematica* (Proposition LI, Theorem XXXIX) in which he considered the motion imparted to a large volume of fluid by the rotation of a long cylinder suspended in it. The hypothesis on which he based his derivation was "that the resistance which arises from the defect of slipperiness of the parts of the liquid, other things being equal, is proportional to the velocity with which the parts of the liquid are separated from one another" (Hatschek's translation). "Defect of slipperiness" (defectus lubricatitis) was the term used to describe what we now call viscosity. This hypothesis emphasizes immediately that in a fluid moving relative to a surface there are laminae slipping on one another and so moving at different velocities. There is thus a velocity gradient in a direction perpendicular to the surface. This gradient is usually called the rate of shear.

Apart from this one theorem Newton did not pursue the subject very far, although in the corollaries to the theorem he did consider the case of the flow between two concentric cylinders. Nor was the problem studied again for more than a century. Nevertheless this first contribution is commemorated in the use of the term New-tonian fluid for simple viscous liquids. The requirement for a Newtonian liquid is one whose viscosity does not vary with the rate of shear, that is to say remains constant at varying rates of laminar flow.

Although the eighteenth century produced many great mathe-maticians, and of these Euler and Daniel Bernoulli devoted much thought to hydrodynamics, the only work that was done was on "ideal" fluids, that is fluids without viscosity. At the end of the century Coulomb studied the damping of the oscillations of a disc suspended in liquids of different viscosities and made the important observation that the smoothness or roughness of the surface of the disc did not greatly influence the drag of the liquid.

The first work on flow in cylindrical tubes appears to be that of Girard in 1813 using brass tubes of from 2 to 3 mm in dia-meter. He obtained the relationship $Q = \dfrac{K.D^3P}{L}$ where Q is the volume flow per unit time, K is a constant, D the diameter, P the pressure drop along L, the length of the tube. Thus he observed that the flow varied directly with the pressure and inversely with the length but thought that it varied with the *cube* of the radius. Ten years later Navier made the first deductions of the theoretical equations for flow of viscous liquids in cylindrical tubes but obtained the incorrect result, already apparently confirmed by Girard's experimental results, that the flow was proportional to the cube of the radius.

The first published experimental work indicating that the flow is proportional to the fourth power of the radius was due to Hagen in 1839. He used brass tubes of a similar size to those of Girard and the results were not very accurate. The exponent of the radius derived from his results was actually 4·12 and he assumed that the real value must be 4·0. Poiseuille published his first results in 1842 although there was not a full paper until 1846. On account of Hagen's priority of publication some reference works use the name "the Hagen-Poiseuille law". Poiseuille's work, however, was much more detailed and precise and it is generally agreed that it is just to name it Poiseuille's law. Poiseuille (1799–1869) had long been investigating the hydrodynamics of the capillary circulation; for example, he was the first to appreciate that the velocity profile was the reason for the varying velocities of individual red corpuscles. Herrick (1942) gives a most interesting account of the physiological observations Poiseuille made on the circulation before he turned to his classic work on the flow of liquids.

Poiseuille may be regarded as fortunate in two respects. In the first place although he had a training in physics he was also a physician who wanted to apply the results of his investigations to the understanding of the blood circulation. Hence he worked with glass tubes of capillary size where his predecessors had been engineers and worked with much larger pipes. The use of minute tubes more easily maintains laminar flow and also greatly facilitates accurate measurement. In the second place he was deflected from his original intention of using blood as a test liquid because no satisfactory way of rendering it incoagulable was known and he was compelled to confine his investigation to water. Blood flowing in capillaries shows anomalous viscous properties that would have introduced great complications in these pioneer studies.

Poiseuille used capillary tubes varying in internal diameter from 0·14 mm to 0·03 mm and his measurements were carried out with an accuracy and completeness that thoroughly deserve the regard which they have been accorded. His results were expressed by the formula

$$Q = \frac{K.PD^4}{L} \quad \dots\dots\dots\dots\dots\dots 2.1$$

where, as above, Q, P, and L are volume flow, pressure drop along the tube and length of tube respectively; D is the tube diameter and K was a constant.

The value of the constant K was determined under various conditions and shown to fall with increasing temperature. This constant is clearly a measure of the viscosity but by purely experimental work it is not possible to define it other than empirically in this way.

The form of Poiseuille's law with which we are familiar is, in fact, dependent on the theoretical solution of the problem. Navier's early work on the equations of motion for viscous liquids were amplified and corrected by Stokes in the 1840s and the Navier-Stokes equations are the general solution of this problem. Stokes, however, did not tackle the particular case of the flow in a tube. The solution of this case was made independently by

Wiedemann in 1856 and Hagenbach in 1860 who both produced the result that

$$Q=\frac{(P_1-P_2)\pi R^4}{8\mu L} \quad \dots\dots\dots\dots\dots \; 2.2$$

where μ is the viscosity so that it can be seen that Poiseuille's constant $K=\dfrac{\pi}{128\mu}$ (as $R^4=\dfrac{D^4}{16}$) or $\mu=\dfrac{\pi}{128K}$. Hagenbach calculated μ from Poiseuille's data and obtained the result in modern units of $\mu=0\cdot013084$ poises at 10°C (modern value $0\cdot013077$P, Bingham and Jackson, 1918, Barr, 1931).

The method of derivation of the solution used by Hagenbach was a simple one and it seems odd to us today to think that it should have taken so long to produce. Compared with the advances made in pure mathematics by the middle of the nineteenth century this is a very elementary problem in applied mathematics and furthermore a problem which had been subjected to experimental investigation for over 40 years.

The basic assumption made for this solution, essentially that made by Newton, is that every particle of liquid is moving parallel to the axis of the tube with a constant velocity v, and the force opposing the flow over unit area is proportional to the viscosity and the velocity gradient in the liquid. In a cylindrical tube the particles travelling at the same velocity will be symmetrically arranged as cylindrical laminae.

Let us consider a cylindrical unit of liquid of length L and of radius r. The viscous force retarding its motion will be the area of its surface $(2\pi rL)$ × its viscosity (μ) × the velocity gradient across the tube $\left(\dfrac{dv}{dr}\right)$.

$$F(\text{visc})=2\pi rL\mu\frac{dv}{dr}$$

The force exerted by the pressure on the end of the cylinder is pressure × cross-sectional area less the force on the far end, so that

$$F(p)=\pi r^2(P_1-P_2)$$

where P_1 and P_2 are the respective pressures at either end of the length (L) of the cylinder considered. The pressure difference per unit length $\dfrac{(P_1-P_2)}{L}$ is termed the pressure-gradient.

These forces are equal and opposite

$$\therefore \pi r^2(P_1-P_2)=-2\pi r L\mu\frac{dv}{dr}$$

$$\text{or } r(P_1-P_2)=-2L\mu\frac{dv}{dr}$$

so that the velocity gradient is

$$\frac{dv}{dr}=-\frac{r(P_1-P_2)}{2L\mu} \qquad \dots\dots\dots\dots \text{2.3}$$

By integration we find that the velocity is

$$v=-\frac{r^2(P_1-P_2)}{4L\mu}+C$$

To determine the value of the constant of integration C it is necessary to make a further assumption of the boundary conditions. This is that the lamina in contact with the wall is at rest, that is when $r=R$, $v=0$

With substitution of these values we see that

$$C=\frac{R^2(P_1-P_2)}{4L\mu}$$

so that $v=-\dfrac{r^2(P_1-P_2)}{4L\mu}+\dfrac{R^2(P_1-P_2)}{4L\mu}=\dfrac{(P_1-P_2)}{4L\mu}(R^2-r^2)$ 2.4

This is the equation for a parabola where $v=0$ when $r=R$ and is a maximum when $r=0$, i.e. at the axis of the tube. (Fig. 2.1.)

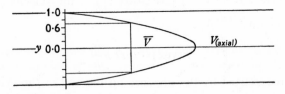

FIG. 2.1. A diagram of the velocity profile in steady laminar flow. This is a parabola whose equation is

$$V=\frac{P_1-P_2}{4L\mu}(R^2-r^2) \qquad \dots\dots\dots\dots \text{(Eqn. 2.4)}$$

The actual equation of the curve shown is $V=10.(1-y^2)$ where $y=r/R$, or the ratio of the radius of the lamina considered to the radius of the pipe.

The average velocity across the pipe ($\bar{V}$) can be shown to be half the axial velocity (see eqn. 2.5 and 2.6).

To obtain the volume of flow it is necessary to determine the volume of the paraboloid which has this parabola as its profile. That is we must determine the volume of the solid of revolution of this parabola. This volume is

$$Q = \int_0^R 2\pi v \; r.dr$$

or substituting the value for v above

$$Q = \frac{2\pi(P_1 - P_2)}{4L\mu} \int_0^R (R^2 - r^2) r.dr = \frac{\pi(P_1 - P_2)R^4}{8L\mu} \quad \ldots \; 2.2$$

To evaluate this equation all units used must be consistent. Thus in the C.G.S. system Q=cm³/sec, P=dynes/cm², R and L=cm and μ is in poises. The C.G.S. unit of viscosity, the poise (P), is named in honour of Poiseuille and is defined as one dyne-sec/cm² or one gram/cm/sec. For convenience the centipoise (cP) is often used. Unfortunately it is more common to express the viscosity of blood as its *relative viscosity*, that is, relative to water. The viscosity of water is very close to $0.01P(1.0cP)$ at 20°C but at 37°C it is $0.007P$ and this should be allowed for when calculating the absolute viscosity of blood from its relative value.

As we saw above (p. 16) the maximum velocity is at the axis of the tube where

$$V \text{ (axial)} = \frac{(P_1 - P_2)R^2}{4\mu L} \quad \ldots \ldots \ldots \ldots \; 2.5$$

The average velocity $(\overline{V})$ across the tube is derived by dividing the volume flow by the cross-sectional area (πR^2).

$$\text{thus } \overline{V} = \frac{\pi(P_1 - P_2)R^4}{8\mu L.\pi R^2} = \frac{(P_1 - P_2)R^2}{8\mu L}$$

so that the average velocity of flow is half the axial velocity (Fig. 2.1). The lamina travelling at this velocity is the one with radius r such that $(R^2 - r^2) = R/\sqrt{2}$, i.e. $r = 0.707R$.

The applicability of Poiseuille's law to the circulation

The conditions under which Poiseuille's law applies precisely are implicit in the method by which it is derived theoretically. In view of its importance in the hydrodynamics of the circulation these conditions should be considered in more detail. They are as follows:

(1) *The fluid is homogenous and that its viscosity is the same at all rates of shear.* Blood is, of course, a suspension of particles but it has been shown that in tubes in which the internal diameter is large compared with the size of the red cells, it behaves as a Newtonian fluid. In tubes with an internal diameter less than 0·5 mm changes in apparent viscosity occur. This is important in the study of flow in small vessels and is discussed more fully in Ch. 3. In the larger arteries and veins, however, blood may be considered as a homogenous fluid with a viscosity that is independent of the velocity-gradient.

(2) *The rate of flow is "steady" and is not subjected to acceleration or deceleration.* If the velocity is altered the pressure-gradient is utilized partly in communicating kinetic energy to the liquid, and the equations do not apply. As the flow in all large arteries and the intrathoracic veins (Brecher, 1956) is markedly pulsatile, it is clear that Poiseuille's law cannot be applied to them. The pressure-flow relationship of flow under these circumstances is considered below in Ch. 5.

(3) *The flow is laminar, that is, the liquid at all points is moving parallel to the walls of the tube.* At rates of flow above a critical value this is no longer true and the flow is turbulent. The deviation from Poiseuille's law that this causes are discussed in the next section (p. 19). Turbulent flow may occur in the largest blood-vessels but as the flow here is also pulsatile condition (2) above is not satisfied so that Poiseuille's law cannot be applied. The evidence available on the occurrence of turbulent flow in the circulation is reviewed in Ch. 3 where it will be seen that laminar flow is almost certainly present in all the vessels where flow is sufficiently steady to consider applying Poiseuille's law.

(4) *The liquid does not slip at the wall.* This was the assumption that $V=0$ when $r=R$ which was made in evaluating the constant of integration in the equations on p. 16. As Poiseuille's law would not be valid if this were not true, the law may be used as a test for the assumption; it is held to be universally true for liquids. Even with gas flows over a solid surface there appears to be no appreciable slip under normal conditions though it may have to be considered with a rarefied gas. These conclusions are derived from the detailed review by Goldstein (1938*b*).

This point is of some importance as it has occasionally been suggested that some of the anomalous flow properties of blood in blood-vessels may be due to non-wettable properties of their endothelial lining with a consequent slip at the wall. Even if the endothelium were shown to be non-wettable the conclusion, that slipping would result, is unjustifiable. For example, Poiseuille's law holds for the flow of mercury in a glass tube so that there must be zero velocity at the wall.

(5) *The tube is long compared with the region being studied.* Close to the inlet of a pipe the flow has not yet become established with the parabolic velocity profile characteristic of laminar flow. The distance required to establish the steady form of flow is known as the "inlet length" and here Poiseuille's law does not apply. Within the inlet length the assumption made in the derivation that there are no accelerations along the axis of the tube, is not true. It is, therefore, a special case of the steady flow condition discussed in (2) above. In viscometers where a flow from a reservoir through a narrow tube is measured a correction for this effect must be applied (Newman and Searle, 1957). In the circulation there is never this condition of a stationary reservoir leading to steady laminar flow so that this correction does not apply. The special problem of the inlet length with pulsating flow in relation to the proximal aorta is discussed below (pp. 47-8).

(6) *The tube is rigid so that the diameter does not change with pressure.* In the smaller vessels where the flow is steady enough to apply Poiseuille's law there is no direct evidence concerning changes in calibre simply due to changes in hydrostatic pressure. Wezler and Sinn (1953) have considered this point in detail and derived a pressure-flow relationship in vascular beds that takes this factor into account. Levy and Share (1953) and Levy *et al.* (1954) on the other hand, found linear pressure-flow relations under a wide variety of conditions. At present it is felt that the experimental information on the behaviour of these small vessels is not sufficient to discuss it satisfactorily in the compass of the present work.

Turbulent flow

It was observed both by Hagen and by Poiseuille that the law relating pressure and flow ceased to be kept when there was a high rate of flow. This was rightly attributed to the breakdown of laminar flow and the onset of turbulent flow. They observed the appearance of turbulence but it was not until the work of Osborne

Reynolds in 1883 and subsequently that the conditions determining the transition from laminar to turbulent flow were described precisely. Reynolds injected a filament of dye in the axis of a tube in which all irregularities at the inlet and of the wall had been eliminated. At low rates of flow the motion of the fluid, as shown by the dye, was smooth and regular. Any disturbance introduced into the fluid was soon damped out. At higher rates of flow the liquid became more sensitive to disturbances. At a critical point a stage was reached when smooth flow could no longer be maintained and "the motion of the fluid becomes wildly irregular and the tube appears to be filled with interlacing and constantly varying streams, crossing and recrossing the pipe". (Lamb, 1932.)

The critical point was found to be dependent on the diameter of the tube, the mean velocity of the flow and the density and viscosity of the liquid. This was expressed as a dimensionless quantity, known as the Reynolds number which, when applied to flow in a circular pipe, is

$$Re = \frac{\overline{V}D\rho}{\mu} \quad \dots \dots \dots \dots \dots \dots \quad 2.7$$

where $\overline{V}$ is the average velocity of flow, D is the diameter of the tube, ρ is the density of the liquid and μ its viscosity. The fraction μ/ρ is known as the kinematic viscosity, written as ν. The C.G.S. unit of kinematic viscosity is the *stokes* (cm^2/sec).

Reynolds' formula is thus often expressed as

$$Re = \frac{\overline{V}D}{\nu} \quad \dots \dots \dots \dots \dots \dots \quad 2.8$$

It will be seen that not only an increase in average velocity causes turbulence, but also that at a given velocity of flow, turbulence will occur in large tubes before it will in small ones.

The fact that the characteristic property of the fluid concerned in determining the stability of laminar flow is the kinematic viscosity, gives rise to some apparently surprising results. Thus a gas like air would appear to be more easily disturbed than blood, or even water. Its absolute viscosity is, of course, much less than water (at 20°C, air—0·0181 cP, water—1·00 cP) but because the density of air is proportionately lower its kinematic viscosity is actually some 10 times as great as water at 20°C (air—10·5 × 10^{-2}, water—1·007 × 10^{-2} stokes). Furthermore as the viscosity of gases increases with temperature while that of liquids decreases the difference is greater at body temperature. The kinematic viscosity of blood at body temperature is about $3\cdot8 \times 10^{-2}$ stokes at 38°C and that of water is $0\cdot686 \times 10^{-2}$ stokes, while that of air (at 40°C) is $16\cdot9 \times 10^{-2}$ stokes (Goldstein, 1938*a*). Thus at body temperature a steady laminar stream of air in a bronchus, for example, would be stable at a velocity four times greater than that of blood in a blood-vessel of comparable size. This also serves to emphasize that in terms of hydrodynamics both blood and water are thought of as liquids of low viscosity.

A certain amount of confusion arises in physiological literature by the use of radius in place of diameter in this equation, especially as quoted figures are often compared without reference to different ways of computing the figures. The general formula for Reynolds number for a channel of any shape is

$$Re = \frac{4m\overline{V}}{\nu} \text{ (Goldstein, 1938}a\text{)} \dots\dots\dots\dots 2.9$$

where m is the "mean hydraulic depth" which is defined as the cross-sectional area divided by the perimeter. Thus for a circle

$$m = R/2 \text{ and } 4m = \text{Diameter.}$$

Hence this formula (2.7 or 2.8) is used throughout in the present work in order to conform to standard hydrodynamic practice and the values of other workers are converted, where necessary, to comparable values.

The critical value of the Reynolds number is usually stated to be 2,000. This, however, is an experimentally determined value and is very dependent on the conditions of the experiment. Reynolds called it the "lower critical value". With very carefully controlled flow from an undisturbed reservoir into the tube, Reynolds himself was able to maintain laminar flow up to a value of 12,000 and much higher values have been attained.

The standard Reynolds number of 2,000 is obtained when there are disturbed conditions in the reservoir. With such conditions it is difficult to cause turbulence in a regular tube at figures below this value. Other disturbances are found, however, at lower values. The period of laminar flow has been described by Schiller (see Goldstein, 1938*a*, Ch. VII) as falling into three regimes. The first is the period of completely undisturbed flow with the streamline running parallel to the sides of the tube. These streams begin to exhibit a wavy motion at higher Reynolds number which is described as the second regime, and these oscillations get larger and vortices start forming at the border and are carried down the tube. The third regime is that with vortex formation, and as they become larger and more frequent this merges into a condition of turbulence. The stage at which these conditions of disturbed flow, heralds of approaching breakdown of the flow pattern, appear, depends on the degree of disturbance in the reservoir or on roughnesses at the entry of the pipe. Naumann recorded a Reynolds number of 280 for the beginning of the second regime with a sharp entrance orifice in the pipe, and White and Davis a similar value with a very disturbed reservoir. The third regime usually begins at $Re=1,600$ but may be considerable earlier with these other disturbing factors at work. This vortex regime at Reynolds values below 2,000 is of considerable importance in the living animal because of the variety of disturbing effects on flow (which are discussed in Ch. 3).

The mere evaluation of the Reynolds number is not, of itself, a proof of the existence of laminar or turbulent flow. The best way to demonstrate turbulence is to measure the pressure-flow relationship and demonstrate that this deviates from that of laminar flow. Whereas with unvarying laminar flow the pressure drop per unit length (pressure-gradient) varies linearly with the rate of flow, when turbulence is present it varies approximately with a higher

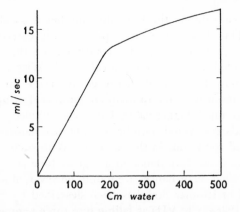

FIG. 2.2. The relation between pressure-gradient and flow in a pipe. At low rates of flow there is a linear relationship and the flow is laminar. The inflection in the curve indicates the onset of turbulence; turbulent flow requires a larger pressure-gradient than the equivalent laminar flow. (*Drawn from data of Coulter and Pappenheimer*, 1949.)

power of the rate of flow. In a pressure-flow diagram this shows as a discontinuity (Fig. 2.2). In other words a greater pressure-gradient is required to maintain turbulent flow than is required for laminar flow. The conditions for turbulent flow have not been precisely determined because it is not possible to give a precise description of the motion of the liquid. The fluid particles, in addition to flowing along the line of the tube, pursue random pathways in other directions and small eddies or vortices are formed. Thus extra energy is required to maintain the increased movement of fluid that does not directly contribute to the flow; that is an increased pressure is required to maintain it. Whereas in laminar flow $Q \propto P$ when the flow becomes turbulent, the relation is $Q^n \propto P$ where n is greater than 1, and increases to 2 with increasing Reynolds number (Goldstein).

Where measurement of the pressure-gradient and flow are not practicable the type of flow may be observed from the distribution of injected dye, as Reynolds did in his pioneer experiments. Whereas such dye will be distributed in a parabolic velocity profile in steady laminar flow, in turbulent flow the dye is seen to be mixed across the stream and the velocity of flow is much more nearly the same across the tube, although there will still be a region of shear near the wall (Fig. 2.3). The extent to which this region of shear

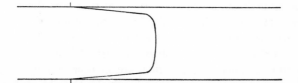

FIG. 2.3. The type of velocity profile seen in turbulent flow. This is very much flatter than the corresponding profile in laminar flow but there is still a marked region of shear near the walls. This example is based on a cinematograph record by McDonald and Helps (1954) where the Reynolds number was about 4,000—at higher values the velocity distribution would become progressively more equal across the tube.

extends and the width of the "flat" front varies with the degree of turbulence. For although the distinction between laminar flow and turbulent flow is relatively abrupt, turbulence, in the sense of disorder of motion of the fluid, will continue to increase with increasing Reynolds number for some considerable time. This is shown by the changing relation of pressure and flow (Fig. 2.2).

The transition from turbulence to laminar flow with conditions of decreasing Reynolds number is even more difficult to define than the onset of turbulence. In general it may be said that in a given tube the restoration of laminar flow will occur at a lower Reynolds number than that at which the onset of turbulence occurred. As variation in the rate of flow is found in all blood-vessels in which the Reynolds number is in the critical region, this point is of considerable interest. As stated above disturbances generated in truly laminar flow will be damped out and this is commonly used to define turbulence as the condition of steady flow where a disturbance, once started, will increase in size until it involves the whole body of the liquid. The consideration of turbulence in pulsating flow such as is found in arteries and the larger veins is, therefore, somewhat difficult. If a disturbance in the flow is short-lasting one cannot know whether its transient character is due to a regime of instability that is too brief to produce turbulence throughout the liquid, or whether the flow is inherently stable and hence has damped out the disturbance.

Thus Helps and McDonald (1954*a*) observed that vortex rings were formed in the thoracic vena cava when flow reversed, but that they were damped out when forward flow was re-established. They thought this could not be considered as true turbulence. Their reasons were that the Reynolds number was well below the critical value throughout the cycle and furthermore the disturbance occurred at a time when flow velocity was minimal. In addition, the vortex rings did not involve all the blood in the vein. They suggested that some term such as "disturbed flow" should be used for conditions such as this which are neither clearly laminar nor clearly turbulent. On the other hand, McDonald (1952*b*) using high-speed cinematography, showed in the rabbit aorta that, while laminar flow with a parabola-like profile could be seen in early systole, the dye pattern was disrupted completely during the peak systolic ejection and the flow appeared to be turbulent (Fig. 2.4). A laminar flow pattern was re-established in diastole although it was impossible to determine at what point it started and streams could not be clearly seen until well into diastole when the flow velocity was very low. In this case it may be more justifiable to call the flow "turbulent" because the disturbance spread right across the artery and was initiated at a time of maximal flow velocity. The "turbulent" phase was very brief, however, and probably did not persist for more than 50 msec. Evans (1955) furthermore, has pointed out that the dye appears to be disposed in the form of helical vortices and is not randomly distributed, but regards this as a usual phenomenon in early turbulence. The Reynolds number in this case, calculated from the peak flow velocity, was at most 1,000 and so considerably below the usually accepted critical value of 2,000. Hale, McDonald and Womersley (1955) however, suggested that the pulsating flow in the rabbit aorta might reach an "effective Reynolds number", calculated on the maximal rate of shear, of 2,000 so that the latter discrepancy may be unimportant. The validity of this reasoning is discussed in the next chapter.

The first example described above (the inferior vena cava) may, therefore, illustrate one group of causes of disturbed flow.

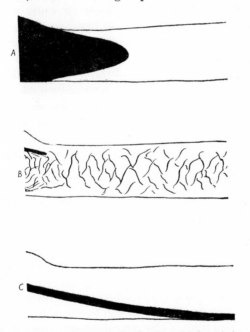

FIG. 2.4. Successive patterns of distribution of injected dye in the rabbit abdominal aorta—traced from single frames of a high-speed cinematograph film.

A, in early systole, the front is approximately that of a parabola (cf. Fig. 3.2) such as that found in pulsating laminar flow.

B, there is a scattering of dye throughout the vessel due to turbulence during the period of peak velocity.

C, a stream of dye reformed during the period of backflow after the end of systole. (*McDonald*, 1952b.)

This type is due to conditions, in this case probably a rapid reversal of flow, that create large vortices which are damped out by the inherent stability of the flow. The second example (the rabbit aorta) would then fall into a second group where a very rapid acceleration may produce a period of true instability that is short-lived because the high velocity is only maintained for a very short time. It should be emphasized, however, that this distinction in circulatory conditions is based on very slender evidence at the present time.

The practical point that arises from this discussion is that the mixing of streams of blood in a vessel, as evidenced by sampling of oxygen content or the dispersion of a dye, may be due to other causes than the existence of turbulence. For much experimental work the most important fact to establish is the presence of adequate mixing, so it may be argued that the cause of such mixing is of little interest. In the study of the hydrodynamics of the circulation, however, it is desirable to know whether the pressure-flow relationship is essentially that of laminar flow, albeit altered somewhat by the creation of eddies, or whether there is fully established turbulence where the pressure-flow relationship may be considerably different. It seems that the assessment of the importance of this last factor by direct experimental measurement will not be made until there is a considerable improvement in the precision of methods for measuring pulsating flow in the circulation.

Bernoulli's theorem

Up to this point we have concerned ourselves with the behaviour of viscous liquids. It was mentioned briefly that Daniel Bernoulli (1700–1782) developed the theoretical behaviour of "ideal" fluids, ignoring the forces of viscosity. One theorem he developed is of importance in the hydrodynamics of the circulation and must be considered briefly here.

Bernoulli's theorem may be deduced from the principle of the conservation of energy (Newman and Searle, 1957). If we imagine a section AB of a tube of changing diameter with a flow of liquid passing through it, then the amount passing into the section of the tube at A must be equal to that passing out at B. If the cross-sections of the tube at the two ends are A_1 and A_2 and the velocities are V_1 and V_2 respectively, then the volume entering per second is A_1V_1 and $A_1V_1 = A_2V_2$.

If the pressure at either end is p_1 and p_2 then the work done on the fluid entering AB is $p_1A_1V_1$ and on that leaving is $p_2A_2V_2$. The fluid also has kinetic energy (which is $\frac{1}{2}mV^2$). At the point A

$$m = \rho A_1 V_1 \quad (\rho = \text{density})$$

so that, assuming that there are no external forces (e.g. the tube is horizontal so that we ignore gravity), the kinetic energy at the point of entry is

$$\tfrac{1}{2}V_1^2.\rho A_1 V_1,$$

so that the total energy at entry, which is equal to that at the point of outflow is

$$p_1A_1V_1 + \tfrac{1}{2}V_1^2.\rho A_1 V_1 = p_2A_2V_2 + \tfrac{1}{2}V_2^2.\rho A_2 V_2 \quad \ldots\ldots \text{2.10}$$

or

$$p_1 + \tfrac{1}{2}\rho V_1^2 = p_2 + \tfrac{1}{2}\rho V_2^2 = C$$

so that if the velocity of flow is increased then the lateral pressure (p) must be correspondingly decreased. This effect is particularly apparent at a constriction in a vessel, and is applied in devices as various as the common water-pump and the orifice or Venturi meter for measuring the rate of blood flow. Provided that the condition of applying the theorem are such that the kinetic energy term is large, the approximation due to ignoring the viscous effects may be regarded as negligible. This approximation, however, limits the appication of the theorem in the circulation.

The effect of change in the size of the vascular bed

We have already considered the relations between the pressure-gradient, rate of flow and internal lumen for steady flow in a straight tube. Changes in lumen of arteries, however, are virtually all associated with the occurrence of branches. These branches are, individually, narrower than the parent trunk but the total cross-sectional area nearly always increases when branches are given off. It is, therefore, of interest to see how a change in the size of the channel due to the occurrence of branches will affect the rate of flow, the Reynolds number and the pressure-gradient. This can be simply derived for steady flow but, of course, this makes it of somewhat academic interest in a consideration of the larger arteries because pulsatile flow has quite different pressure-flow relationships. Using analogous electrical terms we are here calculating the changes in *resistance* in the vascular network, whereas we really need to know the changes in *impedance*. The latter problem is so much the more difficult that it is worth considering the simplest conditions first. These conditions apply in general throughout the venous system and also approximately in small arteries (Ch. 5). The change in impedance at points of arterial branching is considered in Ch. 10.

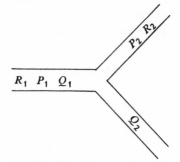

Fig. 2.5. A junction with two equal branches.

Take a main vessel, cross-sectional area A_1, that divides into n branches of equal size and each of cross-sectional area A_2. If the total vascular bed changes by a factor d, i.e. $dA_1 = (n \times A_2)$ we can describe the behaviour of the bed in terms of the ratio d without considering actual cross-sectional areas.

Then if we call the pressure-gradient $\dfrac{(p-p')}{l}$ in the main trunk P_1 and that in the branches P_2, similarly Q_1 and Q_2 for the respective volume rates of flow, R_1 and R_2 for the radii, and V_1 and V_2 the average linear velocities of flow.

The only determining condition is that the rate of flow into and out of the system must be equal or

$$Q_1 = nQ_2$$

Since the rate of flow is the mean velocity times the cross-sectional area of the tube

$$Q_1 = V_1 \pi R_1^2 = n V_2 \pi R_2^2 \text{ or } \frac{V_1}{V_2} = \frac{nR_2^2}{R_1^2}$$

By definition $d = \dfrac{n\pi R_2^2}{\pi R_1^2}$ $\left(\text{hence } \dfrac{R_1}{R_2} = \sqrt{\dfrac{n}{d}} \right)$

$$\therefore \frac{V_1}{V_2} = d \quad \dots\dots\dots\dots\dots\dots 2.11$$

that is to say that the mean velocity of flow in the branches will be less by a factor of d whatever the number of branches.

If the velocity of flow and the radius are both less in the branches obviously the Reynolds number will decrease if the vascular bed increases.

$$Re_1 = \frac{2R_1 V_1}{\nu} \text{ and } Re_2 = \frac{2R_2 V_2}{\nu}$$

or

$$\frac{Re_1}{Re_2} = \frac{R_1 V_1}{R_2 V_2} = d . \frac{R_1}{R_2} = d\sqrt{\frac{n}{d}}$$

$$= \sqrt{nd} \quad \dots\dots\dots\dots\dots\dots \text{ 2.12}$$

As n is always greater than 1 the Reynolds number will remain unchanged only if there is a narrowing of the bed so that $d = 1/n$.

The same reasoning applied to a constriction in an unbranched tube, i.e. $n = 1$ and $d < 1$ the Reynolds number will increase continuously as the tube gets narrower *provided* there is a sufficient head of pressure to maintain a constant rate of flow. In the circulation the maximum pressure drop across the constriction is determined by the arterio-venous pressure difference. When this maximum is reached further constriction will cause a reduction in flow. The Reynolds number thus rises at first and then begins to fall—an effect well demonstrated by Dawes, Mott and Widdicombe (1955) during constriction of the ductus arteriosus (see section on Murmurs, Ch. 4, Fig. 4.3).

In a similar way from Poiseuille's law we may compare the pressure-gradients in the main trunk and the branches

$$Q_1 = \frac{P_1 \pi R_1^4}{8\mu} = nQ_2 = \frac{nP_2 \pi R_2^4}{8\mu}$$

so that

$$\frac{P_1}{P_2} = \frac{nR_2^4}{R_1^4}$$

and as

$$\frac{R_2^2}{R_1^2} = \frac{d}{n}, \frac{P_1}{P_2} = \frac{d^2}{n} \quad \dots\dots\dots\dots \text{ 2.13}$$

from which we see the interesting result that for steady flow the pressure-gradient (the "vascular resistance") remains the same only if
$$d = \sqrt{n} \text{ and increases when } d < \sqrt{n}.$$

As the minimum value of $n = 2$, the pressure-drop will be greater in the branches of a bifurcation unless the cross-sectional area of the vascular bed increases by a factor of more than 1·414.

The average value for d that is often quoted is $1\cdot 26$ at a major arterial bifurcation, and this appears to originate from the work of Blum (1919). In this situation we can see that the velocity in the branches (Eqn. 2.11) will be $1/1\cdot 26$, or $0\cdot 8$, of that in the parent trunk; the Reynolds number will also decrease (Eqn. 2.12) by the factor $1/(2\times 1\cdot 26)$, or $0\cdot 63$; the pressure-gradient on the other hand will increase by the factor $2/1\cdot 26^2$, or $1\cdot 26$.

The relation between pressure-gradient and flow is commonly expressed as the fluid resistance (see following section); if the resistance is expressed as the ratio of pressure and volume flow (Eqn. 2.17), i.e. P/Q and is indicated by K, then $K_1 = P_1/Q_1$, and from Eqn. 2.13

$$\frac{K_1}{K_2} = \frac{P_1}{P_2}\cdot\frac{Q_2}{Q_1} = \frac{d^2}{n}\cdot\frac{1}{n} = \frac{d^2}{n^2} \quad\ldots\ldots\ldots\ldots\ldots 2.14$$

If the resistance is expressed in terms of the average flow velocity and indicated by k we have $k_1 = P_1/V_1$ and from Eqns. 2.11 and 2.13 we obtain

$$\frac{k_1}{k_2} = \frac{P_1}{P_2}\cdot\frac{V_2}{V_1} = \frac{d^2}{n}\cdot\frac{1}{d} = \frac{d}{n} \quad\ldots\ldots\ldots\ldots\ldots 2.15$$

Therefore, the fluid resistance will remain unchanged in an individual branch beyond a subdivision only if the total cross-sectional area of the branches is larger than that of the parent trunk by a factor that is the number of the branches—which at a minimum is two. This applies equally whether the resistance is measured in relation to the volume flow or to the flow velocity. As no one has ever observed an increase in the size of the vascular bed by as large a factor as 2, at any bifurcation it follows that the vascular resistance measured in each branch will always increase.

If, however, the vascular resistance of all branches is taken together then the volume flow is the same on either side of the junction and the corresponding resistance will vary as the pressure-gradient (Eqn. 2.15). As pointed out above this means that at a bifurcation the cross-sectional area must increase by a factor of $\sqrt{2}$ for the resistance (in terms of volume flow) to remain unchanged.

The actual ratio of the cross-sectional area of branches to that of the main stem appears to increase peripherally. The experimental evidence is mainly reported in the older German literature and is reviewed in detail by Hess (1927) and more briefly by

Bazett (1941). For instance, there may be no increase of the vascular bed where the large branches leave the arch of the aorta; in old human beings there may even be a slight narrowing. At the bifurcation of the human aorta Hess (1927) gives the mean ratio as 1·126 in a series of 461 observations. Schlier (1918) analysed the mesenteric system and the ratio he estimated at the first set of arterial branches was 1·7, but rose to about 6·0 over the junctions between the arteries of the villi and the capillary bed; the number of branches, however, increased 47 times.

At some more proximal positions there may be quite marked expansion of the vascular bed. For example, at the beginning of the abdominal aorta the vascular bed has been estimated by Alexander (1954) to increase by a factor of 1·4; the number of branches, however, is five (including the distal aorta) and if these were equal in size the increase in pressure-gradient, and hence of total vascular resistance, would be by a factor of 2·55. This emphasizes that it is not so much changes in cross-sectional area that impose the changes in pressure-flow relationships but the total wall area of the branches (owing to the viscosity of the blood). The wall area is obviously greater the more branches there are. In fact conditions in the body are such that the fluid resistance increases every time that vessels subdivide.

It is interesting to note that, in all the relations worked out above, the only one determined by the total cross-sectional area of the bed alone is the velocity of flow. The measurement of the mean velocity on either side of a vascular subdivision could therefore be used as a measure of the change in the size of the vascular bed in the living animal. In a more general way the changes in mean velocity can be used to indicate where the main changes of size of the bed occur. For example, in the dog the mean velocity in the proximal aorta is usually 15–20 cm/sec and in the femoral artery is about 10–12 cm/sec. This implies that the vascular bed measured at arteries of the same order as the femoral has increased by about 50 per cent compared with the aorta. In the capillaries, however, where the mean velocity is about 0·05 cm/sec there must be an increase of the vascular bed to 300–400 times that of the aorta. Such generalizations are, of course, only approximate as they imply an equal degree of arteriolar constriction in all the main vascular beds so that blood flow is not being shunted preferentially through any one of them.

The consideration of the division of flow between unequal branches cannot be satisfied in such a general way because there are a different set of pressure-flow relations for each branch.

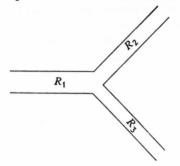

FIG. 2.6. A division into unequal branches.

As before $Q_2 = Q_2 + Q_3$ and from Poiseuille's law we can see that

$$\frac{Q_2}{Q_3} = \frac{P_2 R_2^4}{P_3 R_3^4}$$

P is the pressure-gradient, that is the fall in pressure per unit length and unless we know the length and fall in pressure-gradient in both channels the flow down each branch cannot be predicted. It is usual to assume that as the pressure in each branch will fall to the same capillary pressure $P_2 = P_3$ but this makes the further assumption that the overall lengths of the two branches are the same. If P_2 is equal to P_3 the relative flows in the branches will, of course, be proportional to the fourth power of their radii, R_2 and R_3.

THE MEASUREMENT OF PERIPHERAL RESISTANCE

The application of Poiseuille's formula (2.2) to any set of blood-vessels, in the way it was used in the preceding section, requires a knowledge of the dimensions of those vessels. When considering the vascular system of the body, or of one of its regions, we do not have this information. The formula can, however, be simplified by writing

$$P_1 - P_2 = KQ = k\overline{V} \quad \ldots \ldots \ldots \ldots \quad 2.16$$

and from analogy with Ohm's law the terms K, or k, are called the fluid resistance because the pressure-drop is analogous with the potential difference and the blood flow with the current. It is usual to calculate the resistance in terms of volume flow; but, as was seen in the previous section, it is often more illuminating to compare the velocity of flow in various vessels, so that we will also consider the "velocity resistance". Pursuing the analogy the Poiseuille formula only applies to steady flow, or by analogy, to direct current. In arterial channels where the flow is pulsatile this might be thought to be inapplicable. Pulsatile arterial flow, however, always has a steady flow component—the mean flow—and it is possible to apply the direct current concept to this mean flow. The corresponding pressure-flow relation for the oscillatory flow is, using alternating current theory, called the fluid impedance (see Ch. 10). (In the wider implications of this analogy it is more convenient to take velocity as the analogue and so, at the risk of confusion, it is here also applied to resistance.)

From the Poiseuille equations it can be seen that the resistance in Eqn. 2.16 is expressed by

$$K = \frac{8\mu L}{\pi R^4} \quad \dots \dots \dots \dots \dots \dots \dots \dots \quad 2.17$$

or

$$k = \frac{8\mu L}{R^2} \quad \dots \dots \dots \dots \dots \dots \dots \dots \quad 2.18$$

The length of any vascular channel is virtually constant for anatomical reasons and the mean viscosity of the blood can also be regarded as constant (although as noted in Ch. 3 the viscosity does vary with the radius in small vessels). The vascular resistance is thus very largely determined by the radius of the vessels. In the complete vascular bed of, say, one limb, the total fluid resistance may be regarded as the resistances of, respectively, the arteries, the arterioles, the capillaries and the veins in series. As the resistance is proportional to the drop in mean pressure it is apparent that the resistance of the arterioles constitutes the largest proportion of the whole. Thus the mean arterial pressure is about 100 mm Hg and has fallen very little in the smallest arteries in which it has been measured. In the capillaries it is generally agreed to be about 30 mm Hg at the proximal end and 12–15 mm Hg at the distal end; most of this fall (up to 60 mm Hg) will occur in the 5 mm or so immediately proximal to the capillaries. The pressure in the large veins will only be a few mm Hg so that of a total of 100 mm Hg, up to 60 per cent may occur in the arterioles, about 15 per cent both in the capillaries and the veins and about 10 per cent in the arterial system. The total peripheral resistance is thus dominated by the calibre of the arterioles but the other components of the vascular bed are by no means negligible. The fact that the arterioles can be actively altered in size by physiological mechanisms has focused especial attention on to their contribution to the peripheral vascular resistance. Indeed, under controlled conditions, the measurement of the resistance is a useful and simple way of studying vasomotor activity. Nevertheless, it is regrettable that the term "peripheral resistance" has so often been used as if it were synonymous with "arteriolar resistance".

The value of the concept of peripheral, or vascular, resistance, has been questioned by some authors. The basis of most of their comment has been due partly to the somewhat slipshod way that approximations have been introduced without assessment of the consequent errors, and partly to verbal short cuts such as regarding the arteriolar vessels as the whole of the peripheral resistance. In addition it has been criticized as being an artificial, or abstract idea, useful only for manipulating experimental data. To some extent this is true but only to the extent that the concept of electrical resistance is abstract—for it also only expresses the relationship between the current and potential drop in a circuit. Similarly the measurement of changes in the resistance of a circuit can only give net, or overall, effects and cannot distinguish changes of individual components.

The measurements that need to be made are basically the same in all cases—the mean pressure at the beginning and the end, of the vascular bed to be studied, and the total flow. For the total vascular resistance of the body this means that in place of Eqn. 2.16 we can write

*Mean aortic pressure—mean R. atrial pressure=cardiac output
× total peripheral resistance*

As the pressure in the great veins is very small in comparison with the aortic pressure it is usually taken as zero and the formula is often rendered as   A.B.P.=C.O.×T.P.R.

In smaller regions of the systemic bed the approximation of taking the venous pressure as zero may introduce appreciable errors. In the pulmonary circulation the arterial pressure is much lower and left atrial pressure probably higher; it is then very inaccurate to estimate vascular resistance without measuring the atrial pressure.

The units in which the peripheral resistance is expressed have varied with different authors. The Peripheral Resistance Unit (P.R.U.) introduced by H. D. Green is in the empirical units of mm Hg per ml./min; in practice, this works out in numbers of convenient dimensions in regional vascular beds, but as with all arbitrary units, is difficult to convert or correlate with other dimensions. In standard physical units the corresponding units are dyne.sec/cm^5 if volume flow is used, or dyne.sec/cm^3 if flow velocity is used.

Taking some average figures for the human subject we can calculate some representative values.

(*a*) *Total peripheral resistance.* If the cardiac output is 4·5 *l*./min (75 cm^3/sec), the mean arterial b.p. 100 mm Hg and the mean velocity of flow is 15 cm/sec (i.e. *R* is *c* 1·25 cm)

Then
$$K = \frac{100}{4,500} = 0.022 \text{ P.R.U.}$$

or
$$K = \frac{100 \times 13.6 \times 980}{75} = 1.64 \times 10^3 \text{ dyne.sec/cm}^5$$

or
$$k = \frac{10.0 \times 13.6 \times 980}{15} = 8.20 \times 10^3 \text{ dyne.sec/cm}^3$$

(*b*) *Peripheral resistance of femoral vascular bed.* If volume flow is 225 cm^3/min (3·75 cm^3/sec) and the mean velocity is 12 cm/sec

Then
$$K = \frac{100}{225} = 0.44 \text{ P.R.U.}$$

or
$$K = \frac{10.0 \times 13.6 \times 980}{3.75} = 3.55 \times 10^4 \text{ dyne.sec/cm}^5$$

or
$$k = 11.1 \times 10^3 \text{ dyne.sec/cm}^3$$

(*c*) *Vascular resistance of a single capillary.* Taking the following values for a typical capillary we may obtain comparative values for the smallest vessels: pressure drop 30–15 mm Hg, mean velocity 0·5 mm/sec and a diameter of 10μ.

$$K = 5 \times 10^{11} \text{ dyne.sec/cm}^5$$
and
$$k = 4 \times 10^5 \text{ dyne.sec/cm}^3$$

(From the same figures it may be computed that there must be a total of 2×10^9 capillaries of this size and that their total surface area is 32 sq. metre. The femoral artery values taken above are scaled up proportionately from values observed in the dog.)

Thus the vascular resistance may be estimated for a single channel or for the whole vascular bed (from the point of measurement of arterial pressure to the point in the veins where the pressure was zero, i.e. atmospheric).

The contribution of the various grades of vessels to the

peripheral resistance has been studied by various workers. The estimate given above (p. 33) is, of course, very approximate and the pressure drop across various sections will vary considerably with vasomotor activity. It is also of interest to know whether a change in mean pressure can alter the peripheral resistance by causing a passive change in the calibre of the small vessels. Read, Kuida and Johnson (1958) measured the total peripheral resistance in dogs that were being perfused by a pump so that the total flow was accurately known and found that a rise in venous pressure consistently caused a fall in the resistance. At its largest this was about 20 per cent change in P.R. for an increase of 20 mm Hg in venous pressure and a fall of some 60 per cent with a rise in venous pressure to 60 mm Hg. This is thought to be mainly due to a dilatation of the small venous channels although the arterial pressure increased a corresponding amount. Levy, Brind, Brandlin and Phillips (1954) used the Fick principle to measure the cardiac output and found that, when the baroceptors were denervated, the peripheral resistance remained constant with changes in mean arterial pressure. This suggests that the arterioles do not distend passively with an increase in pressure. When the baroceptors' reflex pathways were intact a rise in arterial pressure caused a marked fall in resistance indicating arteriolar dilatation In the vascular bed of a leg that was being perfused Phillips, Brind and Levy (1955) measured the resistance when both arterial and venous pressures were changed so that the pressure-gradient remained the same but the transmural pressure, i.e. the distending pressure was altered. They found evidence that increase of transmural pressure caused a fall in resistance. In a later paper Levy (1958) found that this change was much more marked when arterial pressures were changed than when the changes were on the venous side. This finding seems to be at variance with the previous finding of Levy *et al.* (1954) that changing arterial pressure did not alter the total peripheral resistance; it also differs from the results of Read *et al.* (1958) where a rise in venous pressure consistently caused a distinct fall in resistance. It is possible that the vascular beds of various regions differ in this respect. Final agreement is far from being reached on this topic as other workers, notably Folkow (e.g. Folkow and Löfving, 1956), have produced much experimental evidence that a rise in arteriolar pressure causes vasoconstriction because of the myogenic response of the smooth muscle in the wall.

Measurement of the peripheral resistance is not, therefore, a very good analytical method for distinguishing the behaviour of individual sections of a vascular bed. For separating the effects of changes in flow or vasomotor activity, however, it is simple and direct. As an example some results of Leusen, Demeester and Bouckaert (1954) may be used. In a series of dogs a fall in the pressure of their isolated carotid sinuses caused an increase in mean arterial blood pressure from 125 to 194 mm Hg (55·2 per cent). At the same time the cardiac output increased from 3·3 to 4·3 l./min (30·3 per cent) and the total peripheral resistance from 3,140 to 3,750 dyne.sec/cm^5 (19·4 per cent). It is clear that the increase in cardiac output played a greater part in increasing the blood pressure than vasoconstriction did. After a haemorrhage of 10 per cent of their estimated blood volume the corresponding increases were: arterial pressure, 72·5 per cent, cardiac output 26·3 per cent and peripheral resistance 38·5 per cent. The rise in pressure was then due more to vasomotor activity than to the increase in cardiac output. These figures alone, however, cannot give any information as to which parts of the vascular bed have constricted. From general knowledge it is assumed that it will largely be in the arterioles, but venous constriction may well play a part in the response to sinus hypotension. Such constriction would cause an increase in cardiac output but would also increase the total resistance, although there is little information on which we can estimate what proportion, of the total increase, this would be.

CHAPTER III

THE CHARACTERISTICS OF BLOOD FLOW IN THE CIRCULATION

The well-defined conditions that are laid down for the laws of liquid flow, which have been discussed in the previous chapter, are clearly not precisely applicable to the circulation. The discussion below will be an attempt to make a compromise in applying the exact results of hydrodynamics to the considerably more complex, and often unknown, circumstances of the circulation. It will be convenient to consider the factors set out (p. 18) as being the necessary postulates for the application of Poiseuille's law.

The viscosity of blood

In the theoretical treatment of liquid flow it was assumed that the liquid we were considering was a Newtonian fluid, that is a homogeneous liquid in which the viscosity was independent of the rate of shear while laminar flow persisted. Blood is not a homogeneous fluid. The plasma, although a colloid solution, behaves like a Newtonian liquid; whole blood however, is a suspension of relatively large particles, the red cells. As a result flowing blood shows anomalous viscous properties. It is not proposed to consider the large body of often conflicting work on this subject. This has been extensively and excellently reviewed by Bayliss (1952). Most of these anomalous properties become important in the flow in capillaries and it is not proposed to deal with this in detail.

The flow of blood deviates markedly from Poiseuille's law in two different ways. (1) At low rates of shear the viscosity increases, and (2) in small tubes the apparent viscosity at all rates of shear is smaller than in large tubes.

The rate of shear in a liquid in a tube depends on the pressure-gradient and the radius of the tube. As the gradient in any given tube increases the apparent viscosity falls. With high rates of flow it gradually approaches a constant value. This "asymptotic value" decreases with the diameter of the tube. Extensive observations on this have been made by Müller and his colleagues (Müller, 1948; Kümin, 1949) and other workers (see Bayliss, 1952). Kümin's data have been analysed in great detail by Taylor (1959a).

When these data are plotted as a pressure-flow curve it appears that, when it is extrapolated to zero flow, there is a positive pressure intercept. This has been compared with the yield-pressure of a plastic solid; that is, a certain pressure has to be applied before any movement occurs. This concept of blood as a semi-plastic body was first suggested by Bingham and has been developed by Lamport (1955). Measurements made with very low rates of flow (Bayliss, 1952; Kümin, 1949; Haynes and Burton, 1959) show that the pressure-flow curve inflects and almost certainly passes through the origin. Thus there is a marked increase in viscosity at low flow rates but no yield-pressure. The rates of shear at which this is marked are so low that it is of doubtful physiological significance.

Close to the wall of the tube there appears to be a relatively cell-free marginal zone, which causes an effective decrease in viscosity. The width of this zone is probably more or less independent of the diameter of the tube and so this effect is only apparent when the diameter is less than 0·5 mm. The existence of this marginal plasmatic zone is now generally agreed although Bayliss (1952) pointed out that most of the earlier observations on which this assumption is based were reported uncritically and are not satisfactory as evidence. The phenomenon was, however, clearly demonstrated by Taylor (1955) who measured the variation in optical density from the wall to the centre of suspensions of red cells flowing in glass capillaries. The confusion over the early evidence is due, in part, to the fact that it has been usual to regard the movement of particles towards the axis of the tube as being self-evident. The analogy used has been the familiar fairground one of a ping-pong ball supported in the centre of a vertical jet of water. The actual analysis of the physical forces involved is, however, very complex and has only recently been satisfactorily achieved (Saffmann, 1956). The predicted forces, however, are very small and it is doubtful if any marked aggregation of the cells occurs toward the axis of the stream apart from the formation of the marginal plasmatic zone.*

The consequences of shear dependent viscosity changes have been investigated in considerable detail by Taylor (1959a). With regard to pulsatile flow, which is the main subject of investigation in later chapters, Taylor demonstrates clearly that the best value of

---

*A recent paper of Bayliss reports that defibrinated blood in a capillary 100 μ in diameter shows a reduced optical density in a zone 5–20 μ wide but any cell-free zone that may exist is less than 2–5 μ wide (Bayliss, L. E., 1960, *J. Physiol.*, **149**, 593–613).

the viscosity to be taken is the asymptotic value, i.e. at high flow rates. Under the conditions that we find in arteries this will not give rise to errors of greater than one or two per cent, either in pressure-flow calculations or in the effects of viscosity on wave-velocity or damping.

Because the rate of flow and the size of the tube influence the viscosity of blood, attention should be paid to the methods of measurement when comparing published values. As the red corpuscles contribute largely to the viscosity it is to be expected that the viscosity increases with the haematocrit value. There is also species variation due to differences both in the normal haematocrit and in the size of the individual red cells. The usual method of measuring viscosity is in a capillary tube viscometer (details of design are given by Hatschek, 1928, and by Barr, 1931). Owing to the anomalous viscous properties shown by blood at low rates of flow—a phenomenon first clearly described by Hess (1911)—a viscometer capable of high rates of flow should be used. Hess himself designed one that is still in common use. In this instrument the viscosity of blood is directly compared with that of water. This ratio is called the *relative viscosity* and is the value commonly given in works of reference. The viscosity of fluid falls with a rise in temperature and it is usually assumed that the relative viscosity is independent of temperature. There is evidence that the viscosity of blood has a temperature coefficient greater than that of water, that is, its viscosity falls more over a given rise of temperature than does water. As viscosities are commonly measured at 20°C the relative change in coefficient between 20°C and 37°C has been estimated by some workers and that of blood falls approximately 1·1 times that of water. The relative viscosity will therefore fall by this amount.

The viscosity of water is 1·0 centipoise at 20°C (more precisely it is 1·00000 cP at 20·2°C (Bingham and Jackson, 1918)) and is 0·695 cP at 37°C. The relative viscosity of blood is reported as being between 2·5 and 4 (Green, 1944) but most reference books give a higher figure—4·7 at 38°C for man and dog (Albritton, 1952), 4·8–5·2 (Whitby and Britton, 1950); 3·9–5·3 (mean 4·7 for males, 4·4 for females, Bazett, 1941); 3·5–5·4 (mean 4·6) (Wintrobe, 1942). In absolute units, at 37°C this gives values from 0·017 P to 0·0371 P. A mean value of the relative viscosity for human blood of 4·6 is supported by the results of a large series by Hess (1908) and Nygaard, Wilder and Barkson (1935) i.e. 4·64±0·025. With dogs' blood Coulter and Pappenheimer (1949) made careful observations on the apparent viscosity in absolute units at varying haematocrits but unfortunately the different experiments were performed over a wide range of temperatures. Calculating the relative viscosities for the experiments with haematocrit values between 40 and 45 per cent their values range from 5·62 to 6·38 which corresponds to absolute viscosities of 0·0391 to 0·0443 P at 37°C. These were all measured at high rates of laminar flow but before the onset of turbulence. It will be seen that they are rather higher than the text-book values quoted above. Whittaker and Winton (1933) obtained values of about 4 with a haematocrit value of 45 per cent in a high-velocity glass viscometer. Using a perfused hind-limb, however, they found that the relative viscosity was of the order of 2·2. This would correspond to a viscosity of only 0·015 P. This result is taken to show that the fall in viscosity in vessels of capillary size is a dominant factor in the effective viscosity in the body.

It is seen that there is no great measure of agreement between various observers concerning the precise value of the viscosity of whole blood. In an animal such as the rabbit with a low haematocrit (Wintrobe, 1942) I have assumed the viscosity at 37°C to be 0·017 P, at the lower end of the range quoted. For dogs and human beings the value would appear to lie between 0·03 and 0·04 P, in tubes of radius greater than 0·01 cm, and such values will be assumed for calculations involving the large vessels.

The viscosity of serum and plasma is lower but in spite of the lack of complication due to the presence of corpuscles there is no very great measure of agreement. Bircher (1921) found the relative viscosity of human serum in the range 1·7–2·0, with whole plasma having values 0·2 to 0·3 higher. Nygaard *et al.* (1935) give the value 1·96±0·004 for serum. Bazett (1941) gives 1·5–1·7 for human plasma.

Pulsating flow

The most obvious characteristic of the arterial blood flow is that it is pulsatile. This has a very large effect on the relationship between pressure and flow, which is one of the major topics of this book. Here we may consider the velocity profiles that will be found in pulsating flow and the effect pulsation has on the stability of the flow (p. 50). We have seen in Ch. 1 that the most convenient way to describe a regularly recurring pulse, such as that created by the

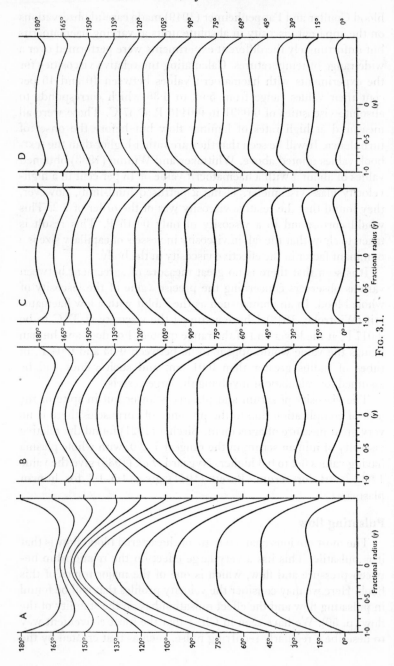

Fig. 3.1.

heart, is by a Fourier series (eqn. 1.1). This will define the wave
by a steady term and a series of sinusoidal oscillations. The simplest
form of pulsation to consider, therefore, is an harmonic oscillation
and Fig. 3.1 shows the forms of the velocity profiles at successive
stages created by a pressure-gradient, cos ωt. The value of ω is
respectively in the ratio 1, 2, 3 and 4 from A to D. The mathematical equations from which these profiles are calculated are discussed in Ch. 5. Similar profiles were predicted by Lambossy
(1952a) and have been verified experimentally by Müller (1954a)
using a Pitot tube which could be moved across the lumen of the
tube.

It will be seen from the illustration that even at the lowest
frequency shown, a true parabolic profile is not formed at any
time. There is a phase lag between the applied pressure and the
movement of the fluid. The laminae that move first are those
nearest the wall and flow successively involves the laminae towards
the axis of the tube. With a simple oscillation of this type there is,
of course, reversal of direction at each half-cycle. Near the wall the
effect of viscosity is high and these laminae always have a low
velocity and hence low kinetic energy. Thus they are reversed
easily. As we move towards the axis the kinetic energy becomes
much higher relative to the viscous drag and so there is a greater
lag between the pressure-gradient and the movement of liquid in
the centre of the tube (see Fig. 3.3). As the frequency increases
there is, as it were, less time in the cycle for the movement to be
translated throughout the axial laminae and the velocity profile
becomes very flattened. Increasing the diameter will, similarly, produce a like alteration in the profile. The liquid in the central part

---

FIG. 3.1 (A) The velocity profiles, at intervals of 15°, of the flow resulting
from a sinusoidal pressure gradient (cos ωt) in a pipe. In this case $a = R\sqrt{\omega/\nu} =$
3·34, corresponding to the fundamental harmonic of the flow curves illustrated
in Fig. 3.2 and 3.3. Note that reversal of flow starts in the laminae near the wall.
As this is harmonic motion only half a cycle is illustrated as the remainder will
be the same in form but opposite in sign, e.g. compare 180° and 0°. (B) A similar
set of profiles for harmonic motion of double the frequency of A ($a = 4·72$). The
amplitude and phase of the pressure are the same here and in C and D as in A.
The effects of the larger a are thus seen to be a flattening of the profile of the
central region, a reduction of amplitude of the flow and the rate of reversal of
flow increases close to the wall. (C) The third harmonic with $a = 5·78$. The effects
of higher frequency noted in B are here further accentuated. (D) The fourth
harmonic ($a = 6·67$) shows the same effects again. The rapidly varying part of
the flow lies between $y = 0·8$ and $y = 1·0$ and the central mass of the fluid reci-
procates almost like a solid core. (*Hale, et al.*, 1955).

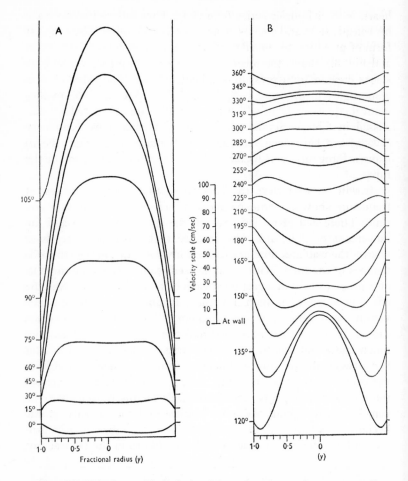

FIG. 3.2. Velocity profiles calculated from the measured pressure-gradient in the femoral artery of the dog. The first four harmonic components with the same values of a as in Fig. 3.1 are summed together with a parabola (axial velocity 30 cm/sec) representing the steady forward flow. The maximum forward velocity occurs in the axis because here the harmonic components are in phase but the maximum backward velocity lies between $y = 0.3$ and 0.4 at 180°. The reversal of flow beginning near the wall is clearly seen.

The variation in velocity of certain of these laminae is also plotted in Fig. 3.3 in a similar way to that of ordinary average velocity flow curves (Ch. 5 and 7). *Average* velocity is used for the average of all laminae across the tube at any moment; *mean* velocity is reserved here for the mean value throughout the cycle, i.e. the steady, or constant, term of the Fourier series (A_o in eqn. 1.1).

The pulse-frequency in this case was 2·8/sec so that the cycle length was approximately 360 ms. One degree of arc is thus approximately 1 millisecond. (*Hale, et al.*, 1955.)

of the tube begins to move more like a solid mass and the lateral variations in velocity become crowded nearer and nearer to the boundary. This increases the rate of shear in the layers close to the wall at high frequencies. The actual form of the profile depends on the value of the parameter a, as explained in greater detail in Ch. 5.

In its simplest form $a = R\sqrt{\dfrac{\omega}{\nu}}$ (R—radius, ω—angular velocity and ν—kinematic viscosity) so that its value increases linearly with the radius and with the square root of the frequency. The profiles shown in Fig. 3.1 A—D were calculated for values of a determined for the femoral artery of the dog. The profiles that would be seen during the cardiac cycle can be derived by adding the curves for the component harmonics together with a parabolic profile representing the steady flow. These profiles are shown in Fig. 3.2. It can be seen that in the fast systolic rush all the harmonics are most nearly in phase and create a profile which approaches the form of a parabola. Then reversal of flow begins in the peripheral laminae and progressively involves the laminae towards the axis. Thus at 135° of the cycle the average velocity across the artery is approximately zero although the axial laminae are still flowing forward. During backflow the harmonics are considerably out of phase with one another and the profile, in contrast to that in forward flow, is very much flattened. Indeed the maximum retrograde velocity does not occur at the axis but in the laminae with a radius of between 0·3 and 0·4 of the tube radius. These effects are also shown in Fig. 3.3 where individual laminar velocities are plotted through the cycle.

These profiles were calculated (Hale, McDonald and Womersley, 1955) on the assumption that blood is an homogeneous liquid. As we saw in the last section there is a tendency for the red cells to move towards the axis of the tube and this region will, therefore, tend to have a higher viscosity than that near the wall. This radial variation of viscosity will tend to cause a blunting of the axial portion of the velocity profile and mathematical descriptions of the effect of various simple conditions of radial variation have been given by Womersley (1955a). In an artery as large as the dog femoral, which has been considered in the graphs above, this effect of the red cells on the velocity profile is unlikely to be very great but there is insufficient evidence available at present to assess it.

In the largest arteries such as the aorta the values of a are much greater than those illustrated. In the proximal aorta the value for the first harmonic will be at least 10 so that the flattening of the velocity profile seen in Fig. 3.1 D where $a=6.67$ will be even more exaggerated and the boundary layer that is undergoing appreciable shear will be confined to a very narrow region close to the wall.

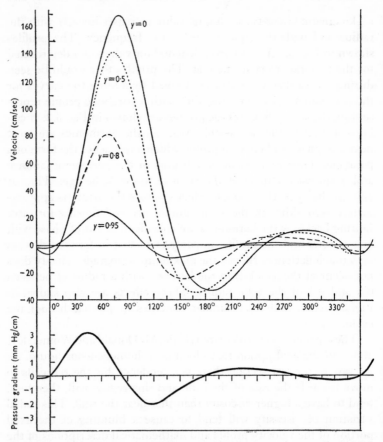

FIG. 3.3. The velocity of pulsatile flow in the dog femoral artery displayed in terms of individual laminae in the stream corresponding to the profiles shown in Fig. 3.2. The position of a lamina is defined by $y=r/R$. Thus $y=0$ is in the axis, $y=0.5$ is midway between the axis and the wall and $y=0.95$ is close to the wall. The measured pressure gradient from which the curves were computed is displayed below. It can be seen that the flow of fluid near the wall follows the pressure gradient most closely and that the phase lag increases to a maximum at the axis. The peak average forward velocity was 105 cm/sec at 75° and the peak *average* backward velocity was 25 cm/sec at 165°. (*Hale, et al.*, 1955.)

Preliminary reports from the Fribourg school (von Deschwanden, Müller and Laszt, 1956) show that with a Pitot tube scanning the velocities across the thoracic aorta a virtually flat velocity profile was recorded. This would appear to agree with the predictions of Hale *et al.* (1955) but in this region the theoretical treatment they used is not strictly valid because in the regions close to the heart we have to consider the conditions which determine the inlet length.

The inlet length

In the consideration of Poiseuille's law (p. 19 section 5) it was pointed out that in a pipe leading from a reservoir, steady flow was not "established" in the proximal part of the tube. The conditions near the entrance may be visualized in this way. At the orifice in the reservoir there is initially the same velocity all the way across. Once inside the pipe the layer of liquid immediately in contact with the wall will become stationary. The laminae close to it begin to slide on it subject to the forces of viscosity and form a boundary layer. The bulk of the fluid in the centre of the tube will move as a mass, affected very little by the forces of viscosity, and will have a flat velocity profile. As flow proceeds down the tube, however, the boundary layer will grow in thickness as the viscous drag involves more and more of the liquid. Finally the boundary layer comes to occupy the whole of the tube and steady viscous flow is established. The velocity profile is then parabolic. The stages of development of the profile are shown in Fig. 3.4. If the Reynolds number is above the critical number then the established flow will be turbulent but up to that point, i.e. within the

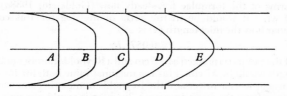

Fig. 3.4. Successive velocity profiles within the "inlet length" between two parallel walls leading from a reservoir—it is assumed that the pattern in a cylindrical pipe would be similar. Near the inlet (A) the shear in the liquid is confined to a boundary layer near the wall and there is no velocity gradient in the centre of the channel. The boundary layer increases in thickness progressively (B, C and D) with a corresponding diminution of the unsheared region. Finally the parabolic profile (E) of steady laminar flow is established. It is of interest to compare the profile such as A with those of oscillatory flow, e.g., Fig. 3.1 D, and of turbulent flow, e.g. Fig. 2.3. (*Redrawn from Goldstein,* 1938a.)

inlet length, the flow is neither strictly laminar nor turbulent. This is only a highly simplified description of a complex problem and reference should be made to Goldstein (1938a, Ch. 2) for further detail.

The conditions determining the magnitude of the inlet length are known for steady flow but have not been determined for oscillating flow. A comparison of the velocity profiles of established oscillating flow where a is relatively large, e.g. Fig. 3.1 D, with the flat fronted profiles seen in Fig. 3.4 near the beginning of the inlet length shows that they are very similar in form. In both cases the region of shear is confined to a narrow boundary layer and the main mass of the fluid in the axial regions of the tube is relatively unsheared. This suggests that the distinction between established oscillating flow and flow in the inlet length is virtually negligible. It also suggests that differentiation of laminar and turbulent flow may be less important in this region than is usually assumed. Clearly this point requires more rigorous investigation, but in view of the large approximations we already have to make in the hydrodynamics of the circulation it would appear that at present a correction for inlet length may be omitted. This approximation has already been used by Fry, Mallos and Casper (1956) in a method for calculating the blood flow in the proximal aorta from the pressure-gradient measured by a double-lumen catheter, but without precise knowledge of the actual flow their results cannot give us an estimate of what correction is needed for the inlet length condition. The interesting implications of Fry's mathematical treatment are discussed more fully in Ch. 5.

In terms of the formulae for steady flow (Goldstein, 1938a) we can estimate what it would be in the aorta of the dog for this condition. For laminar flow the inlet length (x) is

$$x = 0 \cdot 057r.Re$$

so that if the radius (r) is taken as $0 \cdot 5$ cm and a Reynolds number of 2,000 the inlet length would be 57 cm. This is a maximal value both for Re and for r as the aorta grows narrower and the Reynolds number becomes smaller as the distance from the heart increases. Even so it would certainly include the whole length of the aorta.

The minimal size for the inlet length is for turbulent flow starting with turbulence in the reservoir when

$$x = 0 \cdot 693d.Re^{\frac{1}{4}}$$

With the same vessel ($d = 1 \cdot 0$ cm) and Re as 4,000, which may well be attained in the dog aorta (Table I), this would give an inlet length of 6 cm. This would involve up to the proximal half of the thoracic aorta.

Turbulence in the circulation

The theoretical derivation of a relationship between pressure and flow whether it be for steady flow, as in Poiseuille's law, or for the more general solution which includes oscillating flow such as that derived by Womersley (1955*b*) and others (e.g. Lambossy, 1952*a*) depends on the condition of laminar flow. It is, therefore, important to consider whether blood flow is laminar. Unfortunately there is little direct evidence, so that deductions from the Reynolds number are usually our only criteria. The lower critical value for homogeneous liquids is 2,000. The question as to whether this is true for blood has been subject to investigation. Early work is reviewed by Bayliss (1952) but the most precise work is that of Coulter and Pappenheimer (1949). They studied the steady flow of blood through tubes of 0·126 cm internal radius, i.e. similar in dimensions to the femoral artery of the dog. By the orthodox method of recording the discontinuity in the pressure-flow graph they recorded the onset of turbulence at a Reynolds number of $1,960 \pm 160$ (they used the radius in their formula and actually reported the value of 980 ± 80). This is sufficiently close to the accepted value for the critical value for other liquids to indicate that blood does not behave anomalously in this respect. However, they also measured the electrical resistance along the line of flow and found that it did not alter at the onset of turbulence. The electrical resistance was assumed to be a measure of the orientation of the cells in the line of flow, so that they deduced that the turbulence only involved the plasma sleeve, and that the red cells, aggregated in the more axial streams, maintained laminar flow in the centre of the tube. As further evidence that the electrical resistance depended on cell orientation they showed that in oscillating flow there is a marked increase in resistance at each reversal of flow, a point when the corpuscles might be expected to turn through 180° (Coulter and Pappenheimer, unpublished). Nevertheless the conclusion that in flowing blood there can exist at the same time a turbulent "sleeve" of plasma with a laminar central "core", which is physically difficult to conceive, seems hardly to be justified on the evidence. It is probable that the measurement of resistance is a relatively crude way of determining the orientation of the cells and that this orientation is far from complete in laminar flow, and not sufficiently disturbed by the degree of turbulence they created to make a measurable difference. The picture they tended to create of the red cells packed together so that they were perfectly aligned and "floating like a log down the stream" is unrealistic. Taylor (1955), for instance, showed that light transmission is greatest through the axial region of blood flowing in a tube, so that they cannot be very tightly packed. Furthermore, in the transient turbulence observed in the rabbit aorta (Fig. 2.4) it can be seen that the dye distribution is right across the stream and this occurred at a Reynolds number that was certainly not above the critical value of 2,000. In the following discussion it will be assumed that stability of laminar flow in blood is essentially the same as that of other liquids.

The effect of pulsation on the stability of laminar flow is clearly of considerable interest. There seems little doubt that oscillatory flow will become unstable at Reynolds numbers that are less than 2,000, even when these are calculated from the maximum average flow velocities. In the rabbit aorta quoted above, for example, the Reynolds number was less than 1,000 when derived in the usual way. Simple model experiments which we have done, and also those reported by Evans (1955), can demonstrate that rapid alterations in the rate of flow will readily cause a break-up of the pattern of injected dye. Hale *et al.* (1955) considered this question quantitatively and made the assumption that the critical Reynolds number was simply related to the maximum rate of shear in the liquid. By calculating this for oscillating flows they derived the equivalent steady flow velocity that would give the same rate of shear. The ratio of the equivalent average velocity to the actual measured average velocity when multiplied by the Reynolds number would give an "effective Reynolds number". This ratio was dependent on the value of a. The ratio remained at 1·0 for a value of a up to 2·0. When a was greater than 3·0 it increased linearly so that at $a=4·0$ the ratio was 1·2, and at $a=10·0$ the ratio was 2·8. The only experimental evidence in support of the assumption that instability depends on rate of shear was based on a comparison of flow patterns in the rabbit aorta and the dog femoral artery. The maximal Reynolds number calculated in the normal way was about 1,000 for each vessel, yet high-speed cine-films demonstrated turbulence in the aorta of the rabbit but no turbulence in the femoral artery of the dog. The pulse rate of the rabbit is, however, faster than that of the dog, and allowing for this difference in the value of α the effective Reynolds number in the rabbit came close to 2,000, whereas in the dog it was only 1,300. The frequency of the pulse rate would thus be an important factor in determining the stability of arterial flow. The quantitative nature of the effect should, however, be regarded with caution until more precise experimental evidence is available.

It seems likely that the maximum rate of shear is not the only factor causing instability of flow. Prandtl (1952) quotes some theoretical work of Lord Rayleigh which indicated that re-entrant angles in a velocity profile were points of instability, and in more recent work Tollmien has shown that S-shaped inflexions in the profile are in fact the points where stability breaks down. Prandtl suggests that it is the production of such inflexions by small irregularities in the wall that initiate turbulence in steady flow. Certainly in a glass model reversal of flow easily causes vortex rings to appear at the points of backward inflexion that can be seen in the profiles illustrated in Figs. 3.1 and 3.2. The vortex rings that Helps and McDonald (1954a) observed in the inferior vena cava of the rabbit occurred at this situation during reversal of flow. The rate of shear is, of course, zero at the apex of such an inflexion. Evans (1955) has suggested, on the basis of Theodorsen's work, that turbulence originates in such vortices. Against this must be set the fact that in the rabbit aorta the instability of the flow developed during the rapid acceleration phase in systole considerably before any reversal of flow took place, and when the rate of shear would be maximal. This suggests that both high rates of shear and inflexions in the velocity profile may cause instability in oscillating flow when the Reynolds number is relatively high. From the consideration of the probable value of the Reynolds numbers found in the circulation detailed below, it seems likely that transient turbulence during systole will be found in the larger arteries, but that laminar flow should be found in at least part of diastole.

Our knowledge of the Reynolds numbers that are to be found in the circulation is limited by our knowledge of the velocities of blood flow. The available information on pulsatile flow velocity in arteries is limited (see Ch. 6) because volume flows are usually recorded and many authors have not stated the dimensions of the vessel so that one cannot deduce the linear velocity. Spencer and Denison (1956) reported peak systolic velocities as 112 cm/sec for the upper thoracic aorta, 128 cm/sec for the lower thoracic aorta and 141 cm/sec in the abdominal aorta (all in the dog). McDonald (1955*a*) found the peak systolic velocity in the dog femoral artery was about 80 cm/sec, and in the rabbit abdominal aorta (McDonald 1952*a*) about 60 cm/sec.

In the proximal aorta estimates of mean systolic velocity have been made by calculating from the stroke volume, the size of the aortic orifice, and the length of systole. This was done in the human aorta by Prec, Katz, Sennett, Roseman, Fishman and Hwang (1949) using radiography to estimate the diameter of the aorta. Their estimates averaged 40–50 cm/sec (range 21·3–87·4). As the actual size of the aortic orifice is limited by the bases of the aortic valves so that it is more like an equilateral triangle (McMillan, 1955) the velocities through the orifice itself would be double these values. The peak systolic velocity, judging from Spencer and Denison's aortic flow curves, would be at least 50 per cent higher than the mean systolic velocity. The values that Prec *et al.* derived for the Reynolds number are therefore less than maximal. Yet they ranged from 5,000–12,000 in the root of the human aorta, so that we can see that in this vessel very high numbers must be reached in systole even when they are calculated in the standard way. If the "effective Reynolds number" of Hale *et al.* (1955) were estimated it would be over three times as great. There is thus little doubt that there will always be marked turbulence in systole in the human aorta. Similar estimates for the dog have been made by Green (1944) who predicted a *mean* systolic Reynolds number for the root of the aorta of 2,360. From Spencer and Denison's (1956) records the *peak* value in systole is about 3,500 and thus these two estimates are compatible. Generally speaking the velocity of arterial blood flow is apparently of the same order of magnitude for the larger mammals so that the Reynolds number for a particular vessel will vary between species roughly in the ratio of the diameters of the vessel. The influence of the frequency of the pulse on the stability will tend to lessen the difference between larger and smaller species, however, because smaller animals tend to have a faster heart rate.

The values of Reynolds number that have been estimated in the circulation are shown in Table I. Only values to be found in systole are given for arteries as diastolic values are rarely quoted. As there appears always to be zero flow at some point during the

TABLE I.

Estimated Reynolds' numbers in the circulation

Species	Vessel	Diameter cm	Velocity cm/sec	Reynolds No.	Authors
Human	Ascending aorta	2·30–4·35	21·3–87·4 (mean systolic)	5,000–12,000	Prec et al. (1949)
Human	Pulmonary trunk	2·32–3·50	33·1–63·5 (mean systolic)	5,000–10,000	do.
Dog	Ascending aorta	1·0	40 (mean systolic)	2,360	Green (1944)
Dog	Prox. thor. aorta	1·0	112 (peak)	3,000–3,500	Spencer & Denison (1956)
Dog	Distal thor. aorta	0·77–0·82	114–128 (peak)	2,450–2,590	do.
Dog	Abdominal aorta	0·53–0·61	106–141 (peak)	1,710–1,970	do.
Rabbit	Abdominal aorta	0·3	60 (peak)	1,960	Hale et al. (1955)
Dog	Femoral	0·3	100 (peak)	1,300	do.
Dog	Saphenous	0·1	30 (peak)	80	McDonald (see Fig. 7.4)
Rabbit	Basilar	·0·06	40 (peak)	100	McDonald & Potter (1951)
Lamb	Ductus arteriosus	0·24	60 (mean)	750	Dawes et al. (1955)
Dog	Small mesenteric artery	0·005	2·1	0·28	from Schlier (1918)
Dog	Arteriole	0·0025	0·28	0·018	do.
Dog	Capillary	0·0008	0·05	0·001	do.
Rabbit	Small mesenteric vein	0·01	1·0	0·6	Helps & McDonald (1954a)
Rabbit	Abdominal vena cava	0·34	18·0 (peak)	360	do.
Dog	Abdominal vena cava	1·0	15·0 (peak)	930	do.
Rabbit	Thoracic inf. v. cava	0·6	18·0 (peak)	660	do.
Human	Thoracic inf. v. cava	2·0	10·7–16·0 (mean)	1,320–1,980	do.

The range of values for internal diameter and peak velocity for the dog aorta (distal thoracic and abdominal) ascribed to Spencer and Denison (1956) is due to recalculation of the wall thickness on the basis of my own data (see Ch. 8—values of h/R p. 161). The data actually recorded were the volume flow rate and the circumference of the vessel. The values from these authors are in each case for the smaller internal diameter and hence the higher flow velocity.

cycle in all large arteries, and hence a Reynolds number of zero, it can be seen that its fluctuations are very great. It should be emphasized again that the conditions determining the onset of turbulence at a critical Reynolds number were determined experimentally only for steady flow.* The application of this work to pulsating blood flow should be interpreted with reserve. In fact the only justification we have is that, in a field where we know little for certain, any guide is better than none.

*Recent work by Cotton on models indicates that when oscillatory flow is turbulent throughout the cycle the peak Reynolds number ($\widehat{Re}$) and a are related by the following equation giving an "effective" critical value,

$$\widehat{Re}/a \times 532 + 0.009 \ \widehat{Re}$$

As the "mean" a for the root of the human aorta is over 20 and for the dog over 15 it can be seen that none of the values in Table I for large arteries exceeds this effective critical number (Cotton, K. L., 1960, *The instantaneous measurement of velocity of blood flow and of vascular impedance*. Ph.D. Thesis, London.)

In a further study (Cotton, personal communication) he has shown that when the calculations from the data of Hale *et al.* (1955) is corrected by allowing for the momentum gradient a very similar theoretical equation to the experimental one above may be derived.

CHAPTER IV

THE DISTURBANCES IN BLOOD FLOW DUE TO THE CONFIGURATION OF THE VASCULAR BED

Mixing of the blood

In stable laminar flow there is no appreciable mixing of the streams of liquid within the lumen of the vessel. We know that the composition of venous blood varies considerably according to the metabolic activity of the organ from which it drains, so that it is important to know if a sample of blood from a vein is representative of all the blood in it, or whether its composition is dependent on the drainage through one, or more, of its tributaries. The extent of the mixing of dye is also important in dye-dilution methods for estimating blood flow. The easiest way to observe the mixing is to inject a dye into a tributary and watch its flow in the larger vessels. Unfortunately this direct method is only easily applicable to small vessels and we know from the evaluation of the Reynolds number (Table I, p. 53) that these are almost certainly laminar. Observations have amply borne out this prediction. Franklin (1937) reviewed a considerable body of evidence in the smaller veins and Helps and McDonald (1954a) confirmed that there was almost total absence of mixing in veins as large as the rabbit abdominal vena cava where the Reynolds number was about 350. Even so the streamline pattern is easily disturbed and it is probable that inserting a needle or catheter to take a sample would, of itself, cause a certain amount of mixing. An attempt to assess this effect quantitatively is made below.

When the flow becomes subject to pulsatile changes as in the great veins of the thorax, the maintenance of clear-cut streams is very much more difficult. The effect of pulsation on stability of flow has already been discussed, but in a situation like the inferior vena cava, while we can say with certainty on the evidence that considerable disturbance of flow exists (Helps and McDonald, 1954a), it is quite different to assert that *complete* mixing occurs. Even in a condition of turbulence physical admixture will take a

55

certain amount of time to occur, so that near the entry of a large tributary, like the hepatic vein for example, there might well be a difference in composition compared with the blood, say, in the right atrium. Ultimately the evidence from sampling must determine our views on the reliability of such sampling, and general considerations can only act as a guide.

It is unfortunate that the sites where we should most like direct observational evidence mainly concern the large veins and arteries, and that the thickness of the walls makes such direct observations difficult or impossible. A certain number of investigations have been made with cineradiography and these have been very valuable and should be extended. The interpretation of the results is a little limited by the lack of detail in the pictures. Also to obtain better contrast it is usual to inject the radiopaque substance rapidly and this, of itself, will tend to change the normal flow of blood very greatly.

The development of dye-dilution methods to measure blood flow also makes it necessary for us to know the characteristics of the flow in the regions to which they are applied. The details and theoretical basis of these methods have been lucidly set out by Meier and Zierler (1954) and reviewed by Dow (1956) and it is not proposed to consider them again here. Rossi, Powers and Dwork (1953) pointed out on the basis of model experiments that the normal technique will be in error if the flow in the vessels is laminar. If, however, there is a region in the system between the point of injection and the point of sampling where there is fully developed turbulence, or complete mixing from any cause, so that the concentration of indicator is uniform throughout the vessel, then the standard Hamilton-Stewart formula will apply. They did not study, or discuss, the implications of this remark but in so far as the commonest use of the method is for the determination of cardiac output, the heart is clearly the region where such complete mixing is likely to occur. As will be seen in the discussion in the next section, all the evidence suggests that normally the blood is completely mixed on passage through the heart so that the formula is valid. Conversely the general experience that the dye-dilution method gives a reasonably accurate measurement of cardiac output is further evidence for the complete mixing of blood passing through the heart.

Where an indicator-dilution method is used in a peripheral

vascular bed (Meier and Zierler, 1954) the situation is quite different, for we have seen in Ch. 3 that the Reynolds number in these vessels is almost certainly below the critical value. Particular attention has been paid to this problem by Zierler and his colleagues who studied the efficiency of jet-injection in producing complete mixing to the point where the dye was introduced (Andres *et al.*, 1954). In fact injection at a relatively slow rate was found to cause fairly complete mixing as evidenced by the concentration of dye in the radial and ulnar arteries, and was not greatly improved by jet-injection. This again indicates that the disturbances in the circulation, whether they be due to pulsation, the origins of branches or the other causes that are discussed in this and the previous chapter, will always cause a considerable degree of mixing. In the case of an intra-arterial injection the presence of a needle in the lumen would itself be a potent cause of eddy formation, as all such projections are (see p. 65).

Streamline flow may also determine the regional distribution of blood from certain organs. Thus it has been suggested that (as Copher and Dick (1928) showed) as blood from the spleen tends to go to the left lobe of the liver, this might be the reason that yellow atrophy of the liver mainly affects the left lobe. Similarly the distribution of laminar flow has been regarded as the determining factor in the spread of emboli. The portal circulation is a special case in this respect for the blood stream does not have to pass through the heart. It is, therefore, the most favourable site for a streamline pattern to be maintained. While it is very difficult to prove a negative, I regard the hypothesis that streamline flow in the portal vein maintains a regular organ-to-organ pattern of flow in the liver as highly unlikely. In the course of studies on the portal vein in the rabbit (Helps and McDonald, 1954*a*) while streamline flow was undoubtedly occurring, the position of these streams within the vein would change with the slightest movement of the upper abdominal organs, especially the stomach. In addition, respiratory movements caused considerable swirling of the streams. If they were unstable in position in a small animal like the rabbit while it was anaesthetized and immobile, it seems very unlikely that they can be at all stable in an active human being. In radiographic studies of the flow of contrast media injected into the spleen, Dreyer (1954) found evidence of streamlines in the portal vein in only one out of 15 patients and in 2 out of 9 dogs. The presence of a partitioned distribution of blood in laminar flow requires far more stable conditions than those causing incomplete mixing. Any hypothesis requiring the maintenance of such distinct streams through the normal adult heart must be regarded as without foundation.

The Heart

In terms of a hydrodynamic model the heart may be regarded as the reservoir supplying tubes emerging from it. As the standard description of the critical Reynolds number requires disturbed conditions in the reservoir, there is no doubt that this condition is satisfied but is of little consequence in view of the uncertainties underlying the application of the Reynolds number concept to the pulsating flow in arteries (see Ch. 3). The only real concern is with the degree of mixing, of the blood passing through it, that occurs. Treating the heart as a wide channel we can see from comparison with the large vessels that very high Reynolds numbers must be found there. The irregular shape of the channel with the occurrence of valves, and above all the rhythmical contraction of the walls, will cause a very great churning up of the blood within it. No one who has attempted to demonstrate laminar flow in models is likely to have any illusions about the difficulty of demonstrating streamlines through the chambers of the heart. Cineradiographic films of the flow of lipiodol in the dog's heart (Rushmer, 1955a, Ch. 1) show the swirling motion of the blood in the ventricles very clearly. On the question of the degree of mixing of blood in the heart there is a great deal of evidence derived from the standard practice of using an intracardiac catheter to sample mixed venous blood for determinations of the cardiac output by the Fick principle. This evidence can only be summarized briefly here. It is generally agreed that blood is thoroughly mixed, in a normal heart, by the time it reaches the pulmonary artery. In most clinics this is now the standard site for sampling. The catheter is less commonly left in the right ventricle for fear of causing ectopic beats, but here again complete mixing is regarded as occurring (e.g. Warren, 1948). In the auricle however, many workers have suggested that differences between successive samples may be due to the persistence of a streamline pattern of flow. Cournand (1948) has stated, however, that in 75 per cent of catheterizations successive atrial samples do not differ by more than 0·2 vols per cent in oxygen content. My personal opinion, with no practical clinical experience to support it, is that the inadequate mixing is only likely to be in the region of the orifice of the coronary sinus (in hearts where the auricle is beating normally). In the auricle, in fact, the sampling catheter is near the entry of a large vein and incomplete mixing is not a good indication of laminar flow.

In greatly distended hearts in advanced failure where there is a large volume of blood left at the end of systole, even ventricular mixing may be incomplete, and variation may also occur in the composition of samples in the region of septal defects (Wieder-hielm, Bruce and John, 1957). This is due to the fact that, even with fully developed turbulence the mixing of two volumes of liquid can never be instantaneous.* Such mixing cannot be pre-dicted theoretically and the determination of the size of the zones of unmixed, or partially mixed, blood can only be determined experimentally.

The foetal heart may be likened to the human heart with a congenital septal defect in the neighbourhood of which mixing may be incomplete. Barclay, Franklin and Prichard (1944) produced evidence that the blood from the inferior vena cava of the foetal lamb passed through the foramen ovale without mixing much with blood from the superior vena cava. Oxygenated blood from the placenta thus went to the left side of the heart and so preferentially to the head. The venous blood from the superior vena cava would be distributed to the hind-part of the body via the pulmonary artery and ductus arteriosus. In a small heart such incomplete mixing in the auricle might well occur though the separation of the two streams is likely to be far from complete. The phenomenon has been disputed by Dawes, Mott, Widdicombe and Wyatt (1953)

*In this respect it is interesting to draw an analogy, even though it is on a somewhat larger scale, with the distinct "streams" seen in rivers. Where one tributary has clear water, while another is muddy, the waters when they join can be followed distinctly—often for several miles. In former days the examples most quoted were of the Rhône, or the Danube at Vienna; nowadays, when our academic colleagues travel further afield, I am told of the same appearance at the junction of the Blue and White Nile at Khartoum and also in rivers in New Zealand. Unfortunately these are not examples of streamlines in laminar flow as seen in veins for, with Reynolds numbers of the order of millions, these rivers are all turbulent. They are, however, a reminder that even with fully developed turbulence the mixing of large volumes takes a long time. I am indeed sorry to have to demolish this piece of haemodynamic folklore but at least it shows how important scale is in drawing analogies between different systems.

who found no significant difference between the oxygen content of blood from the carotid and that from the distal aorta.

The only hearts in which laminar flow phenomena have been seen are those of some small amphibia such as the frog (Simons and Michaelis, 1953). The conditions here, however, are markedly different from those in the mammal owing to the very small size of these hearts with a low flow rate and low pulse frequency in addition to the anatomical peculiarity of the spiral valve.

In the mammal, especially the human, the evidence about the mixing in the emerging great vessels constitutes the last stage in the consideration of the effect of the heart on the flow patterns in the circulation. Reference has already been made to the results of sampling in the pulmonary trunk. In the systemic circulation sampling is normally done much further peripherally so that we need to consider also the effects of the curvature of the arch of the aorta, the origins of branches and of valves. The effects of pulsatile flow have already been discussed (Ch. 3).

Curves in a tube

The effect of curving a pipe is to increase the stability of flow. The critical Reynolds number increases quite markedly and a lower critical number of 7,000 is quite easy to obtain. The magnitude of the effect depends on the ratio of the curve to the radius of the tube (Goldstein, 1938*a*). The arch of the aorta is the best example of a curved tube in the circulation, but in view of the presence of large branches on it and the proximity of the heart, a simple application of hydrodynamic theory cannot be made.

Studies of steady flow through a full-scale model of the arch of the human aorta have been made by Timm (1942) with very interesting results. For example, at rates of flow that caused turbulence in the descending aorta, his photographs show that the flow in the proximal part of the arch is clearly laminar, although the streams of dye are pursuing a somewhat complex helical course. The velocity of flow at which this occurred in blood was only 28 cm/sec, which corresponds to a Reynolds number of 1,500 at most. Laminar flow is thus less stable in the aortic model than in a straight tube which suggests that the branches may be an important factor in causing a break-up of the flow pattern, for it was just beyond the branches that disturbed flow commenced.

The spiral, or helical, course that streams of dye follow when flowing round a bend can easily be demonstrated in a model. The reason for the generation of motion that is not parallel to the wall, as laminar flow is in a straight tube, is the centrifugal force that is associated with motion in a curve. This force is greatest in the axial streams because they are moving fastest, and least in the liquid near the wall which is moving slowly. Therefore the fluid in the middle of the stream forms a secondary flow towards the outer wall and forces the liquid near the wall to flow towards the inner wall of curvature. Thus there are two minor circulations set up within the tube separated by the medial plane in the line of the radius of curvature.

This pattern of flow around a bend is an integral part of the fusion of the flow of two branches into a parent trunk as seen below in the consideration of the effect of junctions.

Flow at junctions

As the circulation is functionally a distributing system of pipes junctions are a very predominant feature. Yet orthodox hydrodynamics appear to have paid little or no attention to them so that we have no sound basis for discussing the possible effect of branching in the stability of flow in a pipe. Barnett and Cochrane (1956) have published some preliminary experiments on the division of flow in steady flow in various types of model junction. The types of junction to be found in the circulation may be considered in three main types. (1) The division of a main trunk into two, or possibly more, approximately equal branches. This may be called the "bifurcation" or **Y**-junction and the most characteristic example is the bifurcation of the abdominal aorta into the two iliac vessels. (2) The reverse condition where two or more branches of equal size join to form a single trunk. This may be called the fusion junction, or **⋏**-type. This type is almost exclusively found in the venous system, the only arterial example of note being the fusion of the two vertebral arteries to form the basilar artery on the medulla. (3) The "side-branch" where a single branch, usually of much smaller dimensions, leaves the parent trunk at an angle which depends on the anatomical position. In the larger vessels this is the most common group for it contains so many variations.

In the case of the first and third groups the blood is flowing from a region of higher Reynolds number to one of lower Reynolds number. It is well established that the total size of the vascular bed increases at each sub-division and the effect of this in decreasing the Reynolds number has been demonstrated above (eqn. 2.12). The first effect of this will be to increase the stability of flow and conditions of laminar flow are most easily demonstrated in the smaller branches away from the heart. At the point of junction, however, there is a discontinuity in the wall and the effect of this is probably akin to a physical obstacle in the flow, which causes a sudden deflection in the motion of the liquid.

The most striking demonstration of this was shown in a high-speed film of flow at the bifurcation of the aorta in a rabbit (Fig. 4.1). The axial stream of the aortic blood could be seen to impinge on the wall joining the two iliac vessels and rebounded from it so that eddies were set up near the orifices of the two branches. The

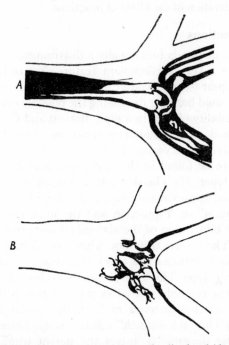

FIG. 4.1. Flow patterns with injected dye at the distal end (the "bifurcation") of the rabbit aorta. These are tracings of single frames of a high-speed film (16 mm) record. A, during the acceleration phase of systole; B, during diastole. There is a marked, but brief, disturbance of flow during systole in the more proximal part of the artery (Fig. 2.4). These drawings, however, serve to show that the presence of a point of branching causes much more marked and prolonged disturbances of flow pattern. The Reynolds number at peak systolic flow in this case was between 800–1,000. (*McDonald*, 1952b.)

dye nearer the walls of the aorta flowed more smoothly around the bend into the branches. In the rabbit (*Re* less than critical) these eddies only persisted through systole and died out early in diastole but in a larger animal would be expected to persist for much longer. The angle of branching will obviously affect the degree of disturbance. In the Fig. 4.1 it can be seen that the beginning of the iliac vessel is almost at right angles to the aorta. This is rather an extreme case but a study of other animals indicates that the angle of branching is always greater at the bifurcation than conventional anatomical diagrams suggest.

The difficulties of making direct observations on the interior of intact arteries are severe limitations in surveying this field. As mentioned above Timm (1942) studied the flow pattern in a glass model which was a faithful reproduction of the anatomical arrangement in the human aorta. Unfortunately he has only published photographs of the flow pattern in the actual arch of the aorta model. From these, however, we can visualize the situation at the origin of the innominate and subclavian branches in his model which will be similar to that of lesser branches leaving a main trunk at right angles. The deflection of the stream causes it to follow a sinuous course, so that the stream entering the branch may first swing over to the far side of the aorta and then curve back into the branch. Presumably the centrifugal force on the curved stream sets up secondary flows at each point where a tributary stream leaves the trunk, and this type of flow pattern will be mainly seen where the velocity of flow in the branch is fairly high, that is in large branches. The sudden creation of transverse motion of the liquid in the main trunk at such branches would tend to cause vortices and ultimately turbulence in the main trunk. Where the branch is very small, on the other hand, the flow into it will be derived almost exclusively from the blood near the wall, which will be the slow-moving laminae. In fact by "milking" off the fluid layers which are undergoing the highest rates of shear, numerous such branches might conceivably contribute to the stability of the flow in the main trunk.

There remains to consider the λ-junction. This differs from the other two types we have considered in that the flow is from a region of lower to higher Reynolds number. We have a little more information on this type of junction because of studies on the basilar artery. McDonald and Potter (1951) showed that in the rabbit the flow at this junction is quite undisturbed (Fig. 4.2). The Reynolds number, however, was only about 100 and the dimensions of this vessel were so small that the pulsatile flow would not raise the effective Reynolds number to any appreciable extent. Helps and McDonald observed similar stability at the junction of the two iliac veins with a Reynolds number possibly as high as 300. Using a glass model they studied the flow pattern up to much higher Reynolds number (McDonald and Helps, 1954*b*). When the Reynolds number was less than 1,000 steady laminar flow was seen. Injected dye formed a typical parabola in the tributary. At the junction the axial stream, that is the tip of the parabola, flowed towards the midline of the parent trunk, but owing to the bend between tributary and trunk a circulating movement developed due to secondary flow. The fluid in the axial stream moved toward

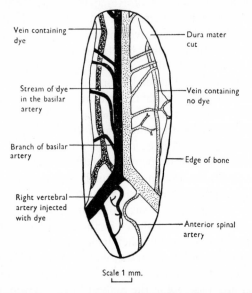

Scale 1 mm.

FIG. 4.2. Streamline flow pattern in the basilar artery of a rabbit shown by injection of dye into one vertebral artery. The unilateral distribution persists through the regions of supply, for it is seen returning only in the vein of the same side. The peak value of the Reynolds number here was less than 100; this low value is the main reason for the stability of laminar flow at this junction compared with that shown in Fig. 4.1.

This figure is a tracing of a still photograph; the phenomenon was also recorded on a colour ciné-film ("Blood streams in the basilar artery"—available from the Wellcome Foundation, London, N.W.1). This film also shows the changes in pattern with partial and total occlusion of the contralateral vertebral artery. (*McDonald and Potter*, 1951.)

the midline on either side and then circulated up to, and outwards by, the wall. There were, in fact, two sets of secondary flow set up in each half of the pipe which persisted for some distance down the parent trunk until a new parabola was formed across the single trunk. In high-speed films (1,500 f.p.s.) of this phenomenon the helical course of the streams can be clearly seen.

At a bend the fluid at highest flow rates tends to move to the outer wall and so in a λ-junction it is the faster flowing laminae that meet. Furthermore, where the curve is not smooth, particularly at the inner angle of the λ there is a zone of "dead water". As this is contiguous to the confluence of the fast flowing laminae, instability tends to occur at this point.

At rates of flow considerably below the critical Reynolds number (600 in branches, 1,000 main trunk) it was observed in the model that vortex rings were formed at this junctional region and were carried down the pipe, and when formed showed no signs of damping out for the length of about thirty diameters that they were followed. This strongly suggests that a λ-junction of this sort lowers the stability of flow across it. The quantitative assessment of this effect is difficult because of the difficulty in making glass junctions without any irregularity of the lumen, and at junctions of blood-vessels the smooth tapering of one tube branch into the other is better managed. It would be interesting to study this problem perfusing an actual venous junction. Disturbances at a variety of junctions in models have been studied by Stehbens (1959).

The effect of projections. Valves

It is common knowledge that an obstacle projecting into a stream will cause eddies to form, but small ones soon die away. If the disturbance is larger the eddies will grow in size and ultimately will cause a complete breakdown of laminar flow. The size of such an obstacle, as a fraction of the width of the channel, that can be permitted before the laminar flow breaks down depends on the Reynolds number of the flow and to a certain extent the shape of the obstacle. Goldstein (1938*a*, Ch. VII, p. 142) states that for a sharp-edged projection of height ε in a pipe of radius r

$$\frac{\varepsilon}{r} < 4/(Re)^{\frac{1}{2}}$$

to maintain laminar flow. For a smooth obstacle of cylindrical cross-section

$$\frac{\varepsilon}{r} < 5/(Re)^{\frac{1}{4}}$$

The commonest natural projection is a valve cusp, and so the formula for a sharp-edged projection is most valid. At a Reynolds number of 400 for example, the tolerated value of ε/r would therefore be 1/5 and at $Re = 1,600$ ε/r would be 1/10.

In pathological conditions such as atheroma the effect of projecting plaques may be estimated by this formula.

Any breakdown that occurs will be an eddy in the first instance and these will form at the free margin and will break away periodically. The formation of vortices at the free edge of a valve cusp will also have the effect of holding the free edge of the valve away from the wall. This has the important functional effect of presenting a considerable surface to flow in the reverse direction, thus closing the valve immediately there is a tendency for back flow to occur. Equally it means that at every valve there is a projection into the stream. The observation of these eddies at valves can very easily be made (for instance, they are seen in the human axillary vein when it is exposed surgically during a radical mastectomy). These eddies will cause mixing of blood in the veins. The obstruction due to a sampling catheter will also cause eddies and so increase mixing, an effect that will be greatest in small veins where the catheter will be large relative to the vessel.

At the aortic orifice the presence of valves adds one more factor to those already considered in producing an irregular flow pattern. In addition the expansion of the aorta, the aortic sinus, immediately beyond the valves will also cause eddy formation. Timm (1942) in the aortic model described above, shows clearly that even in conditions of laminar flow there is a swirling motion of the liquid in this region. The functional significance of eddy formation behind the valve cusps is here not only important for rapid closing, but also prevents the valves from occluding the orifices of the coronary arteries.

A change in calibre of a vessel which is of gradual onset has a considerably different effect from a sudden projection. A tube that is tapering to a narrower diameter causes an increased stability of flow, while an expansion of the tube causes a diminution of stability. This effect of expansion is probably an important factor in diminishing the flow stability of the great veins in the thorax which increase considerably in size during inspiration.

Arteries, of course, also increase in diameter during systole but as this dilatation is small, rarely more than 5–6 per cent, its effect is probably small compared with the effect of the oscillatory flow.

The aorta and large arteries

Blood in the aorta is completely mixed. If it were not then the composition of blood flowing into different branches would vary and withdrawing blood from a peripheral artery would not give a reliable and representative sample of arterial blood. This technique is used so widely in physiology and clinical medicine that the absence of any evidence of variability of samples from different arteries may be taken as proof of this assertion.

We have already seen that passage through the contracting chambers of the heart, together with the disturbances created by the valves, is probably sufficient cause for this mixing. The uniformity of composition does not, therefore, inherently provide any evidence as to whether flow within the arterial system is laminar or turbulent. As this point is of some interest, albeit rather academic, we need more direct evidence.

Cineradiographic investigations by Oppenheimer and Stauffer (personal communication, Stauffer *et al.*, 1955) showed that radiopaque material injected into the root of the aorta of a dog was very rapidly dispersed throughout the vessel. This at least indicates that there is a great deal of radial movement of the fluid in this situation. As we have seen, the aortic valves will create large eddies which could disperse the dye in this manner. In a dog it has also been shown (Table I) that the Reynolds number may reach a value of over 3,000 in the proximal aorta, so that there may be turbulence as well.

Other workers have made observations which suggest that aortic flow may be laminar. The problem of opacity in the aorta of the cat was circumvented by Ralston and Taylor (1945) by inserting a lucite cannula, and watching the flow of injected Indian ink. They reported the presence of streamlines. In view of the disturbances that might be expected to be generated at the margin of a cannula, it is remarkable that they saw no disturbance at all, for the situation may be considered comparable with that in the rabbit aorta where high-speed cinematography showed that there was a brief phase of "turbulence" with each systole (McDonald, 1952*b*). From Table I we see that the Reynolds number here just reached a critical value at peak systolic flow when corrected for the effect of pulsation. Ralston and Taylor did not estimate the Reynolds number and may well have had a considerably lower effective number if the heart rate was slower, as it probably was, than the rabbit's pulse rate (6/sec). On the other hand, simple visual observation may have missed the brief phase of disturbance with each systole and emphasized the longer phase of streamline flow if the alternating patterns were similar to those seen in the rabbit aorta.

In a further study Ralston, Taylor and Elliott (1947) supported these findings by showing that Indian ink injected into the ventricles was not distributed equally to the two renal arteries. This was a similar finding to the classical experiment of Hess (1917) who injected a solution of methylene blue, which was of the same viscosity as the blood, into the arch of the aorta from a cannula inserted down the carotid artery, and found that a higher concentration was found in the left iliac artery than in the right. If these results are correct they certainly show that there is not sustained turbulence in the aorta. This is more impressive in the case of Hess's results because he used a large St. Bernard dog, and although data on velocity of flow and size of vessels were not given, it is certainly to be expected that the Reynolds number would be well above 2,000 during part of each cardiac cycle. If this is always the case it would confirm some of the doubts expressed in the previous chapter as to whether transient fluctuations of the Reynolds number above the critical value do give rise to fully-developed turbulence. It was pointed out that the very flat velocity profiles that will be found in oscillating flow in a vessel the size of the aorta are very similar to those within the inlet length in steady flow conditions. Where the profile is flat there is no shear in the axial direction, and in steady flow terminology the flow is said to be not "established", i.e. one should not call it either laminar or turbulent. If the same restriction is applied to oscillating flow then the disturbances here, and hence the mixing of the blood, may well be less than in the corresponding established steady flow that would be found at these high Reynolds numbers.

Hess also maintained that flow in the thoracic aorta was not turbulent because he could hear no murmurs through a stethoscope applied to the surface of the aorta. The statement that murmurs are simply due to the onset of turbulence is made so frequently in physiological and medical textbooks that it is of interest to discuss the available information on this subject.

The creation of audible murmurs in the circulation

It is an unfortunate fact that relatively little fundamental work has been done by physicists in the generation of sound in liquids so that any discussion of the subject must, of necessity, be speculative. The only relevant work is probably in the field of aerodynamics and the production of noise in high velocity airstreams. This has been briefly reviewed by Wiskind (1957) in a most useful contribution to the Symposium on Cardiovascular Sound held in Cincinnati in 1956. The simpler physiological aspects have been well summarized by Rushmer (1955, Ch. 13) and a much fuller review has been presented in McKusick's (1958) monograph.

Starting with the simplest case, there is no doubt that undisturbed laminar flow is noiseless. Therefore, flow that generates noise must be non-laminar, but this may be due to eddies, or to turbulence. This does not, however, prove the converse case that this type of flow will produce noise, or at least any detectable noise. This is especially so in the circulation where there are considerable losses due to conduction through the tissues of the body. Rushmer (1955) has also emphasized that low-frequency murmurs will not be audible unless they are of considerable intensity because the threshold of hearing is high in this range. This introduces the complication that the appearance of a murmur clinically may only be due to an increase in frequency of a sound that is normally present, but inaudible. However, recording techniques, especially "spectral phonocardiography" as used by McKusick (McKusick, Talbot and Webb, 1954), can eliminate this problem.

An interesting demonstration of the different types of airflow was presented by Gregory, Stuart and Walker (1956). They studied the stability of the boundary layer of air which was moved by the rotation of a flat disk. The speed of flow of this layer depended on its distance from the centre of the disk and they monitored this with a probe microphone. In the central region the flow was laminar and there was no sound produced. Further out on the disk surface a region of spiral vortices was formed and produced a loud note of fairly definite pitch. Beyond this was the region of fully developed turbulence and the sound became a dull, confused roar due to the random turbulent fluctuations. The transition from one zone to another was fairly sharp. My personal impression of the demonstration was that, while turbulent flow in air is accompanied by noise production, the presence of marked vortices, or eddies, created a more audible and easily recognized sound. We may suppose that similar conditions would apply to the generation of noise in liquids. An experiment reported by Robinson (1952) showed a similar result. He created flows of water through a brass-pipe with Reynolds numbers up to 20,000 (i.e. markedly turbulent) without producing any noise. When he divided the tube and inserted a length of polythene cannula a murmur was produced at a Reynolds number of 1,700. This is a value in the transition zone and furthermore the edges of the polythene would accentuate eddy formation. The audibility of the noise might also have been accentuated by the vibration of the more compliant polythene.

If we consider the regions where murmurs occur in the circulation we see, from the discussion of causes of disturbances in flow pattern earlier in this chapter, that they are all situations where there will be a tendency for eddies to form quite apart from whether there is established turbulence or not. The sites of the cardiac valves are all associated with the production of sound and, as shown above, valve margins are almost certainly the site of eddy production. Another type of murmur is found at relatively small orifices through which the blood flows with a high velocity such as an arterio-venous fistula, and in this group we may include the ductus arteriosus as it is a shunt from a high pressure to a low pressure region. The Korotkoff sounds familiar in sphygmomanometry are also related to this type of murmur. Owing to the operation of Bernoulli's law (eqn. 2.10) there will be large eddies formed around the emergence of the jet from the narrow orifice into the wider region beyond. Thirdly, if we regard the first heart sound as a murmur generated within the ventricle there is little doubt that vortices of considerable size are generated within the irregular cavity of the ventricles.

Nevertheless, there are obvious difficulties about accepting vortex-formation as the sole cause of audible noise. The main one, arising from the foregoing discussion, is that there are many places in the circulation where eddies form but which do not create any detectable sound, for example, in the large veins in the thorax. The amount of noise will clearly depend on the energy that is dissipated in the formation of such eddies. In fact, it is as important to consider why murmurs are normally absent in the large arteries as to explain their cause when they are there. As there are always disturbances of flow present in the central regions of the circulation the detection of murmurs is probably a matter of the sensitivity of recording. Thus the popular explanation of the functional murmur in anaemia is that it is due to a lowering of viscosity which causes an increase in Reynolds number. Hence, it is suggested, laminar flow is changed to turbulent flow. In view of the high values of Reynolds number occurring normally (Table I) and their great fluctuation in any cardiac cycle a change in viscosity cannot alone cause any marked change in flow pattern. Already the work of McKusick and his colleagues indicates that there is a considerable amount of low-frequency sound created which we do not hear; with the current development of sensitive intra-arterial microphones (e.g. Rodbard, 1957) we may well learn much more as to the extent to which sound that is created in the blood is merely dissipated in transmission to the surface of the body.

One important factor, that must be coupled with the discussion of the disturbances of the blood-stream, is the vibrational properties of the solid structures of the heart and blood-vessels. In fact it is probably safe to say that no loud sounds will be created unless there is something like resonance of some of these solid structures. Although there will always be coupling effects between the blood and the structures that contain them it is simpler to consider the various factors under two separate headings—

1. Sound generated with the fluid itself
   (*a*) Turbulence
   (*b*) Eddy formation
   (*c*) Cavitation
   (*d*) "Water-hammer" and "shock" waves
2. Sound generated by the vibration of solid structures
   (*a*) Valve margins and chordae tendineae
   (*b*) Jet formation impinging on a wall.

1(*a*) (*b*). The distribution of turbulence and eddies has already been discussed. The acoustic energy that is dissipated in air-streams (Wiskind, 1957) is given by $\eta(V/c)^5$. V is the flow velocity and c is the velocity of sound in air so that V/c is the "Mach" number. At first sight it would appear that the corresponding value in liquids would be the velocity of sound in water so that V/c would be minute. As the blood is contained in an elastic tube the velocity of wave propagation, however, is almost entirely determined by the properties of the wall (Ch. 8). The appropriate value of c is thus the pulse-wave velocity. The factor η is a constant of proportionality which for air-jets is approximately 10^{-4} but I have been unable to discover if it is known for liquids. Wiskind also adds the comment "Workers in underwater acoustics usually regard turbulence as a negligible factor in sound generation." This probably applies equally to eddies considered *per se*.

1(c). Cavitation is a phenomenon where a sharp local fall in pressure causes bubbles to form in a liquid. If the pressure falls below the vapour pressure of the liquid vapour bubbles can be formed and as they grow and collapse they generate noise which has a wide-band of frequencies and which is similar to those commonly recorded by McKusick's technique (McKusick, 1957). It seems highly unlikely, however, that the pressure in the arterial system can ever fall low enough to produce vapour bubbles. Bubbles may also be formed from dissolved gas, and in the case of arterial blood, with its high oxygen content, this would seem a more likely cause. Bubbles of entrained gas, however, only oscillate at their natural frequency and Wiskind (1957) has calculated that oxygen bubbles of 1 mm diameter would have a frequency of over 3,000 c/sec. This is much higher than any appreciable component that has been recorded.

The fact that such bubble formation has not been seen is a drawback though not an insurmountable objection to accepting cavitation as a possible cause of sound generation. These bubbles might be very transitory. Points of pressure drop that might cause them would be in the centre of large vortices or at the point of emergence of a jet through a constriction, such as valve orifices or an arterio-venous fistula. These sites are, of course, commonly associated with murmurs, which makes cavitation an attractive hypothesis, but the drop in pressure required has always seemed improbably large for it to occur in arteries. The type of sound predicted also does not fit in with this idea, but cavitation in liquids in elastic tubes is an unexplored field. I have one personal experience which suggests that it may be easier to cause cavitation in blood than is generally thought. When we were attempting to impose an oscillatory flow from a pump in the arterial circulation (McDonald and Taylor, 1956) we produced cavitation on the pump side of the arterial cannula at frequencies above 6–7 c/sec. Unfortunately we could not record the pressure in this part of the system. The cannula, however, had an internal diameter of about 4 mm and was about 8 cm long; the pressure fluctuation at the arterial end was less than ± 20 mm Hg, which does not suggest that the pressure oscillations in the pump chamber were very great.

The present opinion about cavitation as a cause of cardiovascular sound is that it is extremely unlikely; it does, however, seem to merit further investigation.

1(*d*). A "water-hammer" phenomenon, due to a sudden drop in pressure at the aortic valves as they close, has been suggested by various workers. The relevant equation is discussed in Ch. 9 (9.1). The forces generated are determined by the flow velocity and the wave velocity in the aorta. As these are low there does not seem any likelihood of sound generation from this cause—the comparison with the loud noise produced by the water-hammer effect in domestic water-pipes is misleading because there we have rigid pipes and the wave velocity is that of sound in water.

"Shock" waves have on occasion been speculated about in the circulation. These are of the nature of the noises we have grown accustomed to as aircraft break through the "sound-barrier". This is when the Mach number, i.e. V/c is 1·0. A similar situation might arise in the circulation if the velocity of flow exceeded the pulse-wave velocity. There seems little evidence that this occurs (e.g. the flow curves in Ch. 7) for the fastest velocity of flow recorded appears to be about 200 cm/sec, and the lowest aortic pulse velocity commonly accepted is about 400 cm/sec. However, with high cardiac ejection velocities at a low mean pressure (and hence low pulse-wave velocities) it might occur and is a possible explanation of the "pistol shot" sound recorded by Lange, Carlisle and Hecht (1956). This was transmitted at a velocity of 800 cm/sec which is reasonable for a high-frequency oscillation in the arterial system (Ch. 9).

2. The vibrations of solid structures seem likely to determine the characteristics of cardiovascular sounds even if they are not their

primary cause. Here the frequency analysis of the Baltimore workers has provided invaluable data. The technical details of the method were described by McKusick, Talbot and Webb (1954) and further clinical examples by McKusick, Kline and Webb (1955) and McKusick, Webb, Humphries and Read (1955). Each sound is analysed into its component frequencies which are displayed vertically while the abscissa represents time, and intensity is represented by the density of the record. Normally an electrocardiograph tracing is recorded simultaneously. The great majority of murmurs shows a continuous spectrum of frequencies from almost zero to 500–700 c/sec. One gets the impression that the louder the sound the higher the range of recordable frequencies extend. The most constant and intense part of the range is between 120 and 360 c/sec. Such an amalgam of frequencies is best described as "noise", with no characteristic pitch, to distinguish it from a musical sound, with distinct harmonic components. Noise is what one would expect from the vibration of heterogeneous structures such as the arterial wall, but from a consideration of their elastic properties it is perhaps remarkable how high are the frequencies that are found. Wiskind (1957) states, for instance, that the frequencies commonly found in a tube are of the order of the ratio of flow velocity to diameter. From the recorded values (Chs. 6 and 7) in the dog this is 200 at most and probably nearer 100; for the human where the velocities are probably the same but the diameter greater (2·5 cm as compared with 1 cm as average values) the expected frequencies are even lower.

Much more remarkable, although much rarer, are the "musical murmurs" that have been recorded (McKusick, Murray, Peeler and Webb, 1955; McKusick, 1957) where a pure tone is clearly distinguishable—and the tone modulates with each heart beat so that the trace looks very like a pulse pressure curve, although it is probably a distorted form of the flow curve. One illustrated by McKusick (1957, Fig. 20) varies from 320 c/sec at the end of diastole to a peak value of nearly 600 c/sec in systole. Others (personal communication) have been of the order of 1,000 c/sec. In nearly all these cases, post-mortem examination has shown that there is a structure which can be implicated as the cause of the musical murmur, such as a stenotic aortic valve diaphragm, perhaps with calcification. Unusually rigid structures of this sort might be expected to have a particularly high natural frequency.

2(*a*). Valve margins have long been regarded as a site for the generation of sound. The common analogy between the slamming of a door and the closing of a valve is probably more picturesque than accurate. The studies of valve action that have been made (e.g. Rushmer, 1955, 1957; McMillan, Daley and Mathews, 1952; McMillan, 1955) show that the movement of the free edges of valves are not so extensive as might be imagined. Rodbard (1957) has emphasized the importance of the "flitter" of the free edges (which is due to the eddy formation in the "dead water" between them and the wall) as the source of sound generation. It is probable that something of this nature, rather than simple closure, is the cause of the second heart sound.

The first heart sound similarly owes a good deal to vibrations of the chordae tendineae during ventricular ejection.

2(*b*). Vibration in the wall of a vessel was a predominant feature in the only published example of a detailed investigation of a murmur under experimental conditions—that of Dawes, Mott and Widdicombe (1955) on the murmur in the ductus arteriosus of the new-born lamb. They measured the mean flow through the ductus while it was progressively constricted by an external tape, and recorded the murmurs with a phonocardiograph. From the measurement of the size of the channel through the duct and the mean volume flux, its flow velocity could be deduced. From these data the Reynolds number was calculated. Fig. 4.3 summarizes their results. It will be seen that the velocity of flow through the duct rises continuously with progressive constriction but the Reynolds number rises to a maximum of about 1,500 and then begins to fall. The murmur does not appear until the Reynolds number is greater than 800–1,000 and disappears again when it falls again below this value. The authors suggest that at this value of Reynolds number turbulence was initiated and the murmur was due to turbulence. There are, however, certain difficulties arising from this explanation. Firstly, the murmur was very precisely localized over the junction of the ductus arteriosus and the pulmonary artery, that is, beyond the region of high Reynolds number in the constricted region. Secondly, in addition to the murmur at this site there was also a "thrill" and this was shown remarkably clearly in the pulmonary artery pressure records as a high-frequency oscillation of the manometer. Both these facts suggest that the high-velocity jet into the pulmonary artery from the constricted region was the cause of the murmur and thrill. Such a jet would tend to cause the wall to oscillate, both by forming

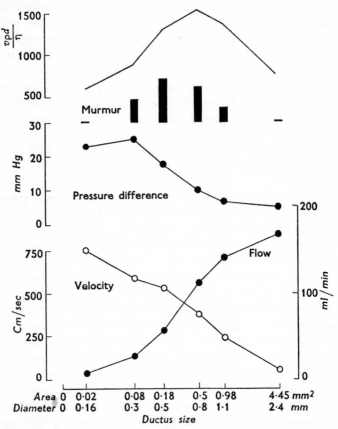

FIG. 4.3. Graphs showing the conditions under which a murmur appears at the pulmonary end of the ductus arteriosus of a new-born lamb. The ductus was progressively constricted by a tape (dimensions as abscissa with complete occlusion on the left).

From above downwards: Top graph—Reynolds number ($vd\rho/\eta$). Next—blocks representing the intensity of the murmur. Middle graph—mean pressure difference between the aorta and the pulmonary artery. Bottom graphs—the recorded mean volume flow (ordinate on right) and the calculated mean flow velocity (ordinate on left).

The Reynolds numbers are calculated for a viscosity (η) of 0·02 poises. They are thus probably a little too high and, of course, only apply to the flow through the constricted region. As discussed in the text it seems probable that the murmur is generated beyond (i.e. on the pulmonary artery side) of this region.

This lamb was of 129 days gestation, with an open chest and positive pressure ventilation. (*Dawes, Mott, and Widdicombe*, 1955.)

vortices, and by impinging on the pulmonary arterial wall, and so produce noise. The argument against this would be that the velocity of the jet is still increasing when the murmur ceases but the volume of fluid in such a jet, and hence its energy, would fall off markedly when the orifice became very small.

In view of the earlier evidence that turbulence of itself is not a potent factor in creating noise, I think that these investigations of Dawes and his colleagues support the contention that we require additional factors, such as the peculiar properties of a jet, to create a murmur. This is supported by the fact that they also showed that there was no murmur in the aorta itself although, from the evidence of the rabbit aorta (Fig. 2.4), turbulence was almost certainly occurring during systole. It is reasonable to suppose that similar conditions to those in the ductus cause the murmur of an arterio-venous fistula which is also normally accompanied by a palpable thrill. Whether jets through the valve orifices can also cause effects of this kind in the heart is a more speculative point.

The conclusions that emerge from a discussion of the causes of heart sounds and murmurs are all depressingly vague and mostly negative. The absence of a murmur is clearly no indication that the flow is laminar, for fully developed turbulence can occur without any detectable sound. Cavitation is one of the principal causes of noise generation in liquids in general, but it seems very doubtful whether it can occur in the circulation. Nor does the type of sound to be expected from cavitation seem to be similar to that found on spectral analysis of cardiovascular sound. The vibrational properties of the heart and blood-vessels themselves seem to be important in determining the characteristics of the sounds, but there is little quantitative information in this respect. However, with the present active collaboration between physicists and clinicians the outlook is quite promising.

CHAPTER V

THE PRESSURE-FLOW RELATIONSHIP OF
OSCILLATORY FLOW

We have seen that Poiseuille's law only applies to flow at a constant rate. Under such "steady" flow conditions in a given tube the volume flow is directly proportional to the constant pressure-gradient, that is the difference in pressure between the two ends of the tube. It is this difference in pressure that is the determining factor and the absolute level of pressure is completely irrelevant.

In an artery it is immediately apparent that the pressure is far from constant but is pulsatile owing to the pumping action of the heart.

This rise and fall of pressure which is distributed throughout the arterial tree represents to some extent a change in the absolute level of pressure in a pipe and so will not, of itself, directly influence the flow. It is not therefore surprising that no simple relationship between the pulse-pressure in an artery and its flow has been discovered. If we record pulsatile flow and pulse-pressure together as in Fig. 5.1 we see that the maximum rate of flow precedes the maximum pressure, which appears odd when one considers that blood must have inertia. The apparent anomaly is due to the fact that, as in the application of Poiseuille's law, it is the pressure-gradient along the artery that is related to the flow of liquid and not the pressure-level.

The pressure-gradient may be easily determined by recording the pressure at two points along the artery and subtracting the pressure from the downstream point from that at the upstream point at each moment. The record of such a measurement is shown in Fig. 5.2 A. As the pressure-pulse generated in the aorta by the expulsion of blood by the heart travels along the arteries the crest of the wave reaches the first recording point a short time before it reaches the downstream point. At this time the pressure is higher at the first than at the second point and the pressure-gradient slopes in this direction. The situation rapidly reverses and when the crest has reached the second point the pressure-gradient is in the opposite direction. Any secondary "bumps" in the wave form will cause similar oscillations. The resultant pressure-gradient therefore is one that oscillates about a mean as shown in Fig. 2 B. As we have a travelling wave in all arteries then all arterial pressure-gradients will be of this form. This gradient is indissolubly related to the flow that is occurring just as are gradient and flow in "Poiseuille" flow.

The factors involved in moving a fluid by a pressure that oscillates in this way is clearly much more complex than those required for steady flow. The mass of the fluid will resist movement when a force is first applied, because of its inertia. Similarly once it is moving its momentum will tend to keep it moving even though

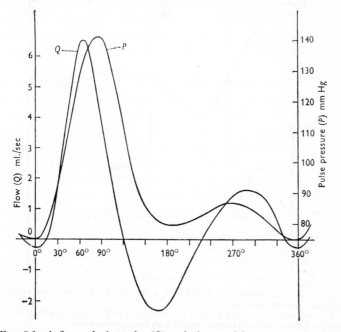

Fig. 5.1. A flow velocity pulse (Q) and the arterial pressure pulse (P) recorded simultaneously in the femoral artery of a dog. The flow velocity was recorded by high-speed cinematography (Ch. 6) but the corresponding volume flow has been plotted as the ordinate (left). Although superficially similar in shape when plotted on a comparable scale, the fact that the peak flow occurs before the pressure peak shows that there is no simple relation between these curves. The flow is, in fact, determined by the pressure-gradient (see text).

The pulse-frequency was 2·75 c/sec in this experiment. The abscissa representing time in this and all subsequent curves is plotted as fractions of the cycle length, i.e. as degrees of arc. As noted in the legend to Fig. 3·2 with pulse-frequencies of this order one degree of arc is about 1 millisecond. (*McDonald*, 1955a.)

the driving force is removed. We have seen in Ch. 2 that the solution of the factors involved in the laws for steady flow could not be determined without an adequate mathematical theory. In

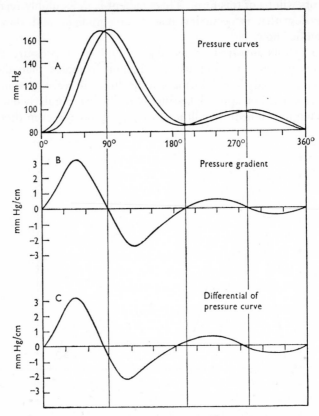

FIG. 5.2. A diagram that shows how a travelling pressure wave creates an oscillatory pressure-gradient.

A: Two waves recorded a short distance apart in the femoral artery of a dog. The downstream wave is here identical with the upstream one.

B: The pressure-gradient (mm Hg/cm) derived by subtracting the pressure at the downstream point from that at the upstream one at $15°$ intervals and dividing by the distance between recording points. (It should be noted that this gives a gradient opposite in sign to the usual mathematical convention for slopes.)

C: The derivative in respect to time of the upstream pressure wave (dP/dt). The form of this curve and that of the pressure-gradient (which in the limiting case of a very small interval is the derivative in respect of distance, dP/dz) is very similar. In this case the only difference is due to the transmission time over the interval necessary to determine the gradient. The vertical lines demonstrate the small phase differences that this creates. In the presence of the usual distortion of the wave as it travels this similarity between time-derivative and space-derivative no longer holds with any precision (see text). (*McDonald*, 1955a.)

the case of oscillating flow it was essential that we should have a mathematical solution of the problem from the start. Such a solution was made by Womersley (1955*b*). The flow in a tube, in which any dilatation is neglected, was considered when the pressure-gradient varied periodically in the form of a sine wave. With a Fourier series the flow related to any oscillating pressure-gradient could then be described.

THE RELATION OF FLOW TO AN OSCILLATING PRESSURE-GRADIENT

The derivation of the equation relating flow to a pressure-gradient that varies with time is essentially similar to the method of deriving Poiseuille's equation (Ch. 2). The conditions set are the same with the exception that the gradient is no longer "steady". The following outline uses that of Womersley (1955*a*, *b*) although it has been derived by previous workers, notably by Lambossy (1952*a*) in connexion with the resistance term in manometer systems (see App 2; Lambossy 1952*b*) and by Schönfeld (1946) who produced solutions for a variety of different shapes of channels. The fundamental equations also appear in a thesis by Witzig in 1914. Womersley, however, was the first to produce a solution in a form that is easily computable.

The equation of motion of the liquid is

$$\frac{\partial^2 v}{\partial r^2} + \frac{1}{r} \cdot \frac{\partial v}{\partial r} + \frac{P_1 - P_2}{\mu L} = \frac{1}{\nu} \cdot \frac{\partial v}{\partial t} \quad \dots \dots \dots \dots \dots 5.1$$

where v is the velocity of the liquid parallel to the axis of the pipe. As in Ch. 2 μ is the viscosity of the liquid and ν the kinematic viscosity (μ/ρ, where ρ is its density). The radius of the tube is R, and r may be written as a fraction $y = r/R$.

If the flow is steady then $\dfrac{\partial v}{\partial t} = 0$ and the solution is that of Poiseuille's equation (2.4).

In the present case where the pressure-gradient is varying in a simple harmonic manner with a circular frequency of ω radians/sec we write
$$(P_1 - P_2)/L = -A e^{i\omega t} \quad \dots \dots \dots \dots 5.2$$

(see Appendix 1 for the explanation of the exponential form of S.H.M.) and eqn. 5.1 is rewritten

$$\frac{\partial^2 v}{\partial r^2} + \frac{1}{r} \cdot \frac{\partial v}{\partial r} - \frac{1}{\nu} \cdot \frac{\partial v}{\partial t} = \frac{A}{\mu} e^{i\omega t} \quad \dots \dots \dots \dots 5.3$$

Let $v = ue^{i\omega t}$ and let the non-dimensional quantity $R\sqrt{\dfrac{\omega}{\nu}}$ be denoted by a. Then the equation for u is

$$\frac{\partial^2 u}{\partial y^2} + \frac{1}{y} \cdot \frac{\partial u}{\partial y} + i^3 a^2 u = \frac{AR^2}{\mu} \quad \ldots\ldots\ldots\ldots \quad 5.4$$

This is a form of Bessel's equation and the solution after replacing v is

$$V = \frac{AR^2}{\mu} \cdot \frac{1}{i^3 a^2} \left\{ 1 - \frac{J_0(ayi^{3/2})}{J_0(ai^{3/2})} \right\} e^{i\omega t} \quad \ldots\ldots\ldots \quad 5.5$$

where J_0 is a Bessel function of the first kind and of zero order. It is this equation that was used to compute the velocity profiles shown in Fig. 3.1.

To obtain the volume flow ($Q = \mathrm{ml/sec}$) it is necessary to integrate, when we obtain

$$Q = \frac{\pi R^4}{\mu} \cdot \frac{A}{i^3 a^2} \left\{ 1 - \frac{2J_1(ai^{3/2}}{ai^{3/2} J_0(ai^{3/2})} \right\} e^{i\omega t} \quad \ldots\ldots\ldots \quad 5.6$$

The function shown in brackets has been termed $(1 - F_{10})$ by Womersley and has been tabulated by him (Table VII in Appendix 1).

If the pressure-gradient is expressed in modulus and phase form (e.g. $M \cos(\omega t - \phi)$) then the flow may be written

$$Q = \frac{\pi R^4}{\mu} \cdot M \cdot \frac{M'}{a^2} \sin(\omega t - \phi + \varepsilon) \quad \ldots\ldots\ldots\ldots \quad 5.7$$

The methods by which either of these forms of the equation may be computed is described in Appendix 1. The modulus and phase form (eqn. 5.7) is the easier one to interpret physically. The terms M' and ε are dependent on the value of a (see Table VI and Fig. A.2) so that in analysing an arterial pulse we write

$$a = R\sqrt{\frac{\omega}{\nu}} = R \cdot \sqrt{\frac{2\pi n f \cdot \rho}{\mu}} \quad \ldots\ldots\ldots\ldots \quad 5.8$$

where R is the radius of the tube, μ and ρ the viscosity and the density of the liquid; f the pulse frequency in c/sec, and n is the order of the harmonic component. Thus a increases linearly with the radius of the tube and as the square root of the frequency. The change in value of M'/a^2 and with an increase in the value of a are shown graphically in Fig. 5.3.

To consider the behaviour of the oscillating components of flow in an artery the best physical analogue is that of a pipe connecting two water reservoirs. If these reservoirs are supported on either end of a beam which is rocked about a fulcrum in the centre, the head of water, and so the pressure-gradient, will vary rhythmically. It is clear that as one reservoir rises water will begin to flow out of it along the pipe into the other receiver. The flow, however, will build up more slowly than the upward movement of the reservoir, i.e. more slowly than the applied pressure, because of its inertia. Hence there is a phase lag $(90-\varepsilon)^\circ$, of flow behind pressure.

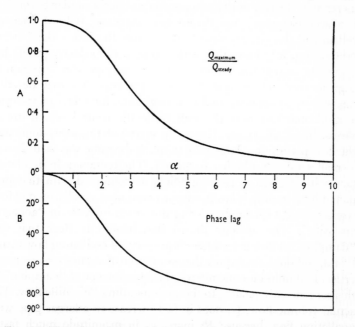

Fig. 5.3. The effect of changes in value of the non-dimensional constant α (eqn. 5.3) on the amplitude and phase of oscillatory flow generated by a pressure-gradient of simple harmonic form.

A: The amplitude as a ratio with the corresponding steady, or Poiseuille, flow. As the Poiseuille formula value (eqn. 5.4) is $1/8$, the ordinate is, in fact, eight times the value of the term M'_{10}/α^2 tabulated in the Appendix, Table VI. For simplicity, M' is usually written in the text for M'_{10}, except where direct comparison with Womersley's papers might cause confusion.

B: The phase lag of the flow with respect to the pressure-gradient. The ordinate here is $(90-\varepsilon_{10})^\circ$ in Womersley's notation.

It will be seen that as α increases the phase lag is tending towards 90° and the amplitude term becomes very small (M' is tending to $1\cdot0$ and ε to 0°—see Appendix figure). At values of $\alpha < 1\cdot0$ however, there is little deviation from Poiseuille's formula. (*Womersley*, 1955b.)

Equally when the movement of the reservoir is reversed the flow will continue in its original direction due to its momentum. As the rate of oscillation increases it is easy to see that the amount of flow generated in the pipe will also become smaller at the same head of water, due to the inertial effect. This is expressed quantitatively by the upper curve in Fig. 5.3. It will also lag more and more behind the changes in the pressure head (lower curve in Fig. 5.3). This is a picture of the change in type of flow when a increases due to the increase in frequency, and will be found in the higher harmonics of the arterial gradient. The reason that an increase in a, due to an increase in the size of the tube, produces effects similar to those of increased frequency, has already been discussed (Ch. 3) when we considered the velocity distribution across the tube—the velocity profile. Fig. 3.1 shows that with a large a the velocity profile becomes flat across the central region of the pipe with a region of disproportionately increased shear at the edge. We may describe this simply as showing that in a large tube the effect of viscosity is most manifest near the wall while the central region moves almost like a solid mass. Hence the inertia of this mass dominates the flow pattern in a large tube in much the same way as it does in a smaller tube at a higher frequency. The reduction in oscillating flow with a given pressure-gradient as compared with that predicted by Poiseuille's law has been noted occasionally by previous workers, and explained as being due to an increase in "apparent viscosity". The analogy drawn here makes it clear that this "damping" of flow is an inherent property of oscillating flow in any liquid, and does not require the assumption of strange viscous properties. It should be remembered that the concept of "damping" in this sense is only relative to the corresponding Poiseuille flow. The actual volume flow, Q, does in fact increase in a larger pipe with oscillating flow because R^4 increases in magnitude much faster than M'/a^2 decreases.

The calculation of flow from the pressure-gradient

With a characteristic arterial pressure-gradient such as that shown in Fig. 5.2 B, measured in the femoral artery of a dog, the first step necessary is to resolve it into its harmonic components by a Fourier analysis. The first four harmonic terms of such a curve are shown graphically in Fig. 5.4 together with their resynthesis to form the original curve. Each pressure oscillation has a correspond-

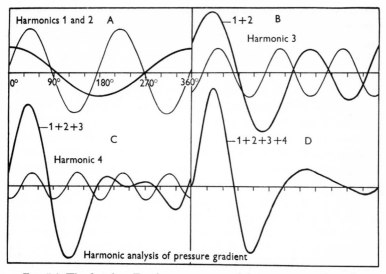

FIG. 5.4. The first four Fourier components of the pressure gradient of one experiment in the form $M \cos(\omega + \phi)$. A: 1 and 2 are the sine waves representing the first, or fundamental harmonic and the second harmonic. The modulus (M) of the second harmonic is 1·32 and that of the fundamental is 0·78. ϕ is $+0°39'$ for the first harmonic and $-82°45'$ for the second. B: $1+2$ represents the sum of the first two harmonics represented in A and the third harmonic (3) is superimposed ($M = -0.74$ and $\phi = +26°30'$). C: $1+2+3$ is the sum of the first three harmonics and the fourth is superimposed ($M = -0.41$, $\phi = -16°39'$). D: $1+2 +3+4$ is the sum of four harmonics.

This figure is slightly modified from Fig. 4 of McDonald (1955a) because there is a small error in the calculated third harmonic. Curve D now represents the correct resynthesis but the other curves have not been redrawn. The discrepancy between the resynthesized curve and the recorded gradient are now mainly, as always with a Fourier series taken to only a few terms, at the points of sharp inflection; it is small but not shown.

ing flow term which is also of sinusoidal form. The conversion factors depend on the values of a for each harmonic term (for a increases as the frequency increases) and are derived from the tables prepared by Womersley. The method of performing the Fourier analysis and calculating the corresponding flows, together with Tables of the function, is given in Appendix 1. Fig. 5.5 shows the relation between individual pressure and flow components.

To derive the total flow due to the pressure-gradient as recorded the harmonic components of the flow are added together and the result is shown in Fig. 5.6. The final curve requires some further explanation because a mean flow has been added to it and this is shown by lowering the line representing zero flow. This is necessary from the nature of the analysis. The harmonic terms are all

Oscillatory Flow

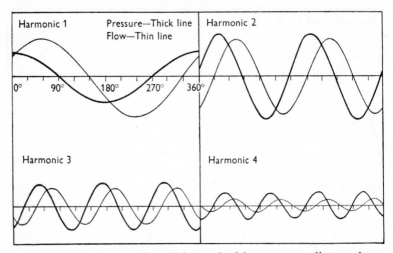

Fig. 5.5. The flow terms for each harmonic of the pressure gradient are shown together. Note that there is a phase shift (ϕ) due to the inertia of the fluid. 1 is the fundamental, 2, 3, and 4 the next three harmonics. ε is $31°14'$ in 1, $19°57'$ in 2, $15°50'$ in 3 and $13°29'$ in 4. The composite modulus (see eqn. 5.2) is $2\cdot4$ in 1, $2\cdot33$ in 2, $1\cdot12$ in 3 and $0\cdot34$ in 4 and the curves show how the resultant flow is progressively damped in the higher harmonics. The ordinates are on an arbitrary scale. (*McDonald*, 1955a.)

sine waves, that is they have a mean value of zero and so the summation of a series of sine waves also can only sum to zero over a complete cycle. Where the mean value is not zero, this is represented in the Fourier series (eqn. A.1, p. 290) by the constant term A_0. The flow through an artery must have a positive mean value of this sort because after all its function is to convey blood from the heart to the tissues of the body. The simplest way of representing this has been to take the mean value of the pressure-gradient over the whole cycle and assume that this generates a steady flow of Poiseuille type which is added to the oscillating term. This method has two defects, one practical and one theoretical. The *practical* difficulty is that the mean positive pressure-gradient is of very small dimensions—in the case illustrated the mean flow is only 1 ml/sec which corresponds to a mean gradient of only $0\cdot13$ mm Hg/cm of artery. It is, therefore, at the mercy of manometric errors for, even measuring over an 8 cm length of artery, this only amounts to a pressure drop of about 1 mm Hg. This accuracy can only be attained by using a good differential manometer. In the illustrations the mean flow has been checked by direct observation. The *theoretical* objection is that there is an interaction between the oscillating flow and the steady flow and so they cannot truly be treated as separate terms. This is discussed in Ch. 9. At the peak of the systolic flow in one case Womersley (1955c) calculated that the alteration in steady flow would be of the order of 15 per cent. In terms of the shape of the pulsatile flow curve this is negligible because the steady flow is itself small compared with the oscillating components of the flow. As regards the steady flow itself the correction cannot be disregarded. As the complexity of the calculation of the correction is coupled with the inherent inaccuracies of the measurement of the mean pressure-gradient we can see that this method is of no practical application in the prediction of *mean* flow in an artery. The work to be surveyed in Chs. 6 and 7, however, shows that important physiological data may be derived from the phasic variations in the pattern of flow and these are well predicted by the calculated curves.

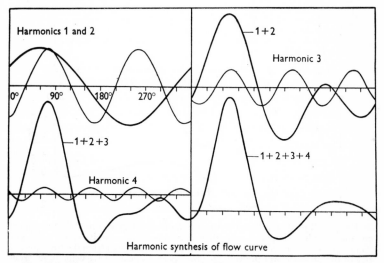

Fɪɢ. 5.6. The flow components shown in Fig. 5.5 are here shown singly and then summed successively as the pressure components were in Fig. 5.4. In the final summation $1+2+3+4$ the zero line has been moved to represent the addition of the mean flow, as the sine waves only represent the oscillating part of the flow. Because of the damping of the flow in the higher harmonics the flow due to the fifth and sixth harmonics is too small to show on this graph.

There is here a correction of Fig. 6 in McDonald (1955a) necessary because of the error in the analysis of the gradient noted in the legend to Fig. 5.4. As these figures are shown only to illustrate the method of calculation only the final curve has been redrawn—this time correctly.

Fig. 5.7 shows the comparison between an observed flow curve and one calculated from the "pressure-gradient" measured at the same time, and it can be seen that the correlation, allowing for experimental error, is fairly good. Mathematically the convincing aspect of these two curves is that the phase relations are accurately predicted. Discrepancies in amplitude may easily arise from experimental error in view of the very precise manometry required. The

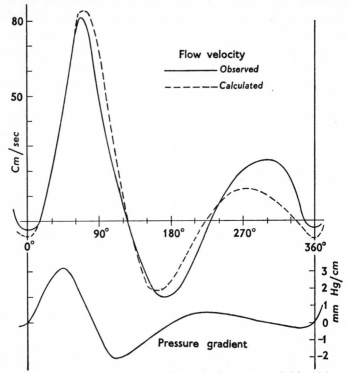

FIG. 5.7. The flow velocity in the dog femoral artery recorded by high-speed cinematography compared with that calculated from a derived "pressure-gradient" (lower curve). The so-called gradient was calculated from the time-derivative of the pressure and the value for the "peak-to-peak" wave velocity recorded in a series of animals by Hale *et. al.* (1955). As discussed in Ch. 10, where the arterial input impedances of this experiment are shown (Fig. 10.9), the amplitude of the calculated flow is almost certainly too great. There are, however, reasons to believe that this method of recording flow also tends to give values that are too high (Ch. 6). The correspondence between the two curves, which is reasonably good, suggests, therefore, that even with these approximations, the equations on which the calculation is based are satisfactory.

The pulse-frequency in this experiment was 2·85/sec. The abscissa is expressed as degrees of arc of a cycle (360°) because of the method of calculation (see Fig. 5.1).

points of reversal of flow are much less subject to error in the observed curve, or in the calculated curve, and these are seen to fit well. Nevertheless the prediction of the diastolic part of the curve is not satisfactory and the explanation of this is discussed below (p. 92).

The effect of the size of the artery on the flow pattern

A return to the formula (5.2) for the oscillating flow shows that it differs from the formula of Poiseuille (eqn. 2.2). For oscillating flow

$$Q = \frac{\pi R^4}{\mu} \cdot \frac{M'}{a^2} \cdot M \sin(\omega t - \phi + \varepsilon)$$

where the pressure-gradient $\dfrac{P_1 - P_2}{l} = M \cos(\omega t - \phi)$

whereas for steady flow

$$Q = \frac{\pi R^4}{\mu} \cdot \frac{1}{8} \cdot \frac{(p_1 - p_2)}{l} \quad \dots\dots\dots\dots\dots \quad 5.9$$

With an oscillating pressure the amplitude of the flow no longer varies linearly with the pressure-gradient but is modified by the term M'/a^2. Furthermore the flow lags behind the pressure by an angle $(90 - \varepsilon)°$. When a is small M'/a^2 approximates to the value $1/8$ which is the constant in Poiseuille's law. At the same time the value of ε tends to $90°$ so that the term $M \sin(t\omega - \phi + \varepsilon)$ becomes $M \sin(\omega t - \phi + 90°)$ or $M \cos(\omega t - \phi)$ i.e. $\dfrac{P_1 - P_2}{l}$. The formula for the flow thus approximates to Poiseuille's law in small vessels. Where a is 0·5 or less for the fundamental harmonic the difference between the two formulae is negligible. The approximation is quite good in a vessel such as the saphenous artery ($a \doteqdot 0·8$) so that in small vessels even if the pressure-gradient varies the flow will vary approximately linearly with it.

With large vessels the oscillating flow deviates very greatly from the Poiseuille formula. When a is 10 it can be seen from Fig. 5.3 that the amplitude of the flow is about 1/15 of that predicted by Poiseuille's formula and furthermore is more than 80° out of phase. The limiting condition as a gets very large is that the flow excursion decreases to a very small value and is 90° out of phase. The phase relation is then analogous to the relation of an alternating voltage to the current it produces in an inductance. Such a situation will be reached in the aorta where the α of the fundamental will be between 10–15 so that the fourth harmonic will reach 30. A calculated flow curve for aortic flow in a dog is shown in Fig. 5.10 and it can be seen that there is an increased lag between flow and pressure-gradient.

The values of α found in the circulation

From values calculated for dogs we have seen that α was less than 1 in the saphenous artery, about 3 in the femoral artery and about 10 in the aorta. These values were for particular individuals and they will show variation in the same individual with changes of pulse-frequency and between individuals because of differences in calibre. It is interesting to compare the range of values found in different species. Because small animals, which have small arteries, tend to have fast heart rates, and *vice versa* the value of α tends to vary over a surprisingly small range at comparable anatomical sites. Some estimated values are given in Table II.

TABLE II

Some values of α in different mammalian species

A: *Site*—Root of aorta (from data in Clark, 1927, relating to heart rates and aortic cross-sectional area)

Species	Pulse rate/min	Radius, cm	α (fundamental)
Mouse	600–730	0·03–0·04	1·19–1·74
Rat	360–520	0·045–0·095	1·38–3·5
Rabbit	205–220	0·17	3·92–4·07
Cat	180	0·2	4·4
Dog	72–125	0·55–0·6	8·27–10·68
Man	55–72	1·08–1·11	13·5–16·7
Ox	43	2·0	21·1
Elephant	40–50	4·47	48–51

The range of average body-weights of the same species ranges from 35 g (mouse) to $2·0–2·5 \times 10^6$g (elephant) (Clark, 1927).

B: *Site*—Femoral artery

Rabbit	210–360	0·06	1·4–1·8
Dog	72–180	0·12–0·15	1·65–3·25
Man	60–72	0·2–0·25	2·5–3·5

The higher range of pulse rates allowed here in the rabbit and dog are based on personal observations in animals anaesthetized with pentobarbitone (nembutal).

Although the larger species tend to have somewhat larger values there is a remarkable correspondence of values. This suggests that the circulation in various mammals has a dynamic, or kinematical, similarity and lends comforting theoretical support to the application of results derived from lower animals to the interpretation of observations made in human beings.

The relationship of the pressure-gradient to the pulse pressure

The pressure-gradient we have considered up to this point is one measured directly by the difference in pressure measured at two points in an artery. It was pointed out earlier in this chapter that it is this gradient that must be considered as the force related to the flow and not the pressure curve itself. Nevertheless the form of the gradient is clearly related to the form of the pressure pulse. In Fig. 5.2 B the pressure-gradient is drawn as the difference in pressure between the two points divided by the distance separating these two points. If the distance is Δz then we may write the gradient as $\Delta p/\Delta z$. If the distance between the recording points is very small the expression for the gradient becomes $\dfrac{dp}{dz}$—that is the differential coefficient, or derivative, of the pressure in respect of distance, i.e. the space-derivative. The pressure curve may be differentiated by putting the output from an electrical manometer through a suitable circuit or by differentiating the Fourier series of the curve. Fig. 5.2 C shows that the differential coefficient of the arterial pressure obtained in this way may be of the same form as the pressure-gradient. By differentiating the pressure we are deriving the coefficient in respect of time, dp/dt. It is, however, clear that the relation between dp/dz and dp/dt is simply

$$\frac{dp}{dz} = \frac{dp}{dt} \cdot \frac{dt}{dz} \quad \dotso \quad 5.10$$

and $\dfrac{dz}{dt}$, or the differential coefficient of space in respect to time, is the velocity of propagation of the pulse-wave — c. The sign convention for slopes of curves also requires that the actual gradient is $-\dfrac{dp}{dz}$ (representing a "downhill" slope) so that the relation is written

$$-\frac{dp}{dz} = \frac{1}{c} \cdot \frac{dp}{dt} \quad \dotso \quad 5.11$$

The rate of flow which is dependent on the pressure-gradient is, therefore, also seen to be dependent on the rate of change of the pulse-pressure although not on its absolute value. The qualitative relationship of flow and the rate of change in pressure was noted by Shipley, Gregg and Schroeder (1943) although they did not determine a quantitative relationship. Indeed it is difficult to see how one could ever be found without a fundamental theoretical analysis, such as has been made by Womersley.

The relationship between the pressure-gradient and the time-derivative of the pressure-wave looks seductively simple but its implications need examining more closely. As it stands it is true for a pressure-wave of sinusoidal form and the value, c, is then called its phase velocity. In a linear system it will also be true of a compound wave in which all its harmonic components are travelling at the same phase velocity. The phase velocity is, however, only independent of the frequency in a perfectly elastic tube filled with inviscid fluid which is so long that no reflection of the wave occurs. The wave will then travel without distortion. When eqn. 5.11 was originally used by McDonald (1955a) and Womersley (1955b) this condition, that it was only valid if the wave travelled without distortion, was stated although its implications were not discussed. Nevertheless, the time-derivative was used for calculating flows. This was not because we imagined that the blood had no viscosity or that the arterial wall was perfectly elastic but because the magnitude of the non-linearity of these two effects was known to be small, especially in comparison with the errors inherent in measuring the pressure-gradient by differencing two manometers. Further work has shown that major errors may be introduced by this method due to the presence of reflection of waves in the arterial tree. The detailed discussion of these factors is deferred to Chs. 9 and 10 and here we are only noting the conclusions presented there.

The effect of the viscosity of the fluid on the transmission of a wave is to damp it in amplitude and also to reduce its velocity. These effects are described mathematically by expressing the wave velocity as a complex number. If the complex value of c is used in eqn. 5.11 the effect of viscosity is, therefore, allowed for. The wave velocity under these circumstances increases with its frequency and in a free elastic tube its limiting value is the velocity that the wave would have in an ideal, non-viscous liquid (see Fig. 9.3). The damping also increases with frequency. From the figure, however, it can be seen that at values of α above 3 the change in velocity is small and for this reason it was considered that the difference in phase velocity of the components of the pulse-wave over the range of a that we have considered in the femoral artery could be neglected. They would only be of the order of 2–3 per cent at most and this is smaller than the errors involved in measuring the velocity of the pulse. The non-linear elastic behaviour of the arterial wall would also cause an increase in wave velocity with frequency (Ch. 8) and, although we do not have such quantitative data for this effect, it also may be regarded as small over the frequency range with which we are concerned.

The possible effect of reflections on the phase velocity was suggested by the fact that predictions of flow curves from the time-derivative of the pressure were very much in error when there was marked vasoconstriction—a condition likely to produce reflection. Conversely, as shown in Fig. 5.8 the fit of the curves in conditions of vasodilatation was very good. Here there is good correspondence even in the diastolic part of the curve, a region where there is discrepancy in the "normal" curve (see Fig. 5.7). Now in a steady-state oscillation (which we assume when we represent the pulse-wave, or a pressure-gradient, by a Fourier series) the reflection of

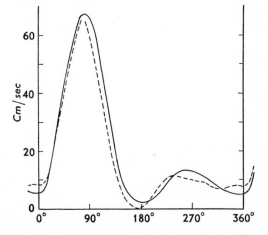

Fig. 5.8. The observed (whole line) and calculated (broken line) flow velocity curves in the dog femoral artery after an intra-arterial injection of 100 µg of acetylcholine, i.e. with marked peripheral vasodilatation. Observed and calculated curves were obtained in the same way as those in Fig. 5.7. The improved correspondence of the curves compared with the figure is attributed to the reduction of reflections (see text). The pulse frequency was $2 \cdot 1$/sec. The input impedance values of the observed curve are shown in Fig. 10.10*b*.

each harmonic wave component will fuse with the incident component of that frequency and one effect will be a shift in phase. Near a reflecting point this will cause an increase in the phase velocity (Taylor 1957 *a* and *b*) as shown in Fig. 10.7. This increase in phase velocity may be very great in some regions, usually due to the proximity of a terminal vascular bed, as shown in the analyses of wave velocity in the abdominal aorta shown in Figs. 10.3 and 12.5. On the other hand, owing to the marked damping that occurs in small arteries this effect may be very small in some vessels.

It is, therefore, necessary to measure the phasic velocity of each harmonic component if it is desired to derive the pressure-gradient from the time-derivative of the pulse. The conditions that cause a significant effect due to reflections are under investigation and the use of the orthodox value of the pulse-wave velocity as the *c* for all harmonics (Figs. 5.7 and 5.8) *can* produce calculated curves which are reasonably satisfactory. The *direct measurement* of a pressure-gradient is, however, the *only reliable* method for the calculation of flow curves because this is independent of factors such as reflection which influence the shape of the pressure curve. The only distortion that is introduced into a pressure-gradient measured directly is due to the fact that we are averaging the difference over a finite interval, but this is of the order of the fraction of half the interval divided by the wavelength, and so is very small.

The interrelationship of flow, wave velocity and the time-derivative of the pulse-wave that this work has revealed is of great interest in assessing the physiological significance of changes of the form of the pulse-wave and will be pursued in greater detail in Ch. 10.

The validity of the Womersley equations when applied to arteries

Any theoretical derivation of pressure-flow relationship must be based on certain basic assumptions and any deviation from these assumptions must be considered as affecting the predictions of the theory just as we did in the case of Poiseuille's law (p. 18). The physical assumptions made in this case were:—

(1) That the flow is laminar. The evidence of the distribution of laminar flow in arteries has already been discussed in Ch. 3. In the case of the arteries specifically studied, namely the femoral and the

saphenous arteries of the dog, direct observation appears to show that flow is laminar. In larger arteries there is some doubt if laminar flow will be maintained throughout the cycle, especially as the oscillating nature of the flow of itself tends to reduce the stability of the laminar flow. To what extent a transient breakdown of laminar flow during the cardiac cycle will affect the accuracy of prediction of flow is not known.

(2) That the fluid is homogeneous and does not have anomalous viscous properties. The anomalous viscosity of blood in steady flow has already been considered (Ch. 3) and it was seen that it was only appreciable in very small vessels where the Womersley equations approximate to those of Poiseuille. This factor will therefore probably be negligible in arteries, although Womersley (1958*a*) has investigated the effects of a plasma sleeve of lower viscosity; anomalous viscosity of blood in oscillatory flow has not yet been investigated experimentally.

(3) That the flow is through a cylindrical tube which does not alter its diameter. Superficially this appears to be a very large approximation that would invalidate the theory. A more critical examination shows, however, that the assumption of "rigidity" is only made for calculating flow in the artery at the point of the observation, while the pressure changes are recorded in the actual elastic tube system. The inaccuracies due to neglecting the changes in radius with pulsation are smaller than might be expected for the maximal change in radius in the femoral artery is very small—of the order of 5 per cent or less, and that is maintained for only a short part of the cycle. The total effect of the elastic behaviour of the wall is considerably more complex than this and has been investigated fully by Womersley (1955*c*). These factors are summarized in Ch. 9 for they are important in the full theoretical analysis of arterial hydrodynamics; it is shown there that this "simple" theory is, in fact, the best approximation for arteries.

(4) It is also assumed that flow may be expressed as a sum of the harmonic components derived from the corresponding individual harmonic terms of the pressure-gradient. With an elastic tube this is not strictly true and there is some interaction between the harmonic components of the flow. This is incorporated in Womersley's theory of the elastic tube (Womersley, 1958*a*) and is considered in Ch. 9.

The remaining assumptions are the same for the theory of oscillating pressure as for Poiseuille's law (Ch. 2) namely

(5) that no "slip" occurs at the wall, and

(6) that the tube is long compared with the region being studied. This is the "inlet length" problem discussed in Ch. 3 and will be involved in considerations of aortic flow, although, as was seen there, the inlet length is probably short with oscillating flow. The work of Fry discussed below suggests that it may be neglected, at least for the present.

In summary, the simple Womersley relation cannot be rigorously applied to arteries but nevertheless it is probably as close, or closer, a practical approximation for oscillating flow as Poiseuille's law is for steady flow in blood-vessels. In both cases it is difficult to provide precise experimental tests of the theory. In the case of Poiseuille's law the inaccuracies derive from the uncertain dimensions of the vascular bed that is being perfused and from the anomalous viscosity of blood in small tubes. In the case of Womersley's theory the principal difficulty lies in the measurement of the oscillating flow for there is still dispute about the design of a meter that accurately records pulsating flow (Ch. 6).

Fry's solution for pressure-flow relations in the aorta

Fry (Fry, Mallos and Casper, 1956) has made an analysis of the pressure-flow relationship in a large artery that is of a simpler form than that of Womersley. This was derived from the fundamental Navier-Stokes equation and considers only movements of flow in the direction of the axis of the artery, as Womersley (1955b) did in the "simple" theory described above. For an oscillating flow in a large artery the velocity profile, as we have seen, is almost flat across most of the lumen and the inertial component is large compared with the viscous component. This latter component is assumed by Fry to be small and so can be reasonably approximated by a term which varies linearly with the velocity of flow. The pressure-gradient was measured as the difference in pressure between two points from 3–5 cm apart recorded with a differential manometer. As the distance over which the gradient was measured is very small in relation to the pulse-wave velocity this gradient was taken as representing the space-derivative of the pressure.

The solution of the equation was expressed as

$$p(t) = \rho \Delta x \frac{du}{dt} + au(t) \quad \ldots\ldots\ldots\ldots \text{5.12}$$

where $p(t)$ is the pressure difference in dynes/cm² between the recording points which were Δx cm apart; $u(t)$ is the velocity in the x axis (along the tube) and a the constant representing the proportionality between the frictional pressure drop and the flow velocity.

The great simplification that is made by treating the flowing blood as, in essence, an inertial mass circumvents the problem of

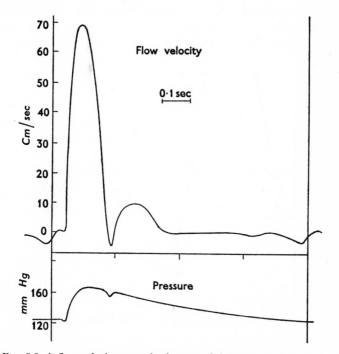

FIG. 5.9. A flow velocity curve in the root of the aorta of a dog derived by Fry's equation (5.7) from the pressure-gradient, measured with a double-lumen cardiac catheter. The simultaneous record of the arterial pressure is shown below.

This curve should be compared with that of volume flow in Fig. 7.1 recorded at the same site with an electromagnetic flowmeter. Taking usual values for the aortic diameter the peak velocity here is less than half of that indicated in Fig. 7.1; however, it is similar to an approximate value obtained in our own laboratory (Fig. 5.10). These differences may be due to biological causes. (*Redrawn from Fry, et al.,* 1956.)

B.F.A.–H

the nature of the flow concerned. Thus it applies equally well to laminar or turbulent flow, and will apply within the inlet length (see Ch. 3). In fact Fry specifically assumes that, in applying the formula to flow conditions in the proximal aorta, entry conditions exist and that laminar flow has not been established. The degree of approximation implicit in this can hardly be estimated theoretically

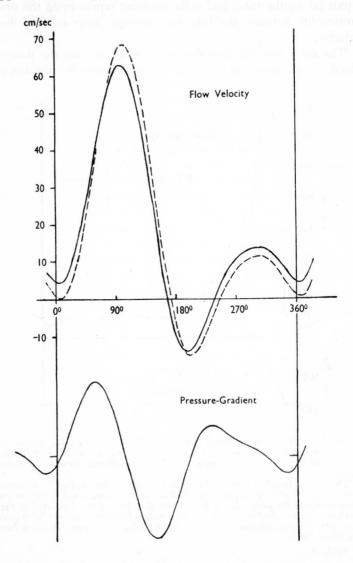

because of our lack of knowledge of the motion of the blood in the root of the aorta. Dissipation of energy by the radial movement of blood due to the formation of eddies at the aortic valves will introduce errors but again these are considered to be small as the measured pressure-gradient did not vary in experiments when the recording catheter was placed at various positions within the artery (Fry—personal communication). As only flow velocity was considered the dilatation of the root of the aorta could be neglected. Fig. 5.9 shows a curve of the flow velocity in the proximal aorta recorded by Fry *et al.* (1956).

The relationship between the pressure and the flow expressed in eqn. 5.12 is independent of frequency. Thus the gradient $p(t)$ may be directly used in the calculation whatever function describes it. Advantage has been taken of this to build an analogue computer which will convert the manometer record of the pressure-gradient into the corresponding flow curve (Fry, Noble and Mallos, 1957*b*). In recording arterial flows the measurement of the constant a in the viscosity term is a problem. It has been estimated by making the assumption that the flow at the end of diastole is always zero. The computer is then adjusted to this condition and so an arbitrary value is assigned to the constant. As the apparatus has only, so far, been used to record flow in the most proximal part of the aorta this assumption is probably justified. As the viscosity term, a, is small in any case in the conditions for which the equation was derived Fry *et al.* (1956) showed that the form of the curve is not very sensitive to alterations in its value.

Fig. 5.10. Flow velocity curves calculated from a pressure-gradient measured in the proximal aorta—the recording points were estimated to lie 2 and 7 cm from the aortic valves. The pulse-frequency was 2·85/sec, i.e. considerably faster than that in the experiment of Fry *et al.* shown in Fig. 5.9.

The *whole line* represents the curve calculated from full eqn. 5.2—a for the fundamental frequency $= 10·7$; the *broken line* shows the calculated curve when the effects of viscosity were neglected and the asymptotic values for M' (1·0) and for ε (0°) were used. The discrepancies between the two curves show that the effect of the blood viscosity is to reduce both the amplitude and the phase lag with respect to the pressure-gradient. In vessels of this size, however, this effect is very small and neglecting it is of little practical importance. The motion of the blood in large arteries is mainly determined by its inertia.

Only four harmonics were used to calculate these curves; this is insufficient to represent accurately a pulse form such as that in Fig. 5.9 so that comparisons of shape are of little value. The mean flow is also arbitrary in this case and was largely determined by setting end-diastolic flow at, or near, zero as in the method of Fry *et al.* (1956).

The nature of the approximations made in the simplified solution here cannot be estimated precisely and the accuracy of the method will emerge as it is tested against other flow records. The authors have demonstrated satisfactory agreement with oscillating flow in a model. In the root of the aorta there is no other method available yet of sufficiently proven accuracy to test it against. A superficial comparison with the Womersley equations suggests reasonable agreement for oscillating flows at large values of a. The frequency dependence of the amplitude of flow and phase lag, illustrated graphically in Fig. 5.3, show that when $a = 10$ or greater (see Appendix 1) these are approaching their asymptotic value slowly, so that for an approximate solution of this kind they could be regarded as not changing with frequency. Fig. 5.10 shows graphically the predicted flow curves from a pressure-gradient measured in the proximal aorta of a dog. In one the full Womersley formula was used (a, fundamental $= 10 \cdot 7$) and in the other the asymptotic values of M' and ε were used. It is seen that there is a slight increase in amplitude and phase-lag in the latter case but they would be difficult to distinguish experimentally. These curves were only calculated to 4 harmonics which is inadequate, close to the heart, to give an accurate description of the wave form.

We can conclude from this that the approximate solution of Fry is a practical method for recording phasic flow in large vessels, and as such is a very valuable contribution. The more general solutions of Womersley remain necessary in smaller vessels and are indispensable for the fuller analysis of circulatory problems.

The "a.c. theory" of flow

Because the behaviour of oscillating liquid flow is not generally familiar we do not have a set of technical terms peculiar to this branch of hydrodynamics and inevitably we have to borrow them from other branches of physics, usually from the language of electricity. In this way we treat an oscillating pressure-gradient as analogous with an alternating voltage and the oscillating velocity of flow as an alternating current. Hence the theory of oscillating pressure and flow outlined in this chapter may be called the "a.c. theory", to contrast it with the "d.c. theory" represented by steady flow. Treated purely as an analogy this makes a useful distinction that emphasizes the fact that phase differences between pressure and flow are important, as they are between alternating voltage and current in electrical circuits. It has already been suggested (McDonald, 1955a) that the term *impedance* should be used when considering pulsatile pressure and flow in arteries and that the term *resistance* should be confined to the steady flow. Womersley has shown that we can proceed to give quantitative expression to these terms from his equations in a way analogous to electrical theory.

For analogy with electrical terms we take pressure as equivalent to voltage and the velocity of flow as equivalent to current. If we rewrite eqn. 5.1 in exponential form then the oscillatory pressure-gradient

$$\frac{P_1 - P_2}{l} = -Ae^{i\omega t} \quad \dots\dots\dots\dots\dots \quad 5.13$$

and the average velocity across the pipe is

$$\bar{V} = Q/\pi R^2 = \frac{AR^2}{i\mu} \cdot \frac{M'}{a^2} \cdot e^{i\varepsilon} \cdot e^{i\omega t} \quad \dots\dots\dots\dots \quad 5.14$$

The *longitudinal impedance*, Z, is the impedance per unit length and so will be defined by the pressure drop per unit length (i.e. the gradient) divided by the velocity of flow.

$$Z = \frac{Ae^{it\omega}}{\bar{V}} = \frac{i\mu}{R^2} \cdot \frac{a^2}{M'} \cdot e^{-i\varepsilon} \quad \dots\dots\dots\dots \quad 5.15$$

$$= \frac{\mu a^2}{R^2 M'} \cdot \sin\varepsilon + \frac{i\mu a^2}{R^2 M'} \cdot \cos\varepsilon \quad \dots\dots\dots\dots \quad 5.16$$

As Womersley (1958a) has pointed out, by analogy with the electrical complex impedance which is

$$Z = R + i\omega L$$

(where R is the resistance and L is the inductance) we may call the real part of eqn. 5.16 the fluid resistance and the imaginary part represents the inductive term (or reactance).

$$\therefore \text{ Fluid resistance} = \frac{\mu a^2}{R^2 M'} \cdot \sin\varepsilon \quad \dots\dots\dots\dots \quad 5.17$$

$$\text{and reactance} = \frac{\mu a^2}{R^2 M'} \cdot \cos\varepsilon \quad \dots\dots\dots\dots \quad 5.18$$

so that, dividing by ω and writing a^2 in full

$$\text{Fluid Inductance} = \frac{\rho}{M'} \cdot \cos\varepsilon \quad \dots\dots\dots\dots \quad 5.19$$

These values are shown in Fig. 5.11 where it can be seen that the inductance falls slowly with increasing a. The fluid resistance, on the other hand, rises steadily and, with $a=10$, is more than double its value when $a=1\cdot0$. Both are thus frequency-dependent, in contrast to the corresponding electrical terms. This emphasizes the necessity for caution in drawing exact analogies for liquid flow from the behaviour of electricity in metallic conductors.

When we are considering a conducting system we also need to define the *input* or *characteristic impedance*, Z_0, which depends both on the longitudinal impedance, Z, and the wave velocity, c.

$$Z_0 = Z.c/i\omega \quad \dots\dots\dots\dots\dots \quad 5.20$$

and if a^2 is cancelled out in eqn. 5.15 we obtain

$$Z_0 = \frac{\rho c}{M'} \cdot e^{-i\varepsilon} \quad \dots\dots\dots\dots\dots \quad 5.21$$

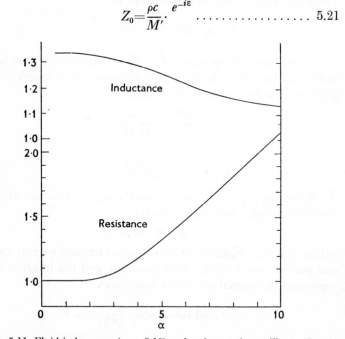

FIG. 5.11. Fluid inductance (eqn. 5.19) and resistance for oscillatory flow in a rigid pipe plotted as a function of a. The values for resistance are given relative to the steady-flow, or Poiseuille, resistance and are 1/8 times that given by eqn. 5.17. As a is a function of the square root of the frequency it can be seen that both these components of the fluid impedance are frequency-dependent in contrast to the analogous electrical quantities. The application of the fluid resistance in oscillatory flow to the manometer equations is discussed in Appendix 2.

Applying the relation between c (the complex wave velocity in Ch. 9) and c_0 the wave velocity determined by the arterial wall (eqn. 8.16) that Womersley (1957) derived for the tethered elastic tube we have

$$Z_0 = \frac{\rho c_0}{\sqrt{1-\sigma^2}} \cdot \frac{1}{(M')^{\frac{1}{2}}} \cdot e^{-i\varepsilon/2} \qquad \dots\dots\dots\dots 5.22$$

It will be shown in Ch. 10 that the input impedance is modified by the presence of reflected waves. The impedance of an artery without reflections calculated from this formula is called the *characteristic impedance* and we reserve the term *input impedance* for the value actually measured in the presence of reflections. It will be seen in Fig. 10.11 that the characteristic impedance calculated from eqn. 5.17 falls with increasing frequency—especially in small vessels. This may, in fact, be offset by the fact that the "stiffness" of the arterial wall, and hence its wave velocity (c_0), increases with frequency (Chs. 8 and 9), so that the characteristic impedance probably remains fairly constant.

It will be noted that the phase of the flow (analogous to current) is always lagging behind the pressure-gradient (potential difference) and so the system is behaving like an inductance. The full electrical analogue of an artery must also include a capacitance to represent the elastic behaviour of the wall. Current flow in a capacitance, of course, leads the potential difference in phase.

If we can measure the characteristic impedance and the complex wave velocity we can distinguish between the resistive, capacitative and inductive components, and Taylor (1959b) has recently published the results of such an analysis in hydraulic models. In the arterial system we can only measure the input impedance and owing to reflections its modulus and phase will be mainly determined by the distance between the point of observation and the reflecting sites. The phase will in some cases be leading by 90°—in reference to the phase of the characteristic impedance. It does not seem helpful or accurate to refer these phase changes to changes in the capacitative and inductive components. In the consideration of arterial input impedance, which is discussed at length in Ch. 10, all calculations are made in the form of modulus and phase. For the sake of simplicity, however, only the measurement of the modulus of the impedance is dealt with in detail. Hardung (1958) has investigated both the modulus and phase of the fluid impedance in long rubber tubes.

CHAPTER VI

THE MEASUREMENT OF PHASIC FLOW VELOCITY

Without a knowledge of the pulsatile fluctuations in arterial flow as detailed as our knowledge of the fluctuations in pressure, we cannot adequately explore the hydrodynamics of the circulation. Accurate measurement of these phasic changes of flow are, however, technically difficult but this difficulty tends to be exaggerated because, in spite of a rapidly increasing volume of work on the subject, the problem has not been attacked with the persistence and vigour that has been devoted to the solution of manometric problems. This is partly due to the feeling that a knowledge of the mean flow is sufficient for physiological purposes. The same argument applies to pressure measurements yet few investigations of circulatory problems would be regarded as complete nowadays if the pulsatile pressure were not accurately recorded. This is in spite of the fact that the significance of changes in the pulse-wave form are far from being understood. The form of the phasic flow pattern is certainly as important as the form of the pressure-wave and, as the discussion below shows, is in many respects easier to interpret. Furthermore the physiological significance of the shape of the pulse-wave will not be fully understood until it can be translated into terms of flow.

The development of an accurate flow meter is, in my opinion, the principal problem in fundamental work on the circulation today. The variety of meters that have been used is, of itself, sufficient comment on their generally unsatisfactory nature. The wide disagreement between published results shows that the first problem is to decide what is meant by accuracy. It is here that the theoretical prediction of the pulsatile flow that is to be expected in arteries has great practical importance. Womersley's mathematical equations admittedly make approximations but he has also shown that these approximations are small, whereas results obtained by different meters may differ by up to 500 per cent. As a consequence we can at least distinguish the meters that give results of the right order of magnitude as a first step towards attaining satisfactory precision in our records.

The principles underlying the phasic flow meters most commonly in use are discussed below. Technical details of the orifice meter (Green, 1948) and the electromagnetic flowmeter (Jochim, 1948) were included in the survey of blood flow recording methods in Volume I of *Methods in Medical Research* and Catton (1957) has, in addition, some comments on the Pitot tube. In other cases reference should be made to the original papers of authors cited.

Differential pressure meters

The types of meters that come into this category most commonly used in physiology are the *Pitot tube* and the *orifice meter*. Both use applications of Bernoulli's theorem (Ch. 2, eqn. 2.10) which states that

$$p_1 + \tfrac{1}{2}\rho v_1^2 = p_2 + \tfrac{1}{2}\rho v_2^2 = C \dots\dots\dots\dots 6.1$$

In the Pitot meter there is a tube in which the tip is bent at right angles so that it points in the direction of the flow. The flow of fluid is dammed up immediately in front of the tip and divides the flow round it, but in the centre of the dammed-up region there is a "stagnation point" where the fluid comes entirely to rest. The pressure, p_1, at this point is called the "total pressure" and

$$p_1 = p_0 + \tfrac{1}{2}\rho v_0^2 \dots\dots\dots\dots\dots 6.2$$

where v_0 is the velocity of flow and where p_0 is the "static", or lateral, pressure in the vessel. The term $\tfrac{1}{2}\rho v_0^2$ or $(p_1 - p_0)$ is called the "kinetic", or dynamic, pressure (Prandtl 1952). The term p_0 is measured by a second tube directed perpendicular to the flow. The difference of pressure between the two tubes is therefore proportional to the square of the velocity of flow. Sometimes the second tube is bent at the tip so that it points directly downstream and so it should theoretically record a pressure p_2 where

$$p_2 = p_0 - \tfrac{1}{2}\rho v_0^2 \dots\dots\dots\dots\dots 6.3$$

so that the differential pressure, $p_1 - p_2$, will be ρv_0^2 and the sensitivity doubled.

One technical difficulty in making a Pitot tube accurate is that the upstream tube causes eddies and so distorts the measurement of p_0 and the problem of design is largely concerned with minimizing this effect (Prandtl, 1952). Green (1948) makes the comment that the Cleveland group abandoned its use for measuring arterial flows on account of the oscillations that developed in their pressure records, and these were probably due to this cause. For the same reason the reduction of pressure at a tip pointing downstream is not equal in magnitude to the rise at the upstream point and separate calibration curves must be made for forward and back flows. Hardung (1957) has discussed the problems connected with the use of Pitot tubes for measuring pulsatile flow.

A second problem is that the velocity, v_0, measured is that of the laminae in the line of the tip and so it is necessary to know the form of the velocity profile and the exact position of the tip within the vessel. This is usually done by centering it in a cannula and inserting the cannula in the vessel. Müller (1954a) has designed a very small Pitot tube that can be advanced across the lumen of the tube in which it is inserted and so establish the shape of the velocity profile before using it for flow determinations. Results obtained in arteries remain to be published although a preliminary report stated that the velocity profile in the dog aorta is very flat (p. 46 above). Baxter and Pearce (1951) also designed a Pitot tube meter which they used in the pulmonary trunk of the cat. It had the elegant addition of a "square-rooting" device so that a linear calibration was achieved. It was however not calibrated with oscillatory flow. In a further paper Baxter, Cunningham and Pearce (1952) compared its mean flow recording with the cardiac output measured by the direct Fick method and found that it averaged some 15 per cent too high, but it seemed a promising instrument.

The orifice meter depends, as its name suggests, on placing a cannula containing a narrowed orifice in the lumen of the tube. This increases the linear velocity of the flow. In the equation (6.1) above v_2^2 is then greater than v_1^2 so that p_2 is less than p_1. The lateral pressure is measured on either side of the orifice and the pressure difference $(p_1 - p_2)$ measured with a differential mano-meter (Shipley, Gregg and Schroeder, 1943). Then

$$p_1 - p_2 = \tfrac{1}{2}(v_2^2 - v_1^2)$$

This principle was used by Broemser (1928) in his "Differential sphymograph" which ingeniously avoided the necessity for cannu-lation by applying an external constriction to an intact artery.

If the radius of the orifice is R_2 and that of the cannula in which it is mounted is R_1 then

$$v_2 = \left(\frac{R_1}{R_2}\right)^2 \cdot v_1$$

and
$$p_1 - p_2 = \tfrac{1}{2}v_1{}^2 \left[\left(\frac{R_1}{R_2} \right)^4 - 1 \right]$$

so that it can be seen that a reduction of the size of the orifice greatly increases the sensitivity of the meter. At the same time, however, it equally increases the impedance of the meter and this is its greatest disadvantage.

In pulsatile flow the pressure difference across the meter, if there were no orifice, would be the oscillating pressure-gradient that is normally present in an artery. As was seen in Ch. 5 this is different in form from the flow curve. The orifice must, therefore, cause sufficient change in velocity for the Bernoulli term to be very large in comparison with the pressure-gradient so that the latter may be neglected. This sets a limit to the extent in which the orifice may be enlarged to reduce the impedance of the meter.

It is not easy to forecast precisely the changes in the flow pattern due to the obstruction of the meter. Gregg and Green (1939) stated that "at flows of 60–80 cc per minute the net loss of head in the stream is not more than 3 to 4 mm Hg". The "resistance" of meters is often defined in this way and in terms of the drop in mean pressure from the large arteries to the capillaries a fall in pressure head of 3–4 mm Hg may seem very small. Looked at another way, however, we saw from the consideration of pressure-gradients in the femoral artery that at a mean flow of this magnitude the mean gradient is only of the order of 0·1–0·15 mm Hg/cm, so that even expressed in terms of steady flow it is as it were, equivalent to introducing an extra length of some 20–30 cm of artery. The effect of a rigid cannula on the oscillating components of the flow will be considered after the description of the electro-magnetic flowmeter as this is a problem common to both. The "resistance" of a meter, used for pulsating flow, defined in terms of a steady flow is not very helpful, for we need to know its impedance for oscillatory flow.

A further point regarding the use of meters in arteries concerns the role of alternative channels. There are two femoral arteries, for example, and the introduction of a meter of appreciable impedance will tend to enhance the flow in the contralateral leg at the expense of the observed leg. With phasic recording this will alter the pattern of the flow curve. Reactive hyperaemia in one leg, for instance, can markedly enhance the backflow phase in the contralateral one. It would be of considerable interest to see if the insertion of orifice meters symmetrically into both femoral arteries altered the flow patterns as compared with those recorded from a single one.

To summarize, the orifice meter is sound in principle and has advantages in relative ease of application. With it Shipley *et al.* (1943) have recorded phasic patterns in a greater variety of arteries than any other workers. Its main disadvantage appears to lie in its relatively high impedance which will cause damping. This damping will not only modify the amplitude of the recorded phasic variations in flow but will also cause a distortion of the shape of the flow curve due to the accompanying shift in phase. Furthermore, a meter with a marked impedance can cause significant alteration in the flow pattern by causing a redistribution of flow into other vascular beds.

A well-designed Pitot tube may be preferable for detailed investigation if its use is restricted to very large arteries such as the aorta so that its impedance can be kept small. The accuracy of the Pitot tube is greatest where the velocity gradient across the pipe is very small and, as we have seen above (p. 46), we appear to have this condition in the aorta. However, there are at present too few published records of flow with adequate Pitot tubes on which to make a judgement.

All types of differential pressure flow meters require accurate differential pressure manometers. The membranes must be sensitive to very small pressure changes and so of a lower "stiffness" than conventional manometers. This tends to lower their frequency response and the compromise this requires in their design raises special problems. Insufficient data have been published to discuss this fully here. Richardson, Denison and Green (1952) have stated that they regard the manometer used by Shipley *et al.* (1943) to be very underdamped. This statement was partly based on the marked discrepancy in their respective flow curves (see Figs. 6.2 and 6.3), but as noted in the discussion below there seems to be very considerable damping in the records of the meter used by Richardson and his colleagues. The Sanborn differential electromanometer has been used by Fry *et al.* (1956) and has satisfactory characteristics. Betticher, Maillard and Müller (1954) have gone to considerable trouble to design and build their own differential manometer for use with the Pitot tube used by Müller (1954*a*). The optical manometer with photo-electric recording designed by

Müller and Shillingford (1954) has been used for recording pulsatile venous flow and it appears that its frequency response is reasonably satisfactory for measuring arterial pressure-gradients (Bergel *et al.* 1958). The conductance manometer designed by Pappenheimer (1954) has a very good performance although it does not appear to have been used in this type of work.

The electromagnetic flowmeter

This meter uses the principle of magnetic induction. When an electrical conductor moves across the lines of force of a magnetic field a potential difference is created. As blood is a conductor of electricity its velocity of movement may be measured by aligning a blood-vessel across a magnetic field and recording the induced e.m.f. Provided that (1) the field is uniform, (2) the conductor moves in a plane at right angles to the field and (3) the length of the conductor extends at right angles to both field and direction of motion then the potential difference is given by the following equation (Jochim, 1948):—

$$E=H.L.V.10^{-8}$$

where E is the potential difference in volts, H the length of the magnetic field in gauss, L the length of conductor within the field in cm, i.e. the internal diameter of the vessel, and V the velocity of the conductor in cm/sec. If H and L are kept constant it can be seen that the potential difference recorded varies linearly with the velocity of flow and, in fact, the velocity recorded is the average velocity across the pipe (Kolin, 1945). The calibration curve is thus a straight line passing through the origin.

The instrument was introduced into physiology independently by Kolin in the United States and Wetterer in Germany (for references see Jochim, 1948). Its apparent advantages are the linear calibration noted above and that it can be applied to an unopened vessel. It also records backflows as well as forward flows.

The problem of creating a uniform magnetic field forms a practical obstacle in applying the meter to some arteries, but with improvement of design small electro-magnets have been developed which can be applied to any reasonably accessible vessel. Interference due to the electrical potentials created by the heart which was earlier thought to limit its use has also been overcome for Wetterer and Deppe (1940) used it successfully on the ascending aorta, and more recently the North Carolina group have used it throughout the aorta (Spencer and Denison, 1956, Spencer *et al.* 1958).

The technical problems have almost all centred round the accurate recording of the very small potential differences that are created in the blood-vessel. The simplest form has a constant magnetic field (the d.c. type) and the recording system has to use a direct-coupled amplifier. Surface potentials formed at the electrodes are relatively large compared with those induced in the flowing blood and it is difficult to discriminate between them in a d.c. system. The d.c. meter is also said to suffer a lot from zero drift. Jochim (1948) attempted to minimize the electrode potentials by embedding them in perspex blocks which fitted closely around the artery. A similar apparatus was used by Richards and Williams (1953). Inouye, Kuga and Usui (1955) and Inouye and Kosaka (1959) have also used this type of meter and found it satisfactory.

Many American workers, however, have abandoned the d.c. type in favour of an a.c. system (e.g. Richardson, Denison and Green, 1952) or more lately for the square-wave type (Denison, Spencer and Green, 1955). In the a.c. meter the magnetic field is produced by an electromagnet using alternating current. The induced potentials also alternate at the same frequency; capacitor-coupled amplifiers are used and the polarization potentials can be eliminated. However the alternating magnetic field induces eddy currents not only in the blood but also in the arterial wall and the surrounding fluid so that it is virtually essential to cannulate the vessel. This discards one of the main advantages of the electro-magnetic flowmeter. The North Carolina group have, therefore, modified it still further and activate their electromagnet by alternating rectangular pulses (the "square-wave type") which, they claim, is immune to the effects of eddy currents and electrode polarization voltages and so may be applied to unopened vessels. It also has an improved linearity and stability over previous models. Certainly the records made of flow in the dog aorta (Spencer and Denison, 1956, Spencer *et al.*, 1958) seem to me among the best phasic flow recordings made with the electromagnetic flowmeter. Those of Inouye *et al.* (1955) and Inouye and Kosaka (1959) with both a.c. and d.c. types, however, also appear to be reasonably satisfactory and it remains to be proved whether the increased complexities of the square-wave type justify themselves by improved performance.

One factor that is common to all types of electromagnetic flow-meter, as well as to others such as the orifice meter, is that either a length of rigid cannula is introduced, or the artery is restrained externally by rigid blocks carrying the electrodes, or by the poles of the magnet. The possible distortion due to this may be due to two causes. One is biological, for insertion of a cannula into the vessel may cause the release of vasodilator substances, as Folkow (1953) maintains is always the case. On existing evidence one must regard this as "not proven"; for example the curve recorded using the orifice meter by Shipley *et al.* (1953) and reproduced in Fig. 6.3 shows a large backflow and is quite uncharacteristic of flow into a dilated vascular bed (e.g. Fig. 5.8). The other effects are due to physical changes in pulsatile flow due to a rigid section in the vessel. Some of these cannulae have an appreciable impedance. For example, that used by Richardson *et al.* (1952) caused a pressure drop of the order of 3 mm Hg with a steady flow of only 30 ml/min, which is greater than that reported for the orifice meter by Gregg and Green (1939).

THE DISTORTION OF FLOW DUE TO A CANNULA

The effect of the insertion of a cannula or of an external restraint due to the poles of a magnet, on the form of the pulsatile flow may be considered at this point. This problem is by no means confined to the use of electromagnetic flowmeters but has been analysed by Womersley (1958*b*) in the case of three meters of this type. Any such device will have an impedance for pulsatile flow, but no workers have measured this in the way that the resistance of meters to steady flow has been recorded. If the impedance is different from that of the artery in which it is inserted then wave-reflection will be created and distortion will occur. Womersley (1958*b*) made some estimations of this effect which essentially depend on comparing the calculated values of the characteristic impedance of the artery with that of the meter assembly. With a short external constraint such as the plastic blocks 1·5 cm long that Inouye *et al.* (1955) used the predicted distortion was very small—about 2 per cent. An increase in length to 2·0 cm, however, could increase this to 8 per cent. In the case of the long catheter assembly used by Randall and Stacy (1956*a*) the reduction in amplitude was predicted to be as high as 42 per cent with 47° of phase shift in the fourth harmonic. The small lateral compression of the artery used by Spencer and Denison (1956) was thought to have a negligible effect.

These results are interesting but a little suspect. For example, the correction calculated by Womersley has been applied to their results by Stacy and Potor (1958 personal communication) and the resultant curve was still very much smaller in amplitude than others recorded in the femoral artery (Fig. 6.2). One difficulty of attempting to apply such a correction is that the measured input impedance of an artery is usually different from the calculated characteristic impedance in the sense that the former is changed by the presence of reflections whereas the calculated value assumes there are none. This is discussed at length in Chapter 10 (Figs. 10.9, 10 and 11) where it is seen that the input impedance can vary greatly with frequency. The distortion due to the meter will almost certainly vary with changes in wave-reflection and hence with vasomotor changes in the peripheral bed. They cannot, therefore, be predicted in a general quantitative way.

The prediction that the shortest cannulae produce the least distortion is undoubtedly true, even though that is a prediction that hardly needs weighty mathematical support. Womersley's estimation of the very small magnitude of this effect is, however, reassuring and indicates that there is no serious physical objection to their use.

The actual performance of various electromagnetic flowmeters is compared in Fig. 6.2 and discussed below. Theoretically the principle is satisfactory and the differences between recordings are probably due to technical problems of design which could be ironed out once it is agreed what are the normal values for arterial flow.

The damping due to the operation of Lenz's law, which was mentioned by McDonald (1955a) as a possible factor in distorting electromagnetic flowmeter records, has been calculated and shown to be far too small to be of any significance.

The hydrodynamic pendulum of Castelli. "Bristle" flowmeters

If a pendulum is suspended so that it is free and lies in liquid then flow in that liquid will cause the pendulum to move. The movement can be used to measure the rate of flow and a device of this sort was first used by Castelli (1577–1644), a pupil of Galileo, to measure the flow velocity of mountain streams. Under the name of the "haemodrometer" an instrument of this sort was used by Chauveau and associates in 1860 (Hill, 1900). It must, therefore, have seniority as a phasic flow recorder. In its simplest form inertia, and hence slowness of response, are obviously its main technical problem. Bergmann (1937) improved it greatly by using a flexible bristle in an instrument known as the "Stromborste". The introduction of thermionic valves that can function as mechano-electronic transducers has made the construction of a very refined version of this type of meter possible. Similar models were introduced independently and almost simultaneously by Scher, Weigert and Young (1953), Pieper and Wetterer (1953*b*), Brecher (1954) and Müller (1954*b*). Brecher has used the instrument extensively in studying venous flow and has named it the bristle flowmeter, presumably to acknowledge its relationship to Bergmann's "stromborste". Müller (1954*b*) gives a full account of the problems connected with this type of meter.

In order to maintain a rigid support for the sensing probe it is necessary to mount the device into a cannula but this can be kept very short. In the valve movements of the external probe move the anode and so cause changes in the anode current. It is thus possible to keep the probe very rigid as very little movement is required, hence the orientation of the probe remains virtually constant. It is, however, very difficult to calculate the forces that a pulsating liquid stream will exert on a structure thrust across a diameter of the tube without precise knowledge of the extent to which the flow is deformed by the obstruction. Scher *et al.* (1953) considered two types. With a streamlined rod the force is in the nature of viscous drag and the deflection varied approximately linearly with the mean flow in their model—more precisely deflection $=k\bar{V}^{1.2}$. In order to increase sensitivity a second type was made with a paddle on the end and with this the deflection is roughly proportional to $\bar{V}^2$. Increasing the size of the obstruction will also obviously increase the impedance of the meter. Brecher (1956) appears to use the latter type exclusively in recording venous flow. He has also used it in the pulmonary artery (Brecher and Hubay, 1954) and Müller and Laszt (personal communication) are using it in the aorta but the only results published to date are in the coronary artery (Laszt and Müller, 1957). One cannot, therefore, compare the results with this meter with others on systemic arterial flow at present. In view of its relative simplicity and the fact that, with the available sensitivity in the tube, a thin probe can be used with approximately linear behaviour, this type of meter deserves much more attention as a phasic meter for use in the larger arteries.

Pieper and Wetterer (1953a) have also introduced a flowmeter which has a cylinder held in the axis of the stream in a cannula. The displacement of the cylinder is detected by a differential transformer outside the cannula.

Taylor (1958b) has made a theoretical analysis of the behaviour of flowmeters of the bristle and pendulum type. This will clearly be dependent on the distribution of flow velocity across the tube which, as was seen in Fig. 3.1, changes greatly in oscillatory as compared with steady flow. From Taylor's results it appears that the true "bristle" meter with a fine probe gives the most satisfactory results. In fact the distortions introduced when applied to a measured femoral artery flow curve produce remarkably little change. The use of a pendulum or "paddle" on the probe greatly increases the distortion; the meter with the axial cylinder (Pieper and Wetterer, 1953a) is shown to introduce very large phase lags in the recorded flow although the amplitude is quite faithfully recorded.

This valuable study emphasizes the necessity for testing the performance of all flowmeters with oscillatory flows of known magnitude and frequency generated by a pump. It would be regarded as peculiar if a new manometer was introduced which had only been calibrated for steady pressures, yet very few proper calibrations of flowmeters designed for recording pulsatile flow have been made. Theoretically the electromagnetic flowmeter should have the same calibration for steady and oscillatory flow for it records the average velocity across the pipe whatever the form of the profile—provided that it is symmetrical about the axis. This is the only meter of the types discussed above of which this is true and even there, in view of the differences between various published results, it would be enlightening to see more calibration curves made with known oscillatory flows, in the way that Ferguson and Wells (1959) have done in their thorough description of meter performance.

High-speed cinematography

The velocity of blood flow can be estimated by filming the movement of some visible discontinuity that moves with the blood.

This has the advantage that it may be used on an intact vessel with no more interference than is required by surgical exposure and the cannulation of a side-branch for injection of a marker substance. Furthermore it is a direct observational method. The rate of filming required to record arterial flow velocities is, however, of the order of 1,000 frames/sec so that a special camera has to be used and observations must be limited to very short periods. It is not, therefore, a method strictly comparable with the use of a meter.

The essentials of the method have been described by McDonald (1952*a*) where bubbles of air were used as the "marker". Oxygen was later substituted for air to diminish the risk of gas embolism. Bubbles of gas can be fairly easily photographed through the wall of arteries up to about 4 mm in external diameter. Larger vessels, in my experience, have walls that are too thick to be sufficiently translucent.

The need to form a clear photographic image determines the choice of marker. Bubbles are by far the best that we have found. Ideally one single spherical bubble filling the lumen of the vessel should be injected in each cardiac cycle. In practice oxygen is injected at the rate of about 0·1 ml/sec with a tuberculin syringe to form a train of bubbles. A bubble just filling the vessel travels at a velocity very close to the average flow velocity (Womersley— unpublished).

Injections of dye, although they might seem preferable, are of little value in measuring flow velocity. With a dye that mixes with the blood the only movement that can be analysed is the "front", or profile, of the dye. Thus for each injection of dye only one observation is possible. Secondly, the profile is seen as a shadow diminishing in density towards the axis and so is impossible to delimit precisely—the optical opacity of the blood renders this especially difficult. Essentially the same problem occurs in cineradiography with radiopaque material and may introduce an error that possibly accounts for some of the extraordinarily high velocities reported by Reynolds *et al.* (1952). Thirdly, there is no simple relation between axial velocity and mean velocity in pulsating flow as there is in a Poiseuille-type flow as we discussed above (Ch. 3). The use of dye is, however, valuable in studying the flow pattern; it is also preferable, possibly, in very small vessels, such as those in the rabbit ear studied by Widmer (1957).

The camera rate at which the flow must be filmed is determined by three factors. 1. The actual length of exposure on the individual frames of film, 2. the degree of optical magnification, and 3. the peak velocity of flow. Of these the exposure on the frame is the most important and is obviously linked with the repetition rate of the camera. With the usual type of high-speed camera a repetition rate of at least 1,000 frames/sec is necessary to avoid visible movement on each frame. This corresponds to an effective frame exposure of about 200 μsec. With the use of synchronized electronic flashes a short frame exposure could be made independent of camera speed but it would still be necessary to film at up to 3–400/sec to follow systolic flow. The power unit for a discharge tube working at that rate would have to be very large. Such a unit would, however, simplify many of the lighting problems. Factors 2 and 3 above are linked together as, although the peak velocities in the smaller vessels are lower, one must magnify them optically to see sufficient detail and the apparent velocity on the film (which determines camera speed) remains much the same. It is desirable for analysis to have the optical field large enough to encompass the movement of a bubble throughout one cardiac cycle. In the dog femoral artery this is of the order of 5 cm but is less in the rabbit aorta.

The camera used in my experiments was the Eastman high-speed camera. This works on the principle of traversing the film continuously behind a revolving block of glass so that the image follows the film. Several different makes of camera are now available on this principle. Some have repetition rates of up to 10,000 frames/sec and more but the lowest effective speed for the purpose should always be used as the length of the event that can be photographed is inversely proportional to the camera running speed. While the camera is accelerating to its steady speed the film cannot be used for analysis and this wastage increases with the speed used. When the effective film run becomes less than 1 sec the problems of synchronizing the injection become very difficult (16 mm film has 40 frames per foot length so that a 100 ft reel has 4,000 frames).

When the exposure of the individual frames is about 1/5,000 sec a high intensity of incident light is required. I have used continuous lighting with a Mazda MEC/U compact source mercury/cadmium high pressure arc in a quartz bulb. On continuous running this is rated at 1 kW but it can be overrun at 3, 5 or 10 kW for short pulses coincidentally with the running of the camera. It is rarely necessary to use more than 5 kW. With this setting the lens aperture was usually *f*.8. The film used has been Kodak positive reversal Super XX or preferably Super X for its finer grain. Faster films with acceptable grain size are becoming available.

Blood-pressure is recorded simultaneously through a second cannula in a side-branch with a capacitance manometer and synchronized with the film by a flashing light in the picture area whose pulses are recorded on the second beam of a double-beam cathode-ray oscilloscope.

To analyse the results precisely the film is projected on to a motor-driven drum rotating at 90° to the line of the artery. The movement of the bubble is then traced manually on to the moving paper (McDonald, 1955*b*). The resultant curve (Fig. 6.1) has time as the abscissa and the distance travelled by the bubble (which is what the film record shows) as ordinate. This curve, in fact, represents the distance the blood has flowed throughout the cycle, and for many purposes, such as the study of hyperaemia, is the most valuable form of the flow curve. However, the conventional representation of phasic flow is in terms of a velocity curve and, to derive this, the total flow curve must be differentiated. Graphic differentiation has usually been used. If the slope at any point is $\frac{y}{x}$ then

$$\text{Velocity} = \frac{y}{x} \times \frac{\text{camera speed (f.p.s.)}}{\text{projector speed (f.p.s.)}} \times \frac{\text{drum paper rate (cm/sec)}}{\text{magnification of projected image}}$$

The mean velocity throughout the cycle is easily determined from the slope of the line joining the beginning of two successive systoles. The differentiation of the curve may be performed by a Fourier series if the ordinates are measured from the sloping abscissa representing the mean flow.

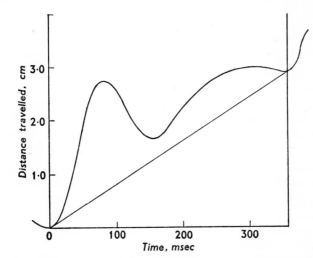

Fig. 6.1. An example of the method of analysing a high-speed ciné film of oxygen bubbles in an artery. The film is projected so that the axis of the artery lies vertically on a rotating paper-covered drum (see McDonald, 1955*b*). The movement of the bubble is then traced and the resultant curve represents distance travelled (vertically) in respect to time (horizontal movement of the drum). The slope is, therefore, a measure of the velocity of the bubble and, hence, of the blood carrying it. Reversal of slope indicates backflow. The slope of the straight line represents the mean velocity; it can be seen that the total travel of the bubble in one cycle is about 3 cm.

The record shown here is from a dog femoral artery while there was an occluding cuff at 40 mm Hg obstructing the venous return. The backflow phase is very marked.

The errors inherent in the method are small. They may be due (1) to the introduction of bubbles of gas into the circulation or (2) to the discrepancies between the rate of travel of the bubble and the rate of flow of the liquid. The main factor under the heading (1) is gas embolism. Under the heading (2) are (*a*) the possibilities of the bubble being carried in the axial streams, (*b*) the flow characteristics of large bubbles and (*c*) surface tensions effects causing "sticking" of the bubble.

(1) Gas embolism of any significant amount can be avoided by injecting only very small volumes of gas. Ideally one bubble is needed in each cardiac cycle. If the femoral artery has an internal diameter of 3 mm then a spherical bubble filling it has a volume of 0·014 ml. It can be seen that the amount of gas injected, even if 4 or 5 bubbles are injected per cycle, is rarely more than about 0·2–0·25 ml in the course of a film run which lasts about 1 sec. Furthermore, only a small fraction of this will reach the minute vessels, where embolism occurs, within the short time of the film run. If this caused a significant difference then there would be a change in shape of the flow curve in successive cardiac cycles, and this has not been observed. The danger of embolism lies in the accumulation of gas in the capillary bed due to successive injections. When air was used (McDonald, 1952*a*) it was found that after several runs there was an alteration in flow pattern which was attributed to embolism. Since then oxygen has been substituted for air and no such effect has since been observed. As film runs are rarely made at intervals of time shorter than 20 min it appears that the oxygen is totally absorbed. In large arteries the use of oxygen, in small injections at considerable intervals of time, does not cause any modification of flow pattern due to obstruction of the vascular bed. In much smaller vessels the possibility of gas embolism causing an alteration in flow would be greater.

2(*a*) and (*b*). The rate of travel of bubbles in flowing liquid has been studied in relation to the use of the bubble flowmeter (Bruner, 1948). A small bubble will tend to move into the centre of the tube and so will travel faster than the average velocity because the axial velocity is higher than the average. Bruner states that a large cylindrical bubble also travels at a higher velocity than the average for the blood because the viscosity of air is less than that of blood. Both these effects are avoided by rejecting any film analyses of bubbles that are not spherical and filling the lumen. In pulsatile arterial flow I have never seen the formation of very small bubbles. Large ones are only formed when an injection is made too fast in error.

2(*c*). The "sticking" of bubbles in tubes is a familiar phenomenon in physiological apparatus. It is, however, virtually confined to bubbles that are small in size compared with the tube in which they are found. In these cases they commonly float to one wall and the apparent "sticking" is due largely to the fact that the laminae close to the wall have a low velocity. In the flow records made with this technique the pulsatile velocities have, as shown in Figs. 6.2, 6.3, been usually higher than those recorded by other methods so that this factor, which would cause a low recorded velocity, cannot be the cause of the discrepancy.

The errors that arise in practice are due to the technical problem of obtaining a good photographic image. Extraneous highlights on the artery and changes in the translucency of the artery may make analysis of some films very difficult, and inaccuracies may be introduced which are hard to eliminate. This often necessitates the rejection of a proportion of the records. The method of analysis by tracing the movement of the bubble also implies an observational error which can only be minimized by repeated analyses by more than one observer. The character of the image makes it impossible to use a photographic method of recording the rate of travel of the bubble as seen in the projected film. These factors constitute practical limitations to the usefulness of the method as a technique for the experimental recording of blood flow. McDonald (1955a) showed that the velocities of flow recorded by this method (e.g. Figs. 5.7 and 5.8) were in good agreement with those calculated from the pressure-gradient, or the time-derivative of the pressure curve. This gives us confidence in the method as no other has been simultaneously checked in this fashion and few different meters have shown much agreement one with the other. It should be remembered, however, that the direct measurement is of *velocity* of flow and that where *volume* flows have been reported they are derived secondarily. Some volume flow curves previously reported (McDonald, 1955a) have undoubtedly been too high due to overestimation of the internal radius of the artery.

As regards the cinematographic method of recording flow velocity, the peak values may be rather high—possibly as much as 25 per cent in some cases. This doubt is based on current estimations of arterial impedance (Ch. 10) and may prove to be unjustified. During the present stage of search for a satisfactory phasic flowmeter I feel that high-speed cinematography has a place in providing a direct observational technique for the calibration of meters *in vivo*.

Calculation of phasic flow from the pressure-gradient

In a rigid tube steady flow is commonly measured by recording the pressure-gradient and using Poiseuille's law to calculate the flow. As was shown in Ch. 5, it is now possible to calculate pulsatile flows in a similar way. This is not considered at length in the present chapter as an independent experimental method because the calculations involved are somewhat lengthy, although with increased use of computers this may soon be a small objection. Also the estimates of mean flow are subject to error. The oscillatory terms may be predicted with fair accuracy but the steady flow is dependent on such a small pressure-gradient that manometers at present available are not able to measure it precisely. All the calculated curves presented have had the mean flow checked by direct observation. For the measurement of arterial impedance the measurement of the gradient has been used by Bergel *et al.* (1958).

The method of Fry *et al.* (1956) for computing flow curves in the root of the aorta from the pressure-gradient has already been discussed and it is a very promising application of the method to a special region. The assumptions on which it is based make it equally applicable to recording flow in the pulmonary artery.

Other meters

A few other principles have been applied in the design of flowmeters although they are not yet in general use.

The ultrasonic flowmeter. The velocity of sound in a flowing liquid is the algebraic sum of the velocity of sound in that liquid and the stream velocity. For flow in an elastic tube very high frequencies have to be used so that the velocity of transmission is determined exclusively by the properties of the fluid. This principle has been used for the measurement of the velocity of fast-flowing liquids but it was usually felt that the velocities of flow found in the blood stream were so small relative to that of sound as to make it technically impossible to build an apparatus that was sufficiently accurate. The impossible in this case has been achieved by the Mayo Clinic group (Haugen, Farrall, Herrick and Baldes, 1955).

The degree of precision required is illustrated by the fact that even with a flow velocity of 100 cm/sec the difference in transit time to be detected is only 2×10^{-8} sec. At the ultrasonic frequency used (300–400 kc) this represents a phase shift of 3 degrees. To obtain an accuracy of 1 cm/sec it is therefore necessary to measure a phase shift of 0·03 degrees. Such very great precision requires extreme stability in the transducers etc., and it is a triumph to have achieved it. No records have yet been published of phasic flow curves but ultrasonic transducers have been designed which can be fitted around arteries with very little interference. The meter has been used by Marshall and Shepherd (1959). It may, however, prove necessary to insulate them acoustically from the surrounding tissues to reduce ultrasonic vibration transmitted through parts of the body other than the blood-vessel.

There would seem to be no theoretical objections inherent in this meter. The vessel is intact and with the small transducers developed by the Minnesota group there is very little external restraint.

Rushmer and his group (Franklin, Ellis and Rushmer, 1959) have recently developed a different ultrasonic flowmeter which has been fixed around the thoracic aorta of dogs which were allowed to recover. Continuous records of aortic blood flow in conscious dogs have thus been possible. The principle used in their meter has been the alteration in the transmission time, of single ultrasonic "pips", by the blood flow velocity. The recorded curves agree quite well with those made with the electromagnetic flowmeter.

The hot-wire anemometer is capable of recording rapid fluctuations of flow. Machella (1936) used an instrument of this type to record pulsatile flow in the carotid artery. His records show a close correspondence of the form of the flow and pressure curves which indicates that there was an appreciable phase lag in his flow records.

The Thermostromuhr has been used extensively in the past for recording mean flows in unopened or cannulated arteries. In its conventional form it has been criticized because reversals of flow are apt to be recorded as increases in forward flow (Gregg, Pritchard and Shipley, 1948). Rein's original model, which used diathermy current to provide the heating, has been modified, and is said to be sufficiently rapid in response to record pulsating flows (Aschoff and Wever, 1956; Wever and Aschoff, 1956). There appears to be insufficient data at present to assess its value in this respect, although the diathermy model has been tested critically for recording mean flows as compared to the bubble flowmeter and rotameter (Janssen *et al.* 1957).

The comparison of the behaviour of various meters

It is of interest to discuss briefly some of the various records of pulsatile flow patterns that have been published. The femoral artery of the dog has been chosen for a comparison of the curves shown in Figs. 6.2 and 6.3 because there are more records available for flow in this vessel than any other. Such a comparison cannot give precise details as to the respective behaviour of the meters because there is no doubt that the amplitude of the pulsatile flow variations will be different in animals and in changing dynamic conditions. In view of the possible errors in meters that have been discussed above we may reasonably indicate causes for the large differences that are seen.

Fig. 6.2 shows flow curves recorded with electromagnetic flowmeters compared with a typical curve of my own based on the cinematography of a travelling oxygen bubble. Fig. 6.3 shows some flow curves recorded by Shipley, Gregg and colleagues with the orifice meter compared with the same flow curve of my own. This curve which is used as a comparison fits well with the curve calculated from the pressure-gradient. Where the other authors have reported details of the arterial pressure these have been checked and indicate that in all these cases the animals were in a similar circulatory condition.

In Ch. 5 it was pointed out that the pulsatile flow in an artery can be usefully considered as a steady flow (the mean flow throughout the cycle) with an oscillatory flow superimposed on it. The measurement of the steady term should present no instrumental problems other than that of accurate calibration. The consideration of the fidelity of the instrument in recording rapid fluctuations of flow should, therefore, concentrate on the amplitude and phase of the whole of the oscillating component in respect to the value of the mean. Where comparison of results has been made by some authors the presence or absence of a backflow, for example, has been taken as a criterion. By itself the absence of backflow may be of no significance unless the mean flow rate is considered. An increase of mean flow, as in reactive hyperaemia, commonly causes

---

* A symposium devoted to "Blood Flow Measurement" was held in Omaha, Neb., in June 1959.

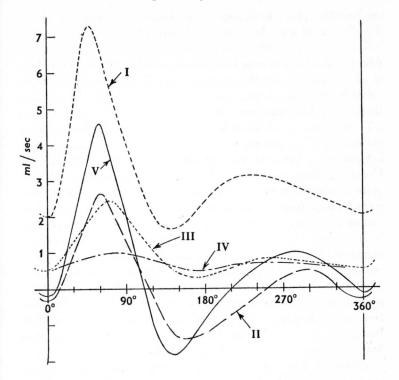

F<small>IG</small>. 6.2. The pulsatile flow in the dog femoral artery as recorded by four different electromagnetic flowmeters (curves I–IV) compared with a reference curve (V) of my own, recorded by high-speed cinematography and checked by calculation from the pressure.

I—from Richards and Williams (1953)

II—from Inouye and Kosaka (1949)

III—from Richardson, Denison and Green (1952)

IV—from Randall and Stacy (1956a).

The drawing is only approximate as the original records were mostly too small to plot accurately. However, the maximum and minimum values alone emphasize the tremendous variation in pulsatile amplitude recorded by various meters. The extent of the normal physiological variation in flow pattern is not known; the mean flows are, however, very similar (c. 1.0 ml/sec) in all curves except I (which is over three times as great—3·0 ml/sec). It is doubtful if a similar variation (the pulsatile flow amplitude differs by about 1200 per cent) in recorded arterial pulse pressures at the same mean pressure would be accepted as accurate. Comparison with Fig. 6.3 shows that the variation of these meters compared with the orifice meter is even greater.

The records of flow curves published by Ferguson and Wells (1959) are most similar in form to curve V in this diagram. Their peak systolic flows were between 5 and 6 ml/sec and peak backflow between 1·7 and 2·1 ml/sec (mean flow 0·8 ml/sec). These maxima occurred somewhat earlier in the cycle than those shown in curve V.

the backflow phase to disappear (see Fig. 5.8 and also Ch. 7). On the other hand a marked damping in the recorded oscillatory flow will also eliminate backflow. In this case, however, the forward flow will also be seen to be markedly less. In Fig. 6.2 the mean flows of all the curves with the exception of I (Richards and Williams, 1953) is about the same, that is 1 ml/sec or slightly less. In all Richards and Williams records the mean flow rate is of the order of 2·5–3·0 ml/sec which is far higher than anyone else has recorded under normal conditions, and is in excess of the recorded flows in hyperaemia I have recorded or those reported by Randall and Horvath (1953). As Inouye and Kosaka (1959) have said, this suggests a calibrating error. The phasic fluctuations in flow in their record range from a minimum of 1·5 ml/sec to a maximum of almost 7·5 ml/sec and so, if the calibration is correct, is larger than in any other record of femoral artery flow made with an electromagnetic flowmeter. The curves are all similar in form to the reference curve, in that there is a peak flow in systole followed by a minimum in early diastole and a second maximum in the latter part of diastole. The curves II, III and IV (due to respectively Inouye and Kosaka, 1959; Richardson, Denison and Green, 1952; Randall and Stacy, 1956a) which, as noted, have similar mean flows but show progressive degrees of damping in the oscillating components. The transcription of the form of these curves is only approximate, but it is fairly clear that with reduction of amplitude the peak values are progressively retarded. This fits in with the assumption that this is due to damping in the meter. The case of curve IV due to Randall and Stacy has already been shown to be heavily damped owing to the length of rigid cannula in the system. The discrepancy between curve II and the reference curve V is difficult to assess with certainty and may well be due to biological variation. Damping due to the rigid enclosure of the vessel has been shown to be negligible because it is short in length. Some records with the bubble method do show an oscillatory amplitude that is almost as small as this, with a similar mean flow. On the other hand this represents a curve with one of the greatest amplitudes of oscillation in the records of Inouye and his collaborators. This suggests that even this meter may record less than the real phasic variation. This should be checked against curves calculated from the pressure-gradient, but insufficient data are available to do this at present. If this curve represents the phasic changes in flow rate inadequately then it can be seen that curve IV (Richardson *et al.*, 1952) is even further damped. The recently published femoral flow curves of Ferguson and Wells (1959) appear to agree closely with that of curve V in Fig. 6.2. In view of the careful calibration of their instrument it would seem that we can regard, with some confidence, this as the normal form of the curve. In curve IV it seems likely that the amplifier system is over-damped. Unfortunately the square-wave meter, which was developed after the one used by Richardson *et al.*, has not yet been used to record femoral flows. The records of flow in the aorta (Spencer and Denison, 1956) are qualitatively similar to those recorded in the rabbit aorta (McDonald, 1952*a*). These authors did point out that they found no backflow in the thoracic aorta in comparison with the curves showing backflow reported in my paper. These curves, however, were all in the abdominal aorta and the single curve of abdominal aorta flow published by Spencer and Denison similarly shows a backflow. The evidence they advance, that they could only reproduce curves similar to mine by creating a partial obstruction downstream to their recording point is, therefore, irrelevant. Curves of thoracic aorta flow in the rabbit were not published in this paper (McDonald, 1952*a*) because only a few successful recordings had been made, but it was reported in the text that very little or no backflow was seen in the thoracic aorta. More recently Spencer *et al.* (1958) have recorded distinct backflows in the thoracic aorta. The development of a backflow phase in the abdominal aorta was, at that time, related to the fact that the large visceral arteries were creating a run-off upstream. Evidence on this point is developed in the next chapter.

Fig. 6.3 shows the two curves of femoral artery flow published by Shipley *et al.* (1943) compared with the same reference curve of my own as in Fig. 6.2. The forms of the curve II and of curve III are very similar although the oscillatory amplitude of the former is greater. This amplitude is very similar to that illustrated in McDonald (1955*a*, Fig. 8), which, for reasons discussed above, is now thought to be too high. The amplitude in curve I is quite close to that of curve III but the pattern is somewhat different in that there is a marked forward flow (approximately equal to the mean flow) at the end of diastole. In my own records I have only found this with marked vasodilatation (e.g. Fig. 7.6). It should also be noted that, in an accompanying paper, the Cleveland group

(Pritchard *et al.*, 1943) have recorded normal femoral artery flows that are much smaller in amplitude (peak forward flow *c.* 2·5 ml/sec) than those illustrated here. The form of these latter curves is similar to those shown here and always has a backflow phase. This suggests that the variation in oscillatory flow amplitude in "normal" dogs under experimental conditions may vary by over 100 per cent, and so is much more variable than the pulse-pressure. In my own series, admittedly smaller, the variation in the amplitude of velocity oscillation has been much less than that of the Cleveland group and the variation in arterial calibre in dogs

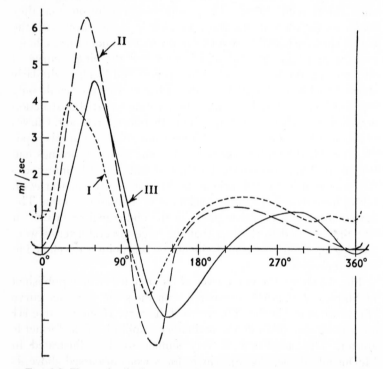

FIG. 6.3. Two pulsatile flow curves (I and II) recorded in the dog femoral artery with an orifice meter by Shipley *et al.* (1943); curve III is the same reference curve as shown in Fig. 6·2, V. Curve II appears to have the largest total amplitude of any published record in this artery with this, or any other, meter; the variation from +6 to −3 ml/sec is some eighteen times greater than that shown in curve IV and five to six times greater than in curve III (of Fig. 6.2). It is surprising that such differences have previously escaped critical comment.

The orifice meter records seem to show a consistent tendency to lead all other records in phase; the possibility that this is an artifact is discussed in the text.

of different size (which has not always been clearly stated) may contribute in large part to the variation in volume flow.

In general, I regard the orifice meter records of these workers as giving some of the most useful measurements of femoral artery flow fluctuations that we have at present. Nevertheless, the orifice meter records do seem to show a considerable divergence in their phase relations from my own—a divergence which is too great to be accounted for by errors in copying. Both curves I and II lead curve III in phase throughout the cycle; at the end of the backflow this lead is nearly 60°. These phase relations are reminiscent of those between the pressure-gradient and flow shown in Fig. 5.7. This suggests that the differential pressure in the orifice meter is not wholly dependent on the kinetic energy term (eqn. 6.1) but that the pressure-gradient itself is forming an appreciable fraction of it and is being recorded as flow. This point could perhaps be elucidated by calibration of the meter with oscillatory flow and taking account of the phase relations as well as the amplitude of the meter record.

The general agreement between the orifice meter curves, the curves derived from films of bubble travel and the calculated flow curves does reinforce the view that the amplitude of the variations in the rate of flow in the femoral artery during the cardiac cycle is large. In curve III Fig. 6.3, for example, the flow varies from $+4 \cdot 5$ ml/sec to $-1 \cdot 9$ ml/sec which is over seven times the value of the mean flow ($0 \cdot 86$ ml/sec). On present evidence any meter which records phasic changes which are less than half this must be suspected of inaccuracy. As we have seen the flow curves recorded by most electromagnetic flowmeters show a smaller oscillatory component than the orifice meter and the cinematograph records. Therefore, in spite of biological variation, that is undoubtedly large, it must be suspected that they show the effects of damping. A comparison of flow curves recorded by the best electromagnetic flowmeters with those calculated from the pressure-gradient at the same time is very desirable as a step towards the perfection of the design of this type of meter. Womersley (personal communication) reported reasonably good agreement between calculated flow curves and the curves recorded in the thoracic aorta by Spencer and Denison (1956). However, there appears to be a considerable difference between their results which indicate a peak flow of less than 100 ml/sec and those of Wetterer and Deppe (1940) and

Wetterer (1954) with a peak flow of 170 ml/sec, although the latter were recording more proximally. The peak velocity (assuming an aortic diameter of about 1 cm in a 15 kg dog) in Wetterer's results is about 200 cm/sec, in Spencer and Denison's 112 cm/sec, and in those of Fry *et al.* 70 cm/sec. This further illustrates the need for further work on the determination of normal values. Spencer *et al.* (1958), however, have published flow curves recorded in the ascending aorta which seem almost identical in form and amplitude with those of Wetterer and Deppe (1940).

CHAPTER VII

THE PULSATILE FLOW PATTERN IN ARTERIES

We will now consider the available evidence about the different forms of the pulsatile flow pattern that are found in various regions of the arterial tree, and the changes in flow that are caused by vasoconstriction and vasodilatation. Unfortunately, this evidence is meagre compared with the information about the form of the pressure pulsations and much of it has to be interpreted with reference to the possibility of the flowmeter artifacts which were discussed in Ch. 6. If accurate and simultaneous measurements of flow and pressure were available it would be a much easier task to give an account of the physical behaviour of the arterial circulation in terms of the input impedances of the component vascular beds. At present most of this discussion has to be based on the analysis of the pressure-waves and is considered later in Ch. 10 and 12. The present review of pulsatile flow patterns will first consider them in relation to different anatomical sites and secondly in relation to changes in the vascular bed.

THE "NORMAL" FLOW PATTERN IN VARIOUS ARTERIES

The nature of the pulsatile flow varies greatly according to the position and size of the artery. By "normal" is meant flow in an animal under standard conditions of anaesthesia, and on which only the operative procedure necessary to record flow has been performed. In my own experiments pentobarbitone (Nembutal Abbott) 30 mg/kg i.v. has been used initially in dogs. In most cases morphia (0·5 mg/kg) was given subcutaneously 1 hour before the induction of anaesthesia. In rabbits either pentobarbitone (25 mg/kg) i.v. followed by ether inhalation, or morphia (0·5 mg/kg) and chloralose (120 mg/kg intraperitoneally) was used. Gilmore (1956) has reported that pentobarbitone in dogs does not change the cardiac output or blood-pressure significantly from the values in the unanaesthetized animal but does increase the heart rate. The latter effect does not occur if morphia is used.

B.F.A.–K 129

The normal values of arterial blood-pressure are still sufficiently in dispute for us to realize that "normality" in terms of pulsatile flow, on which so little work has been done in comparison, is unlikely to be generally agreed on for a long time.

Reference to the flow curves illustrated previously (Figs. 5.7, 6.2, 6.3) shows that it may be described as two successive oscillations dying away rapidly towards the end of the cycle. Thus in the femoral flow curve in Fig. 5.7 we see a large systolic peak followed by a period of backflow, then a smaller forward flow maximum in mid-diastole and finally a very small backflow at the end of diastole. This type of curve represents a condition where there is a large oscillatory fluctuation superimposed on a relatively small mean flow. Descriptively we may compare other flow curves in other arteries with this pattern.

In the *ascending aorta* pulsatile flow curves were first recorded by Broemser (1928) but the later records with an electromagnetic flowmeter by Wetterer and Deppe (1940) (see Wetterer, 1954) are probably much more accurate and one of their curves is shown in Fig. 7.1. Recently Spencer, Johnston and Denison (1958) have published a very similar record. It will be noted that nearly all the outflow is during systole when flow rises very rapidly to a peak and then declines rather more slowly. The maximum flow velocity is approximately 2 m/sec. There follows a short, sharp backflow which is synchronous with the incisura in the pressure curve. This is attributed, e.g. by Spencer *et al.* (1958), solely to reflux through the aortic valves, but the surge into the coronary arteries at this period of the cycle must also be considered. During the remainder of diastole only a very small flow is recorded. The curve recorded by Fry *et al.* (1956) and illustrated in Fig. 5.9 shows a very similar pattern although the flow velocities recorded are markedly less (the comparison is only approximate because the aortic cross-sections in the relevant experiments are not precisely known). The short period of backflow corresponding to the incisura is much smaller in Fig. 5.9 and is followed by a more definite diastolic forward flow than shown in Fig. 7.1. Green (1950) has also published one flow curve made in the proximal aorta with an orifice flowmeter. This shows two backflow phases, one at the end of systole and the second in mid-diastole.

A flow curve recorded in the *thoracic* aorta by Spencer and Denison (1956) is shown in Fig. 7.2. The main differences between this curve and that shown in Fig. 7.1 are that the short but marked backflow phase has almost disappeared and that there is quite an appreciable forward flow in diastole. Later recordings in the same region by Spencer *et al.* (1958) show a larger backflow phase than this but never as fast, or as sharp in form, as that in the ascending aorta. The peak flow velocity (112 cm/sec in Fig. 7.2) is also markedly less than in the ascending aorta.

In the few observations that I have been able to make, a backflow phase has not been seen in the rabbit thoracic aorta. Otherwise the curves were similar in form to that seen in Fig. 7.2.

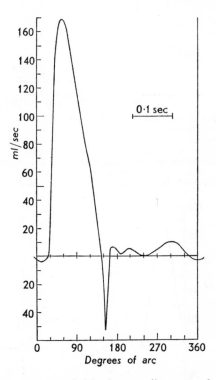

Fig. 7.1. A flow curve recorded in the ascending aorta of a dog (Wetterer and Deppe, 1940) with an electromagnetic flowmeter (redrawn from Wetterer, 1954).

Forward flow is virtually confined to the period of systolic ejection, the end of which is marked by a sharp, but brief, backflow. The cross-sectional area of the ascending aorta is probably 0·8–1·0 cm², so that the peak velocity is about 200 cm/sec. This may be compared with the curve (Fig. 5.9) recorded by Fry *et al.* (1956). A very similar curve to the present one has been reported by Spencer *et al.* (1958).

The *abdominal aorta* shows a flow curve which is rather different in shape (Fig. 7.3) and more resembles the form seen in the femoral artery (e.g. Fig. 5.7). The systolic peak is followed by a marked backflow phase. In a few personal observations, however,

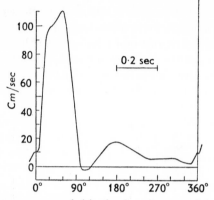

FIG. 7.2. A flow curve recorded in the thoracic aorta of the dog. Replotted from Spencer and Denison (1956) as average velocity to facilitate comparison with other flow curves.

The main differences seen in this curve as compared with the ascending aorta is the marked reduction in the backflow phase and an increase in forward flow in diastole. The systolic peak velocity was 112 cm/sec. Note that the pulse frequency is considerably slower that in most other curves illustrated.

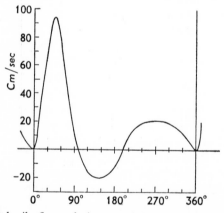

FIG. 7.3. Pulsatile flow velocity recorded in the rabbit abdominal aorta (distal to the renal arteries) using high-speed cinematography.

There is a marked backflow phase of much longer duration than that seen in the ascending aorta. Forward flow in late diastole is also well established. The curve is now similar in shape to that seen in the femoral artery (e.g. Fig. 7.4 and 5.7). Pulse frequency was 5 c/sec.

this backflow has been very small. Diastolic flow is usually faster than in the thoracic aorta, but occasionally (McDonald, 1952a) there may be no diastolic flow. Backflow in late diastole has not been recorded as it has in the femoral artery. Fig. 7.3 represents a typical curve recorded in the rabbit aorta with a mean arterial pressure of about 100 mm Hg and a pulse-pressure of about 30 mm Hg. The earlier curve with zero flow in the latter part of diastole appears to be related to the low mean pressure and small pulse-pressure reported in that series of experiments. Flow patterns similar to that shown in Fig. 7.3 have also been reported in the abdominal aorta of the dog (Spencer and Denison, 1956; Spencer *et al.*, 1958).

In major arterial branches we have a considerable number of records of flow in the *femoral artery* of the dog. These have been considered in detail in Ch. 6 comparing the fidelity of various types of meter. In my own observations there has always been a post-systolic backflow phase under normal conditions, but the late diastolic backflow has only been seen in about one-third of cases. Where there is no backflow, however, the flow velocity always falls to zero at the end of the cycle. This is not found in all the records of other workers—the curve of Shipley *et al.* (1943) which is often reproduced, for example, records an end-diastolic flow approximately equal to the mean value.

The *common carotid artery* has also been studied by several workers. Shipley *et al.* report curves similar to those found in the femoral artery with the principal difference that the backflow phase is sometimes absent. They also reviewed previous work on this artery. Recently Inouye and Kosaka (1959) have only rarely found a post-systolic backflow in flow records in this artery in rabbits and dogs. In a small (unpublished) series I also found that backflow was rarely found in the common carotid artery of the rabbit, but that flow fell to zero at the end of systole and then accelerated again in the forward direction during diastole.

Compared with the "type" curve of the femoral artery discussed above it can be seen that the fundamental pattern with velocity maxima in systole and mid-diastole and with minima at the end of systole and at the end of diastole, is found in all these major arteries. The relative amplitude of these maxima and minima differs considerably, however, with anatomical position.

In smaller arteries the shape of the curve becomes qualitatively different. In the *saphenous artery*, the typical flow curve has a peak in systole with a continuous deceleration throughout the remainder of diastole. The comparison of velocity of flow recorded simultaneously in the femoral artery and its saphenous branch in the dog is shown in Fig. 7.4 A. The main variations that have been recorded in my own experiments have been related to the amplitude of the peak systolic velocity and the velocity of flow in late diastole. In the curve illustrated (Fig. 7.4 A) there is a period of zero flow, in others a slow forward flow persists almost to the end of diastole, or it may terminate earlier (Fig. 7.4 B).

Shipley *et al.* (1943) have recorded the pulsatile flow in the *superior mesenteric* (see Fig. 7.8), *hepatic* and *renal* arteries of the dog. These are all similar to that illustrated in the saphenous artery in that there is a systolic maximum and a progressive slow-

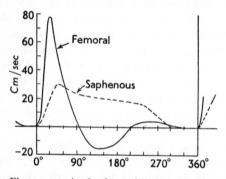

FIG. 7.4. A. Flow curves in the femoral and saphenous arteries of the dog recorded simultaneously by high-speed cinematography.

The flow pattern in the saphenous artery is very different from that in the femoral artery and is attributed to a marked reduction in the oscillatory flow components in the small vessel. This is in part due to damping caused by viscosity but is mainly determined by the large increase in the input impedance especially of the lower frequencies (see Fig. 10.11).

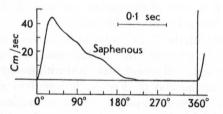

B. A flow curve recorded in the saphenous artery of another dog. Pulse-frequency 2.5 c/sec in both cases.

ing of flow throughout the remainder of the cycle, albeit with some minor secondary oscillations superimposed. There is one marked difference in that in all the records of Shipley and colleagues of the visceral arteries the velocity of flow never falls to zero at any period in the cycle. As the vascular bed of the abdominal viscera has a relatively low peripheral resistance the visceral arteries probably have a higher mean flow velocity than the saphenous artery, which has a cutaneous distribution and so a higher peripheral resistance. A difference in the amplitude of the mean flows could explain the difference in their respective phasic flow curves.

The rabbit *basilar artery* is the smallest artery in which I have recorded a flow curve (Fig. 7.5, Potter and McDonald, 1950). This can be seen to be similar to those in the smaller arteries discussed above. There is maximum velocity in systole falling to a low value

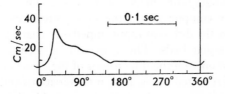

FIG. 7.5. Pulsatile flow velocity recorded in the basilar artery of the rabbit (*ciné technique—Potter and McDonald*, 1950).

in diastole although never coming completely to rest. Widmer (1957), also using high-speed cinematography, has recorded flows in the arteries of the rabbit ear. The main artery is approximately the same size as the basilar artery but he also studied small branches down to some 30μ in diameter. These are the smallest arteries in which flow velocities have been recorded. The mean values during systole were 19–24 cm/sec in the central artery (i.e. comparable with that in the basilar and saphenous arteries) and 4–5 cm/sec in the smallest branches. No backflow phase was seen at the end of systole and there was a steady forward flow during diastole of between 10 cm/sec (in the larger artery) and 2–3 cm/sec (in the smallest). Widmer used dye injections and measured the rate of travel of the dye "front". This shows very interesting variations in pattern during the different phases of the cardiac cycle. Unfortunately these variations also make it very difficult to determine the average velocity across the vessel, which is recorded by all other methods. During systole he recorded very rapid oscillations of flow velocity, even including apparent backflows. I cannot envisage any physical forces that could cause such high-frequency oscillations in a liquid of the viscosity of blood in tubes of such small diameter. Therefore, for the present, their occurrence should be regarded with reserve as they probably represent the relative velocities of different laminae in the stream which are being picked out by the changing distribution of dye.

The average diameter of the basilar artery in the rabbit is 0·5–0·6 mm; that of the dog saphenous artery is 0·8–1·2 mm, while the superior mesenteric and renal arteries of the dog are probably 2·0–2·5 mm. These last-named branches are of the same order of size as the femoral artery, and it is clear that the marked difference in the shapes of their respective flow curves cannot be explained simply in terms of the changes in pressure-flow relations due to the changing dimensions of the vessel. These differences in the oscillatory components of the flow pattern are undoubtedly determined by the different input impedance characteristics of the respective vascular beds. These, as will be seen in Ch. 10, are dependent not only on the dimensions of the vessel but also on the occurrence of reflected waves at their terminations and the distance from the recording site to these terminations. Until determinations of input impedances, in such vessels as the renal and superior mesenteric arteries, have been made, no profitable quantitative comparison of their flow curves and those recorded in the femoral artery can be made.

There is also a considerably larger mean flow in the renal artery than in the femoral artery. This, is of course, an important factor in determining features of the phasic flow curve as the evidence presented in the following section shows.

CHANGES OF FLOW PATTERN DUE TO CHANGES IN THE VASCULAR BED

It is clear that an increase of the mean flow will alter the form of a flow curve because, in effect, it shifts the whole curve upwards. Now a change in mean flow is usually considered entirely in terms of a change in the peripheral resistance *distal* to the recording point. It must also be remembered, however, that the rate of flow in one section of the circulatory bed is also profoundly modified by the "run-off" into branches proximal to it. Although changes in the vascular bed distal and proximal to any region we are studying will occur simultaneously in the intact animal, it is easier to consider them independently.

(i) The distal vascular bed

Vasodilatation confined to the vascular bed of the leg will cause an increase in mean flow in the femoral artery. In our experiments vasodilatation has been studied either by creating a reactive hyperaemia, or by an intra-arterial injection of acetylcholine. Reactive hyperaemia was created by compressing the whole thigh with a pneumatic cuff (3–4 cm wide) inflated to 200 mm Hg for one minute. Flow records were made 30–45 sec after release of the cuff when the hyperaemia was expected to be maximal (Randall and Horvath, 1953). A typical result is illustrated in Fig. 7.6. Flow records were made with the cinematograph technique. The use of a cuff to produce hyperaemia with this recording method was technically awkward so that the use of acetylcholine as a vasodilator drug was tested (Fig. 5.8). Flow recordings were made 5–10 sec after completion of intra-arterial injection (100 μg) into a femoral branch and completed before the drug had reached the heart. It is seen that the modification of the flow curve is similar in both cases. The most obvious change from the normal curve is the disappearance of the backflow phase. There is, however, still a point of minimum velocity at the end of systole corresponding in time to the backflow phase in the normal. The peak systolic velocity is increased and also the flow velocity at the end of diastole (which is

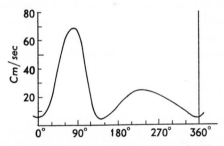

FIG. 7.6. The flow velocity curve recorded in the dog femoral artery during reactive hyperaemia. There has been an increase in mean flow which is largely responsible for the disappearance of the backflow phase normally seen in this artery (e.g. Fig. 5.1). Changes in the shape of the curve also occur but are usually only appreciated after numerical analysis. This curve should be compared with the flow curve during vasodilatation due to intra-arterial acetylcholine (Fig. 5.8). The pulse-frequency in this experiment was 2·4/sec.

no longer zero). As a simple approximation the change may, in fact, be accounted for by a shift upwards of the whole curve due to an increase in the mean flow rate.

Pritchard, Gregg, Shipley and Weisberger (1943) have made the most extensive report so far available on the action of vasomotor drugs on the flow pattern in various arteries. As in the accompanying paper by Shipley *et al.* (1943) the flow was recorded with an orifice meter. In the period immediately after the intra-arterial injection of a vasodilator drug the mean flow was increased in all cases as would be expected. Usually the intrinsic shape of the curve appears unchanged and, as in my results, the backflow was reduced or disappeared. In some cases the oscillatory components were augmented and they noted that a backflow phase, previously absent, might appear or an existing one be increased. From their records it appears that this latter condition only occurs when general vasodilatation resulting from recirculation has taken place, judging by the fact that the mean flow has fallen below its early maximum. This is only a tentative suggestion to account for this one marked difference in our observations, but it may well be one type of response to a marked vasodilatation.

Localized vasoconstriction was produced by intra-arterial injections of adrenaline (10 μg) or nor-adrenaline (10 μg) and the film records made before the drug had time to return to the heart. This caused a marked reduction of mean flow. The systolic forward flow was markedly reduced and the backflow increased so that they became comparable in size (Fig. 7.7). These changes in the oscillatory component were considerably greater than could be accounted for by the reduction in the mean flow. The observations of Pritchard *et al.* (1943) on the effect of intra-arterial injection of vasoconstrictor drugs are very similar to my own. The effects of vaso-

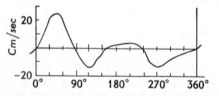

Fig. 7.7. Flow velocity recorded in a dog femoral artery during marked vasoconstriction—recorded in the same animal as the curve shown in Fig. 5.8. The double oscillation seen is not characteristic and was also present in the pressure record. The impedances found in this experiment are displayed in Fig. 10.10*b*.

dilatation and vasoconstriction on the shape of the flow curve are probably due, at least in great part, to the alteration in wave-reflection that they cause and hence a change in the input impedances of the various frequency components of the pulse-wave. These changes are illustrated in Figs. 10.9 and 10.10 where the dependence of the input impedances of the femoral flow curves illustrated in Fig. 5.1 (normal) and Fig. 5.8 (vasodilatation) and Fig. 7.7 (vasoconstriction) are displayed. Detailed discussion, which strongly suggests that the reasons for this frequency distribution are due to wave-reflection, is deferred until Ch. 10 but the main effects of vasomotor changes may be briefly noted here. With a moderate (i.e. "normal") degree of arteriolar constriction the input impedance of the low frequency components recorded in the femoral artery, notably the first two harmonics, is raised above the value of the characteristic impedance. The input impedance of the higher frequency components falls progressively, reaching a minimum value for between 13–14 c/sec. With vasodilatation the distribution of impedances tends to become more equal for all frequencies, that is, it falls for the lower frequencies but increases for the higher frequencies. As the amplitude of the pressure and flow pulsation is mainly determined by the amplitude of the first and second harmonic components this fall in amplitude tends to cause an increase in the flow oscillation. The reason that this is often not seen, as for example in Fig. 5.8 as compared with Fig. 5.7, is that the pressure oscillations, i.e. the pulse-pressure, tends to fall when there is vasodilatation.

The change of impedances due even to maximal vasodilatation (such as acetylcholine may produce) appear to be considerably smaller than the converse changes produced by maximal vasoconstriction (with intra-arterial nor-adrenaline). In the former case it is apparent that the anatomical arrangement of arterial and arteriolar branches must always produce an irreducible minimum of reflection however much the arteriolar bed is opened up. In the case of vasoconstriction reflection can presumably be increased, at least theoretically, to the point of complete closure. As this greatly increases the input impedances of the low frequency components the result is a marked reduction in the amplitude of the main oscillatory flow component so that the total flow pulsation is reduced. As the mean flow is also greatly reduced by the arteriolar constriction the flow pattern is almost all described in terms of its oscillatory components, and its dissimilarity from the normal curve is easily seen. With the flow curve in conditions of vasodilatation the change in shape is less apparent.

Venous occlusion also alters the phasic flow pattern in a similar way to vasoconstriction. Flow records have been made on film (see Fig. 6.1) while pressures of 40 and 80 mm Hg were applied to the thigh with a narrow pneumatic cuff. The changes in the flow curve were very similar to those reported by Gregg, Pritchard and Shipley (1948). The systolic forward flow was reduced and the backflow phase increased. The similarity of these changes to those due to vasoconstriction indicates that the net effect of an occluding cuff is to increase the vascular impedance of the bed.

(ii) Changes in the proximal vascular bed

One of the most striking things to be noted in Fig. 7.4 is that at a junction there is blood flowing distally in the small saphenous branch during the period of backflow in the femoral artery. Earlier a similar observation had been made with regard to the renal artery and the abdominal aorta (McDonald 1952*a*). This relationship is illustrated by Fig. 7.8 in which an abdominal aorta flow curve (in the rabbit) is superimposed on a superior mesenteric flow curve as recorded by Shipley *et al.* (1943) (in the dog). In the thoracic aorta,

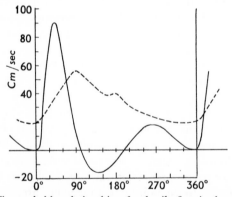

FIG. 7.8. The probable relationship of pulsatile flow in the abdominal aorta and the main visceral branches—although the curves were recorded in different species. The aortic flow is that seen in a rabbit (Fig. 7.3) while the other curve is a representation of the flow in the superior mesenteric artery of the dog recorded by Shipley *et al.* (1943). A situation of this kind, where there is forward flow in a branch during backflow in the main trunk, has been observed, qualitatively, in the abdominal aorta and renal artery of the rabbit, and recorded in the femoral and saphenous arteries of the dog (Fig. 7.4A).

as we have seen, there is little or no backflow. This difference in flow pattern may be considered as being due to the run-off into the visceral vascular bed from the whole aorta, which, once the aortic valves are closed, functions as a reservoir. If the main run-off is into the viscera this blood will be flowing forward out of the thoracic aorta but flowing back from the distal aorta. When studying the flow in one specific region the presence or absence of backflow will be determined by local conditions, that is by the magnitude of the flow into the proximal branches relative to that in the distal vascular bed.

The effect of altering the flow pattern in the abdominal aorta by changing the visceral blood supply has been reported in a preliminary communication (McDonald, 1954). In a rabbit the phasic flow pattern in the abdominal aorta distal to the renal arteries was that shown in Fig. 7.3. The coeliac and superior mesenteric arteries were then occluded by haemostats close to the aorta (the left renal artery was cannulated and therefore occluded throughout the experiment). Mechanical obstruction of vessels was preferred to the use of vasoconstrictor drugs as it ensured that the effect was confined to a specific part of the vascular bed. The resultant change in flow pattern is illustrated in Fig. 7.9. It can be seen that it is

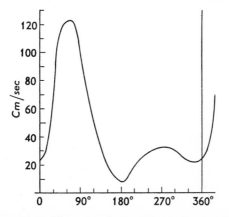

Fig. 7.9. The pulsatile flow pattern in the abdominal aorta, of the same rabbit as in Fig. 7.8, after clamping the coeliac and superior mesenteric arteries. The peak velocity has increased and the backflow phase has disappeared—these changes are mainly attributed to the considerable increase in mean flow velocity through the aorta as a result of preventing the run-off into the two large vascular beds supplied by these arteries. The change in pattern is similar to that caused by "downstream" vasodilatation (Fig. 5.8 and 7.6).

similar to that seen in reactive hyperaemia in the femoral artery
(Fig. 7.6). There is a marked increase in the systolic flow and the
backflow has been eliminated although the minimum velocity still
occurs in mid-cycle. Occlusion of two large visceral branches will,
of course, cause a considerable increase in the mean flow through
the abdominal aorta and this accounts in part for the difference
between the curves illustrated in Figs. 7.8 and 7.9. The shape of
the curve, however, has been changed as well. On releasing the
occlusion (after 1½ min) of the coeliac and superior mesenteric
arteries, the flow pattern seen in Fig. 7.10 was recorded. The most
marked effect is the very prolonged backflow which persists
throughout diastole. This would appear to be due to a marked
degree of reactive hyperaemia in the vascular beds of the coeliac
and superior mesenteric arteries. The curves in Figs. 7.9 and 7.10
show the extremes of modification of the arterial flow pattern in
that the major visceral arteries were completely occluded and later
released. They serve to emphasize the marked effect that can be
caused by changes in the flow in proximal branches. The form of
the curve in Fig. 7.10 may be compared with that of Fig. 7.7
showing the effects of vasoconstriction in the distal vascular bed.
In both cases there is a marked reduction of the mean flow but the
oscillatory components are very different in the two cases. This
indicates that a detailed investigation of the shape of the phasic
flow curve could be valuable in differentiating changes in mean flow

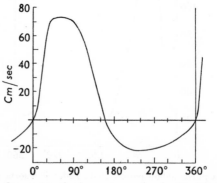

Fig. 7.10. The flow pattern in the same vessel as in Fig. 7.9 shortly after the
removal of the clamps from the coeliac and superior mesenteric arteries. The
marked changes in the shape of the curve, especially the prolonged backflow, is
attributed to a greatly increased run-off into these upstream branches as a result
of reactive hyperaemia in their vascular beds.

The pulse-frequency in this rabbit was 5/sec.

that are due to alterations in the run-off into proximally situated branches from those that are due to changes in the distal vascular bed.

Similar experiments have been performed in dogs. The cinematograph technique for recording flow velocity cannot, unfortunately, be used in the dog aorta as the wall is too opaque. Studies were made, as before, in the femoral artery. The superior mesenteric artery was occluded as in the experiments recorded above. Comparison with normal flow curves showed a change of the same type as in the rabbit aorta but much smaller in degree. For example, the backflow was diminished but remained present. As the superior mesenteric artery flow forms a much smaller proportion of the upstream run-off with reference to the femoral, this difference in degree is to be expected. A more marked change in flow pattern was caused by occluding, and subsequently releasing, the contralateral common iliac artery. In relation to one femoral artery the other iliac-femoral blood flow is an upstream run-off. This emphasizes the general principle that the arterial tree is a branching network of parallel channels and increasing the impedance in one vascular bed will, under steady conditions of cardiac output, cause a shift of flow into other parallel channels. The alterations in mean flow may be relatively slight but the changes in the form of the flow curve may be considerable. As noted in the discussion on the design of meters (Ch. 6) this is a factor which must be borne in mind in the use of meter with an appreciable fluid impedance.

The experiments reported briefly here are, as it were, only a pilot investigation. The hydrodynamic problems concerned with the distribution of pulsatile flow in a branched network are among the most difficult to treat theoretically. We could obtain much useful data from a careful study of flow patterns in the aorta and one or more branches simultaneously together with the associated changes in the pressure-wave. In these experiments only flow has been studied because of the technical difficulties of the flow recording method used. Alexander (1953) and later Ryan, Stacy and Watman (1956) have made valuable observations on the changes in the form of the pressure pulses due to occlusion of visceral arterial branches. A combination of both approaches is needed and should be feasible with flowmeters, such as that of Denison *et al.* (1955) now available.

CHANGES IN FLOW PATTERN DUE TO EXTRA-VASCULAR FACTORS

The *coronary arteries* represent the clearest example of the way in which flow is modified by the movement of the tissues, in this case the contraction of the ventricular muscle. The phasic flow pattern was recorded by Gregg and Green (1939) with the orifice meter. There are several striking differences compared with the other peripheral arteries that have been described above. The maximum flow velocity occurs in diastole and the major part of the volume flow into the cardiac muscle occurs during the period of diastole. This is to be expected as a result of compression of the small vessels within the contracting muscle. There is, however, an appreciable flow during systole with a peak velocity of similar amplitude to that in diastole. A feature not seen in other vessels is a sharp reduction of flow in the left coronary artery, usually forming a backflow, during the isometric phase of contraction in early systole. A second minimum of flow occurs at the end of systole. The backflow during isometric contraction is attributed to the intramuscular tension which is then at a maximum. This minimum of flow is much less marked in the right coronary artery. The difference in pattern is due to the lower intramural pressure developed in the right ventricular muscle. A similar investigation has been recently reported by Laszt and Müller (1957). They used the "bristle" flowmeter designed by Müller (1954b) and described in Ch. 6. The flow patterns recorded are similar to those of Gregg and his colleagues (Gregg, 1950). Small differences are shown in that Laszt and Müller did not record any backflow in early systole and the systolic maximum flow velocity is very much lower than the diastolic maximum. The general agreement between the records made with two completely different types of flowmeters is reassuring in view of the discrepancies between the responses of various meters that were discussed in Ch. 6.

Changes in flow pattern in arteries supplying skeletal muscles when they contract will also undoubtedly be seen but have not yet been investigated. The studies on coronary artery flow are only mentioned briefly here because they are outstanding examples of the valuable information to be gained by accurate recording of phasic flow patterns. The physical complexities introduced into the hydrodynamic study of arterial flow by the contracting muscle are better left until the solution of simpler systems is thoroughly understood.

CONCLUSIONS

The evidence at present available on the shape of the flow pulse is insufficient to make any firm generalization. It appears quite clear, however, that the total excursion of flow during the cardiac cycle diminishes progressively as we make observations further away from the heart. This is illustrated in a qualitative way in Fig. 7.11 which is derived from the figures in this chapter and those of Spencer *et al.* (1958). This marked diminution of the size of the flow pulse makes an interesting contrast to the increase in size of the pressure pulse as it travels from the heart to the small arteries (Ch. 12). The inference is that the reduction in flow pulsation is not solely, or even mainly, due to damping but is due to the greater impedance in the small vessels of the periphery. This is discussed in greater detail in Ch. 10.

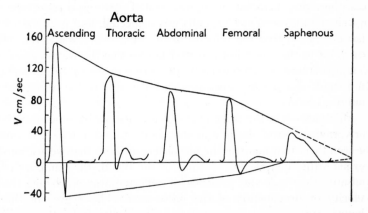

FIG. 7.11. A diagrammatic display of the change in form in the pulsatile flow pattern recorded in arteries of the dog from the heart towards the periphery. These curves are based on Figs. 7.1–4 but that for the abdominal aorta has been derived from Spencer *et al.* (1958) recording with an electromagnetic flowmeter in the dog.

It is apparent that there is a progressive decrease in the total amplitude of oscillation as far as the saphenous artery; the broken lines beyond suggest the decrease that probably occurs in the smallest arteries until all oscillatory flow is damped out in the arterioles. The mean velocity also falls progressively. With a relatively low mean value in vessels such as the abdominal aorta or femoral, where the oscillatory terms are still large, a backflow phase appears. It disappears again with progressive damping in the saphenous artery (the very brief backflow in the ascending aorta is probably due to reflux of blood through the aortic valves).

B.F.A.—L

CHAPTER VIII

THE PHYSICAL PROPERTIES OF THE ARTERIAL WALL

In the consideration of the pressure-flow relationships of pulsatile flow in arteries (Ch. 5) the vessel was treated as a simple tube of unvarying diameter. This neglects the fact that an artery is an elastic tube and a pulsating flow will cause it to vary in size. Another property of an elastic tube is that it will propagate a wave, in this case created by the ejection of blood from the heart, at a certain velocity which is largely determined by the elastic properties of the wall. In considering the relation of the pressure-gradient to the form of the pulse-wave it was shown that this involved the velocity of travel of the wave. The model of the artery was, therefore, inconsistent. It was treated partly as a rigid tube, in that the movement of its walls was neglected, and partly as an elastic tube, in that the velocity of the pulse-wave was given its real value in the body. For it is well known that the wave velocity in a pipe is largely determined by the elastic properties of its wall. In a rigid tube the pressure-wave would travel at the velocity of sound in blood.

Full analyses of the behaviour of pulsatile flow have been made for various types of elastic wall and are described in Ch. 9. It will be seen there that many of the physical conditions that we are concerned with such as the viscosity of the blood, the damping of pulsatile flow and the presence of reflected waves, change the velocity of propagation of the pulse-wave. The degree of this change can only be measured experimentally if the "natural" velocity, that is the wave velocity in the arteries being studied due to the properties of the wall alone, is known. To study the hydrodynamics of the arterial system a knowledge of the elastic constants of the arterial wall, from which one can predict this "natural" wave velocity, is of fundamental importance. The evidence that is selected for review is, therefore, biased by this consideration. The literature reporting various aspects of the elastic properties of arteries is large, but in few fields of physiology has so much research been done that is valueless to other workers because in-

146

sufficient data have been recorded. For this reason it is necessary first to consider briefly the physical definitions on which studies of elasticity should be based to allow quantitative comparisons to be made.

THE PHYSICAL CONSTANTS OF AN ELASTIC BODY

No solid body is completely rigid. When forces act on it without displacing it they will deform it, that is, cause a movement of the various parts of the body relative to one another. When the force is removed, if the body regains its original form exactly it is said to be *perfectly elastic*. If the body retains the deformation then it is said to be *plastic*. The fundamental description of elasticity is not, therefore, concerned with the amount of deformation caused by a given force in contrast to the non-technical use of the term which usually implies that a very elastic substance is one, like rubber, that is easily altered in shape. This confusion has been emphasized by Burton (1954) in his stimulating review of the elastic properties of the arterial wall where he suggests that "extensible" and "extensibility" better describe the popular use of "elastic" and "elasticity".

No substance is perfectly elastic when very large forces are applied but for smaller forces it is found that the deformation is proportional to the magnitude of the force applied. This proportionality is known as Hooke's law for it was first described by him in the famous phrase *Ut tensio sic vis*. The point at which Hooke's law ceases to apply is known as *the elastic limit* and when the solid has been deformed beyond this point it cannot regain its original form and has acquired a *permanent set*. With larger loads still the *yield point* is reached when the deformation continues to increase without further load and usually leads rapidly to breakage.

The deformation produced in an elastic body is called the *strain* and the force causing it is the *stress*. In the general case we also assume that the body has the same elastic properties independent of the direction of any stresses, that is it is *isotropic*. The types of strain that are distinguished are (1) longitudinal, caused by the longitudinal component of a tensile stress, (2) compression, or distension, that is a change in volume and (3) shear, or angular deformation. The relation of stress to strain of each of these is defined by a modulus of elasticity and the relations between the three moduli describe the elastic properties of the body.

The deformation most commonly considered is that of a longitudinal strain due to a longitudinal tensile stress (i.e. the amount it stretches as a result of pulling). The modulus that describes this is Young's modulus (usually designated by E or Y). By definition

$$E = \frac{\text{Applied load per unit area of cross-section}}{\text{Increase of length per unit length}}$$

If F is the load, A the cross-section, L the initial length and ΔL the extension then

$$E = \frac{F/A}{\Delta L/L} = \frac{F.L}{\Delta L.A} \quad \ldots\ldots\ldots\ldots\ldots\ldots 8.1$$

and its dimensions are of a force per unit area (e.g. dynes/cm^2) per 100 per cent elongation. When applied to biological materials the term modulus may give a spurious air of scientific precision because they are not homogeneous. Only some components of the tissue are elastic in behaviour and yet, as has been shown with collagen, their "elastic" properties are greatly modified by the other components of the tissue. If, however, it is accepted that by using the term modulus we qualify it as "effective modulus" we can describe the stress-strain behaviour of a tissue like the arterial wall in a quantitative way that allows comparison between vessels irrespective of their dimensions. An agreed basis for comparisons of this sort is urgently needed and I am here following Burton (1954) in adopting this familiar physical term even though it cannot be rigorously applied. One alternative is to describe the elastic properties of these materials by their *stiffness*. This is more acceptable to some workers for inhomogeneous materials but is not, I think, so generally familiar and its technical use is easily confused with the common non-technical use of the word.

Other terms have become familiar, especially in respiratory physiology. Thus the ratio of volume increase in the lung to an increase in intratracheal pressure is spoken of as the *compliance* and its reciprocal as the *elastance* (Bayliss and Robertson, 1939). In a system of such complex geometry as the lung it is clearly impossible to reduce these ratios accurately to the dimensions of stress and strain. It does not seem, however, that it is always appreciated that a pressure-volume curve of this sort will be non-linear quite apart from deviations from linearity due to the properties of the tissues involved. In arteries which have a simple geometric form there seems to be no reason for using these terms.

When a body is stretched it also gets thinner; that is, the production of a longitudinal extension produces a lateral contraction. The ratio of the lateral strain (decrease in width per unit width) to the longitudinal strain (increase in length per unit length) is called the *Poisson's ratio*, σ. This ratio is an important characteristic of an elastic substance. It is clearly connected with any volume change that may result from the stretching. If the ratio is 0·5 the total volume of the elastic body remains the same when it is stretched. If the value of the Poisson's ratio is less than 0·5 the total volume will increase on stretching, this volume increase obviously being maximal when $\sigma = 0$ for then the volume will increase proportionally to the increase in length. The Poisson's ratio thus has the possible range of values 0 to 0·5 (a value greater than 0·5 would necessitate a *diminution* in volume on stretching). The usual value for india-rubber is $\sigma = 0\cdot48$ (Newman and Searle) while for most metals it lies between 0·25 and 0·4. The measurement of this constant for biological materials is difficult but Hardung (1952) states that it is very close to 0·5 for the wall of the thoracic aorta and Lawton (1954) has shown that the same tissue extends almost isovolumetrically which as seen above indicates that $\sigma \doteqdot 0\cdot5$.

The other two moduli of elasticity are not often considered in physiological investigations. The "bulk modulus" (k) defines the "compressibility" (the ratio of change in volume to a compressing, or distending, force). The "modulus of rigidity" or "shear modulus" (n) describes the ratio of a tangential force to the angular deformation. The shear modulus should be considered when bending stresses are applied to materials under test. In experiments on arterial loops, for example, loading with small weights is putting both a tensile stress on the vertically disposed parts of the artery and a shearing stress at the regions near the points of support.

These four elastic constants are interrelated in such a way that from the values of two of them the others may be deduced.

For example $$E = 2n(1+\sigma) \dotfill 8.2$$

so that if $$\sigma = 0\cdot5$$
$$E = 3n$$

This gives the same relationship as that quoted by Burton (1954) from

$$E = \frac{9nk}{(3k+n)} \dotfill 8.3$$

where Burton points out that if k is very large compared with n, as he says it is in tissues, then
$$E \doteq 3n$$

which is the same result as assuming the Poisson's ratio to have a value close to 0·5. I do not know of any direct measurement of the bulk modulus of tissues. I assume that Burton's assertion is based on the fact that as tissues have a high water content then their bulk modulus, or compressibility, will be of the same order as that of water which is about 2×10^{10} dynes/sq. cm (Newman and Searle). Taking Burton's value of $E=1 \times 10^9$ dynes/sq. cm for collagen this gives it a Poisson's ratio of 0·48 and for elastin (even taking the high figure of $E=2 \times 10^7$) a value of at least 0·4998. The previous evidence that σ is close to 0·5 suggests that this assumed bulk modulus for the elastic tissues is of the right order of magnitude.

As we have seen it is necessary, even if we treat an artery as a simple elastic structure, to know at least two of its physical constants. The Young's modulus is the most easy to measure directly and is the only one for which we have much data. The Poisson's ratio has, in effect, been measured by Lawton (1954) so that these two constants (E, σ) will be used as the most direct description of the ideal elastic properties of the arterial wall in the analyses discussed in Ch. 9. The deviations from ideal behaviour will be considered below after describing the behaviour of elastic material when it forms a cylindrical tube like an artery.

THE PROPERTIES OF AN ELASTIC TUBE

Within its elastic limits the increase in length of an elastic substance is proportional to the tension applied to it. In the case of a tube this tension is the circumferential tension, which cannot be measured directly. When an internal pressure is applied to a closed tube its volume will increase due to lengthening and distension. The distension creates the circumferential, or tangential, tension.

This tension is simply related to the pressure by Laplace's law for a cylinder
$$T=P.R \quad \dots\dots\dots\dots\dots\dots\dots\dots \text{8.4}$$

where T is the tension in dynes/cm, P the internal pressure in dynes/cm² and R the radius. As R increases with P it can be seen that the tension does not increase linearly with P. Therefore even if the wall of the tube is perfectly elastic the relation between the pressure and the increase in circumference will not form a straight line. Thus if the increase in circumference or the volume of the tube is plotted against the internal pressure deviations from Hooke's law cannot easily be seen. The resultant curves need to be compared with those which would be followed if the Young's modulus remained constant throughout the range of distension. As it is a common practice to plot the elastic behaviour of an artery by means of a volume-pressure curve this should be emphasized. Burton (1951, 1954) has already made this point with much force and it is to be hoped that his advice will be taken by future workers in this field so that unnecessary confusion may be avoided. As some interesting points arise from his more detailed analysis of this relation it is repeated here with some modifications.

As $T = Pr$

a small increase in P, δP will cause an increase in tension δT so that

$$\delta T = r\,\delta P + P\,\delta r \quad \dots \dots \dots \dots \dots \quad 8.5$$

from the definition of Young's modulus (eqn. 8.1) we also have

$$\delta T = E.A.\frac{2\pi\,\delta r}{2\pi r} \quad \dots \dots \dots \dots \dots \quad 8.6$$

assuming that we are distending a length l which is held constant then $A = hl$ where h is the wall-thickness, and equating 8.5 and 8.6 we have

$$r\,\delta P + P\,\delta r = E.h.l.\frac{\delta r}{r} \quad \dots \dots \dots \dots \quad 8.7$$

so that at the limiting value

$$\frac{dr}{dP} = r \Big/ \left(\frac{E.h.l}{r} - P\right) \quad \dots \dots \dots \dots \quad 8.8$$

In terms of volume we have

$$\frac{dV}{dP} = \frac{dV}{dr}\cdot\frac{dr}{dP} = 2\pi r.\frac{dr}{dP} \quad \dots \dots \dots \dots \quad 8.9$$

so that

$$\frac{dV}{dP} = 1 \Big/ 2\pi\left(\frac{E.h.l}{r} - P\right) \quad \dots \dots \dots \dots \quad 8.10$$

From this it is clear that if the modulus of elasticity remains constant the rate of increase in volume with pressure will increase until at the point when

$$P = \frac{E.h.l}{r} \quad \dots \dots \dots \dots \dots \quad 8.11$$

it will become infinite, and, as pointed out by Burton, this represents the "blow-out" point of an elastic tube. If the elastic modulus, however, also increases as the tension increases, as is the case with an artery, the tube can remain stable over a wide range of pressures.

The shape of the curve is a complicated one because h/r is also a function of the pressure, and decreases with increase of pressure because r increases and h decreases *i.e.* the wall gets thinner. Furthermore the assumption that the length l does not change is unjustifiable in an isolated arterial segment (see p. 159) unless special precautions are taken.

To set out results that can be easily interpreted in terms of the elastic behaviour of an artery that is being distended, it is clear that tension should be plotted against length (i.e. circumference) that is, as a stress-strain diagram. Direct comparison can then be made between the results obtained by distending an artery and by loading strips with weights and measuring the elongation. If the relationship is a straight line it is following Hooke's law and the Young's modulus is constant and is represented by the slope of the line. A curve which is concave towards the tension axis indicates an increase of Young's modulus with increase of tension. This form of curve is characteristic of arteries as illustrated by the thoracic aorta in Fig 8.1. The reasons for this non-linear elastic behaviour remain to be discussed.

DYNAMIC BEHAVIOUR OF ELASTIC MATERIALS

The properties of a "perfect" elastic body take no account of the rate at which the stress is applied. In many materials, and this includes all living tissues, the time factor is important. With such a substance it is found that if it is rapidly extended the tension also increases rapidly, but while the material is held at the new length the increase in tension gradually falls to a steady value. This phenomenon is known as *stress relaxation*. Similarly if a load is applied to the material it will increase in length immediately and then slowly continue extending until it reaches an equilibrium state. This is known as *creep*. Clearly the two phenomena are fundamentally of the same nature and only differ according to the way they are defined. Creep and stress relaxation are described as *visco-elastic* behaviour. This implies that the stress-strain relations of the body are determined by some components that are elastic in the sense defined in the preceding sections but that other components are behaving as if they were flowing like a viscous fluid.

The resultant behaviour will differ according to the arrangement of these components which may be in series, or in parallel or a combination of both. This is lucidly set out in the textbook of Stacy, Williams, Warden and McMorris (1955).

Arterial wall has visco-elastic properties. One aspect that has received considerable attention is the form of tension-length curve that results from first stretching a segment of artery and then allowing it to relax. Owing to the creep these curves form a hysteresis loop. The size of the loop depends on the rate at which the specimen is stretched and relaxed. This has been studied in detail by Remington (1955). The same properties can be described more quantitatively by subjecting the arterial wall to an oscillatory stress and determining the *dynamic modulus* of elasticity. The viscous properties of the wall will then cause a phase lag between force and extension, and if a loop is recorded, will determine its width. The clearest quantitative way of expressing this visco-elastic behaviour appears to be that used by Hardung (1952a, 1953), who expressed the dynamic elastic modulus (E') in complex form so that

$$E' = E_{dyn} + i\eta\omega \quad \dots\dots\dots\dots\dots \quad 8.12$$

where

$$E_{dyn} = \frac{\Delta P}{\Delta l} \cdot \frac{lm}{qm} \cdot \cos\phi \quad \dots\dots\dots\dots \quad 8.13$$

$$\eta\omega = \frac{\Delta P}{\Delta l} \cdot \frac{lm}{qm} \cdot \sin\phi \quad \dots\dots\dots\dots \quad 8.14$$

ΔP and Δl are the amplitudes of stress and strain respectively; lm and qm are the average values of the length and cross-section of the specimen; ϕ is the phase difference between force and extension; η is the coefficient of viscosity of the viscous element in the wall and ω is the circular frequency ($2\pi f$) as in Ch. 5. Hardung measured the stress-strain behaviour of strips of rubber, synthetic polymers and the wall of the thoracic aorta. As discussed below the use of strips, although convenient, is open to objection. A similar investigation has been undertaken in our own laboratory by Bergel (1958) in which an isolated segment of artery is subjected to an oscillatory internal pressure. The segment is first pulled out to its *in vivo* length and kept at that length; the diameter of the specimen is then measured photoelectrically. From the pressure and diameter the tangential tension (stress) and elongation of the circumference (strain) can easily be calculated.

In a simple visco-elastic material it is to be expected that the term E_{dyn}, which represents the elastic element, would be constant in spite of changes in frequency but that the term $\eta\omega$, representing the viscous element, would rise linearly with frequency. In this case the increase in this second term would be the cause of increasing "stiffness" with frequency for the dynamic elastic modulus is the mathematical modulus of the complex term E', i.e. $\sqrt{E_{dyn}^2 + \eta\omega^2}$. (It is unfortunate, but unavoidable without new nomenclature, that the word "modulus" has to be used in these two different senses in "elastic modulus" and in "the modulus of a complex number" as in Appendix 1.)

Hardung (1953) finds results of this kind in strips of thoracic aorta except that the constant value of E_{dyn} is always higher than the value of the static modulus—a rise that occurs at very low frequencies. Also the term $\eta\omega$ is very small compared with E_{dyn} over the range of frequencies, say 0–20 c/sec, which are of most physiological interest. The dynamic modulus is thus largely determined by the term E_{dyn}. The preliminary results of Bergel using a complete segment of artery are rather different and, if confirmed, show that the simple visco-elastic model is inadequate to describe the properties of the wall. These are illustrated in Fig. 8.4 and discussed more fully on p. 171. Briefly they show that E_{dyn} not only rises sharply at very low frequencies (as in Hardung's results) but thereafter remains fairly constant with increasing frequency. The value of $\eta\omega$ rises slightly but also shows a sharp initial rise at low frequencies.

These visco-elastic properties of the arterial wall, although not as simple as we would wish, are similar to those of rubber and most synthetic polymers. These latter are classed as *elastomers*. The terms *elastomeric* and *visco-elastic* tend to be used interchangeably but this is somewhat imprecise. It appears certain that elastomeric substances all have visco-elastic properties but the converse is not necessarily true and tissues showing visco-elastic properties are not necessarily elastomers. The analysis based on eqn. 8.12 is, however, easier to handle than the equations of elastomer behaviour developed by King and discussed in the next paragraph, and are probably adequate as a working description of the arterial wall.

Elastomers are defined (Stacy *et al.*, 1955) by the properties they have in common. (1) They have a low Young's modulus, of the order of 10^7 dynes/cm^2 compared with most solids which have moduli of the order of 10^{11} dynes/cm^2. (2) They can be stretched to comparatively great lengths before the breaking point is reached. (3) The stress-strain curve is usually S-shaped. King has suggested that elastomeric theory can be applied widely to the behaviour of living tissues and has explored its possibilities in a series of papers (King 1947*a*, 1950, King and Lawton 1950). A review of his analysis also appears in Stacy *et al.* (1955). The mathematics, unfortunately, becomes complicated and will not be reproduced here. Lawton has used it to describe the behaviour of strips of arterial wall and King (1947*a*) has deduced an equation for describing the pulse-wave velocity in an elastomeric tube and calculated examples for application to arteries. This, however, is difficult to compute in the form that he gives it and it is to be hoped that a simpler approximation may be derived. Morgan and Kiely (1954) have attempted to do this and a similar approach has been used by Womersley (1958*a*).

THE VELOCITY OF WAVE PROPAGATION IN AN ELASTIC TUBE

As we know, the elastic behaviour of the wall of a tube plays an important part in determining the velocity of propagation of a pressure-wave. The study of this problem is closely related to the physics of sound and was first studied by Newton. Its application to the physiology of the arterial pulse was first due to Thomas Young (1808, 1809) and later E. H. Weber (1850), and is the subject of a stimulating historical review by Lambossy (1950).

The simplest equation for the velocity of propagation of a pressure pulse is that due to Moens (1878) who from experimental evidence established the formula

$$c = K\sqrt{\frac{E.h}{2R\rho}} \quad \dotsb \quad 8.15$$

where c is the wave velocity, E and h are the Young's modulus and thickness of the arterial wall, ρ the density of the fluid and R the mean radius. K was an arbitrary constant which Moens set at 0·9. The same formula was derived theoretically for a tube of perfectly elastic material at about the same time, and apparently independently, by Korteweg and Resal without the constant K so that it is usual for the formula to be written

$$c = \sqrt{\frac{E.h}{2R\rho}} \quad \dotsb \quad 8.16$$

The equation is only true for a thin-walled vessel, i.e. with h small compared with R. It assumes that the fluid within is incompressible, i.e. that its bulk modulus is high compared with E, and that it has no viscosity. The first two assumptions are reasonable approximations for blood in an artery for the value of $h/2R$ is less than 0·1 (see p. 161 below) and the bulk modulus of water is from 10^3 to 10^4 times greater than the Young's modulus of the arterial wall. The solution of the wave propagation with a viscous fluid has only recently been analysed and is discussed more fully in the next chapter. The effect is great in small tubes and at low frequencies, but in tubes comparable with the larger arteries has the effect of reducing the predicted velocity by 5–10 per cent. This is equivalent to setting Moens' constant K at 0·9–0·95, and the viscous effect is probably the reason he found it necessary to introduce this constant. In the mathematical treatment of elastic tube the wave velocity (c) as expressed in eqn. 8.16 is frequently used to describe the elastic properties of the tube. Where it is necessary to distinguish this from the modified wave velocity the term c_0 will be used.

To eliminate the experimental difficulties of measuring the wall-thickness and the Young's modulus the equation (8.13) was modified by Hill (Bramwell and Hill, 1922) so that the elastic behaviour of the tube was expressed in terms of its pressure-volume distensibility.

The formula can then be reduced to

$$c = \sqrt{\frac{V}{\rho.\,\delta v/\delta P}} = \sqrt{\frac{V.\,\delta P}{\rho.\,\delta v}} \quad \dots\dots\dots\dots \text{8.17}$$

then substituting $\rho = 1\cdot055$ and converting P from dynes/cm² to mm Hg this becomes

$$c = 0\cdot357\sqrt{\frac{V.\,\delta P}{\delta v}} \quad \dots\dots\dots\dots \text{8.18}$$

which is the form familiar in most textbooks.

It should be noted that it is essential to know the initial volume V, as well as the increments of volume with pressure to make any estimate of the elastic behaviour of a tube. Failure to record the actual volumes rather than the proportional change in volume alone robs a great number of published observations of their value, as was pointed out long ago by Clark (1933). In this derivation the increase in volume also is assumed to involve no change in length. The volume increment due to elongation in excised arterial specimens is often considerable and either it should be allowed for in the calculation from experimental results, or the length must be held constant, and this should be at the natural length of the specimen in the body. As pressure-volume curves are liable to error through leaks from the arterial specimen it is preferable to work in terms of tension and radius. Increases in radius can be measured directly, or derived from the increase in distances between markers on the wall. Tension is calculated from the relation $T = PR$ and eqn. 8.17 then becomes

$$c = \sqrt{\frac{R \cdot \delta T}{2\rho \cdot \delta R}} \quad \dots\dots\dots\dots\dots \quad 8.19$$

From eqn. 8.16 we can see that the velocity of wave propagation will increase when the elastic modulus of the wall increases and as seen from Fig. 8.1 this occurs as the distension increases. This results in the finding that the velocity of the pulse-wave depends on the mean arterial pressure.

From the results of Hardung (1953) and Bergel (1958) discussed above we saw that the dynamic modulus increases with the frequency of oscillation of the wave, so that it is to be expected that the wave velocity will increase as a function of the frequency.

EXPERIMENTAL INVESTIGATIONS

The comparison of the isolated specimen and its behaviour in the body

For technical reasons it is much easier to measure stress-strain relationships in an excised artery than it is to measure them in the living animal, and nearly all the data we possess have been obtained in this way. It is, therefore, necessary to consider briefly the validity of these observations. From general principles the most obvious reason for doubting their value is a post-mortem change commonly seen in biological tissues. Attention has been paid to this point but there is no evidence that the physical properties of collagen and elastin alter with the cessation of the blood supply. This is not surprising in view of the fact that chemically they are two of the most stable proteins known. Any changes that may occur in elastic properties in the isolated segment of artery will be due to loss of viability of smooth muscle. As previous work is virtually confined to the study of large arteries, which have very little smooth muscle, it is reasonable to neglect this factor. Nevertheless it is clearly desirable to maintain the arterial segments so that the muscle remains viable. Furthermore with a little ingenuity it is possible to measure elastic properties *in situ*, as Alexander (1954) has done, by recording pressure-volume changes in thoracic aorta segments, and so avoid any possible artifacts.

The important misconceptions that may arise from the study of isolated segments are mainly due, in my opinion, to the alteration of dimensions that result from removing an artery from the body.

(*a*) *The length of an arterial segment.* Arteries in the body are naturally under a condition of longitudinal tension. This is demonstrated by the familiar experience that if any artery is severed the vessel retracts. What does not appear to have been generally noted, however, is that dissection of a severed artery will allow it to retract much farther. In a series of my own observations on the dog femoral artery it was noted that a marked 5 cm length of artery retracted some 3–5 mm when it was severed at both ends. When it was removed from the body its excised length was only 3·0–3·4 cm (i.e. a total retraction of 16–20 mm). This occurs to the same order of magnitude in all arteries and indicates that the connective tissue exercises a *tethering* effect in the longitudinal direction. The fact that they are tethered in extension, as it were, may seem odd until we remember that these measurements are necessarily made with no internal distending pressure. When inflated, arteries show an increase in length as well as a radial distension; by the time that normal mean arterial pressures is reached the length of an isolated segment more closely approximates to its natural length. In my experience, however, it rarely, if ever, fully elongates to its length in the body which suggests that a certain proportion of the natural longitudinal tension is due to other causes, possibly different rates of growth.

This simple fact indicates that, as arterial wall is a complex structure, any measurements of elastic properties that are to have application to their behaviour in the body should be made with the isolated segment extended to its natural length. In measuring the relation of radial expansion to internal pressure this suggests that the arterial segment should be pulled out, and held, at the physiological length. This has the further advantage in that under these conditions changes in volume (where pressure-volume curves are recorded) are entirely due to changes in circumference, which is the assumption usually made but commonly left uncontrolled.

A considerable proportion of studies of arterial elasticity have been made on longitudinal strips of arterial wall. This provides a specimen which is technically easy to handle as tension can be applied by direct loading with weights or measured with a strain-gauge at different degrees of extension. The information this gives as to the behaviour of the artery in response to longitudinal stresses in the body can only be limited because the initial length, as we saw above, of an excised artery is usually only 60 per cent of its natural length (thoracic aorta specimens may be as little as 50 per cent). Furthermore I have never seen a report of this type of experiment that has recorded the natural length, although Remington and Hamilton (1945) refer to it in relation to experiments on rings of arterial wall. The elastic properties of the artery in the longitudinal direction at low extensions, therefore, represents conditions that are never found in the body. In one of the most thorough investigations of this nature Lawton (1955) recorded the Young's modulus of thoracic aorta strips up to extensions 80 per cent longer than the excised length; in my experience the natural length of thoracic aorta is 70–100 per cent longer than the excised length, so that the behaviour of Lawton's strips at their greatest extensions probably represents their physiological conditions.

The use of this type of record to describe the elastic properties of the arterial wall in general assumes that it behaves as a homogeneous material so that the stress-strain relation is independent of the direction in which it is stretched. This is sometimes termed *isotropic* behaviour. This assumption has never been explicitly defended in relation to the measurement of the longitudinal modulus. Indeed the observation, mentioned above, that when an internal pressure is applied to an excised segment (blocked at both ends) it lengthens, as well as distending, has been emphasized by Fenn (1957) as a reason for assuming that the longitudinal modulus of such a specimen is lower than its tangential modulus. An isotropic cylinder of an elastic material with Poisson's ratio of 0·5 should remain at a constant length under these conditions. If the wall is isotropic then Fenn calculated that the Poisson's ratio is about 0·3 in his specimens. This is extremely unlikely and the evidence that it is in fact close to 0·5 has already been discussed (p. 150 above) and is further discussed by Fenn (1957). In a retracted excised segment there is, therefore, little doubt that the artery is *anisotropic* and that the modulus in a longitudinal direction is less than that in a tangential direction. Lawton (1956— personal communication) has made some observations, discussed below, which lead him to believe that one can regard the thoracic aorta, at least, to be virtually isotropic.

At, or slightly above, their natural (*in vivo*) length it can be seen (Fig. 8.2) that many arteries show a sharp increase in their longitudinal elastic modulus. Coupled with the tethering effect discussed above, which provides an external constraint, this means that functionally the artery is much less extensible in the longitudinal direction than it is circumferentially. Thus it may be described as markedly anisotropic *in situ*, but now with a much higher modulus in the longitudinal direction. The effect this has on its physiological behaviour, especially in relation to the pulse-wave velocity is discussed in Ch. 9. The indirect evidence presented there supports the simple observations above that the main arteries in the body behave as if they were almost rigid in the longitudinal direction. It is fortunate that the physical behaviour of waves in such a system is simpler mathematically than those in a free elastic tube. These findings do, however, emphasize how important it is to control precisely the conditions under which isolated segments are studied.

(*b*) *The thickness of the arterial wall.* From eqn. 8.16 we saw that the relative thickness, the ratio of wall to the diameter $(h/2R)$, is a determinant of the wave velocity. It is also necessary to measure the thickness to calculate the Young's modulus of the wall. Our usual ideas on the thickness of the arterial wall derive from the appearance of histological sections. It is usually appreciated that with the distension provided by the blood-pressure the wall of the living artery will be thinner than this. The shortening that takes place in the excised artery actually causes a larger difference between the apparent thickness and that in the living artery than does the radial distension. Tables based on histological sections such as that recently published by Noordergraaf and Horeman (1958) should be regarded with caution.

The real thickness of the arterial wall under physiological conditions may easily be measured by making use of the fact that it stretches isovolumetrically, i.e. that the Poisson's ratio is close to 0·5 (p. 149). The mean external diameter is measured *in situ* and a measured length is excised and weighed. Its density is also measured. In my experiments the density of arterial wall was close to 1·06. The volume (V) of the wall of the specimen is thus known from the weight (W) and the density(Δ). From this the wall-thickness in its extended state may be calculated easily for

$$V=\frac{W}{\Delta}=L \cdot \pi(R^2-r^2) \ldots\ldots\ldots\ldots 8.20$$

and as W, Δ, L and R are known, the wall-thickness $(R-r)$ may be derived.

In a series of 8 dogs I have found that the value of the ratio $h/2R$ remains remarkably constant in all arteries studied from the ascending aorta to the saphenous artery. The mean value for this ratio is 0·08. This obviously varies with the arterial pressure and it is technically difficult to measure the dimensions of a large number of arteries at identical mean pressures in the same animal owing to the extensive surgical dissection required. This value for the wall-thickness ratio of arteries is close to that determined by Hürthle (1920) and by Kani (1910). Bergel (personal communication) finds rather lower values, with $h/2R$ about 0·05–0·06 (dog—thoracic and abdominal aorta; carotid and femoral arteries).

The relative constancy of this ratio is contrary to the general conception, based on histological evidence, that arteries get relatively thicker walls as they pass to the periphery. It might be anticipated, however, from their physical properties. The mean pressure is approximately the same throughout the arterial tree. The wall tension, which is the product of pressure and radius in a cylinder (eqn. 8.4), will therefore decrease linearly with the radius. As the elastic properties of the wall are similar throughout the arterial tree it is to be expected that to maintain the wall tension arteries will only require a wall that also decreases linearly with the radius (this was pointed out by D'Arcy Thompson in *Growth and form*, 1942). This will cease to apply, of course, when the vessel acquires other tissues, such as the smooth muscle coats of arterioles, with functions other than maintaining the tension in the wall.

The composition of the arterial wall

For a full interpretation of the elastic behaviour of the arterial wall it is necessary to know what proportion consists of elastic material and how that material is arranged. The elastic materials to be considered are collagen, elastin and smooth muscle. Most estimates of their distribution have been made by histological techniques using differential staining. These have little more than qualitative value. Recently chemical methods have become available that enable collagen and elastin to be estimated. The collagen content may be measured very accurately; the technique for elastin has a more uncertain chemical basis but is reasonably accurate. Harkness, Harkness and McDonald (1957) have used these methods to survey the proportions of collagen and elastin to be found in various parts of the arterial tree of the dog. In brief, their results show that about 50 per cent of the wall is made up of collagen and elastin, the remainder presumably being non-fibrous connective matrix and the relatively small amount of muscle. This fraction was based on the dried weight, the water content being 70 per cent, but there is no evidence that collagen and elastin fibres contain less water than the other components. In the thoracic aorta the elastin constituted some 60 per cent of the total fibrous material (elastin and collagen) and hence about 30 per cent of the wall. This ratio changed rapidly over short transition zones in the 5 cm above the diaphragm and in the proximal parts of the large branches leaving the arch of the aorta. In all other systemic arteries outside the thorax the proportion of elastin formed only 30 per cent of the total elastin plus collagen. This remained the same down to the smallest arteries they were able to study, such as the saphenous and internal mammary arteries. This evidence thus conflicts with the traditional histological classification of "elastic" arteries which is usually regarded as including all the major arteries, whereas it can be seen that the thoracic aorta is unique, in that it alone contains more elastin than collagen. Furthermore the extra-thoracic arteries show no gradation of composition. The biological causes of such a distribution are obscure. The large pulsations in vessels close to the heart does not appear to be the cause for it because the pulmonary arteries have a collagen-elastin ratio similar to the peripheral arteries. The low intrathoracic pressure appears to have no relation to it for the characteristic distribution is present at birth.

It is interesting to note that the thoracic aorta, if we accept the value of 30 per cent elastin, has approximately the same proportion of elastin as ligamentum nuchae which is the standard tissue of reference for a tissue of pure elastin. The ligament however has only about 9 per cent collagen as compared with 20 per cent in the thoracic aorta.

The structural distribution of the collagen and elastin has been the subject of much histological description. The collagen fibres are probably arranged in a symmetrical helical pattern so that a reticulated arrangement results. This was demonstrated very elegantly by Franklin (1937) in the walls of veins, and the arterial wall is likely to be similar in this respect. The elastin probably forms a more irregularly arranged network and the elastic laminae have been described as a sort of perforated membrane (Ham, 1950).

Muscle fibres are present even in the thoracic aorta in considerable numbers. In the larger arteries, in which nearly all studies of elasticity have been made, there does not appear to be any sort of muscular continuum but each fibre is separate.

THE ANOMALOUS ELASTIC BEHAVIOUR OF THE ARTERIAL WALL

All investigators of the elastic behaviour of the arterial wall have agreed that it deviates markedly from Hooke's law if studied over a considerable range of extension (Fig. 8.1). The most commonly described form of the elastic diagram is a sigmoid curve. At the smallest extensions the effective modulus is relatively high, but falls as the extension increases. The curve may then approximate to linearity for some distance, but as the extension increases the modulus begins to rise fairly rapidly. Fig. 8.2 (modified from Wezler and Sinn, 1953) shows a typical curve of this kind. The region of relatively increased stiffness at the beginning of the curve is not agreed by all workers, some of whom such as McWilliam and Mackie (1908) have stated that it is an artifact in excised arteries in which postmortem contraction of the arterial muscle has been allowed to occur. In considering the behaviour of arteries under physiological conditions it seems clear that the extensions at which this phenomena occurs are too small to be of importance in their functional behaviour, so that it is not proposed to review the evidence on this point. The remainder of the curve in which the effective modulus increases with increasing extension is not in dispute. It should be remembered, however, that most arterial walls can be stretched to over twice their unstressed length and so are very different from the relatively rigid materials, such as metals, which are discussed in textbooks of physics as examples illustrating the laws of elasticity we have discussed above. We have seen that elastomeric substances (p. 155) have properties similar to arterial wall and it is likely that most of the anomalous elastic behaviour of arteries can be explained in the light of our knowledge of the behaviour of elastomers. An alternative explanation, based on the fact that the arterial wall is composed of elastin and collagen with a variable amount of smooth muscle, has been advanced by Burton (1954). As the experiments performed to measure the

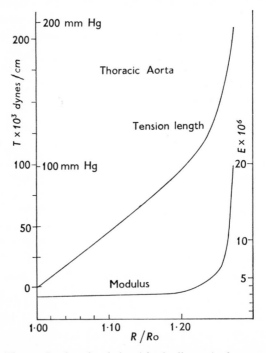

Fig. 8.1. The tension-length relation (elastic diagram) of a segment of the thoracic aorta of a dog subjected to various distending pressures. Ordinate—left, tension in dynes × 10³/cm (from eqn. 8.4); right, elastic modules. Abscissa—relative increase of radius (and hence of circumference).

The curve for the Young's modulus is plotted from the slope of the elastic diagram (tangent modulus). If the modulus were calculated with reference to the resting length the value at 200 mm Hg pressure would be about $4 \cdot 2 \times 10^6$ dynes/cm². This discrepancy between the two methods only becomes noticeable (see Table III) when there is a marked departure from linearity—for pressures up to 100 mm Hg the elastic behaviour, in this case, is remarkably linear.

elastic constants of arteries have varied, according to the concept various workers have held, it is necessary to try and form some opinion of their respective merits.

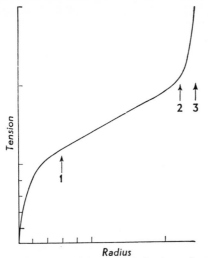

FIG. 8.2. Schematic diagram of the elastic behaviour of an artery to illustrate the hypothesis that the three main components successively determine the form of the curve. Up to point 1 the contracted smooth muscle is the only element being extended; from point 1 to point 2 the elastin is determining the extent of the elongation; at point 2 it is assumed that the collagen fibres are straightened out and, therefore, between points 2 and 3, the collagen (having a much higher modulus than elastin) is determining the tension-length relation.

Some difficulties in accepting this simple hypothesis are discussed in the text. In particular, I have never seen an exhibition of relative rigidity at low extensions such as that illustrated here (e.g. Fig. 8.1). The ordinate and abscissa are in arbitrary units (*redrawn from Fig. 1, Wezler and Sinn, 1953*).

The arterial wall as a mixture of various elastic elements

This view of the arterial walls is not altogether novel for it is implicit in much of the older literature which attempted to relate the behaviour of arteries to their histological structure. Wezler and Sinn (1953) used it in a qualitative way to describe the shape of the elastic diagram (Fig. 8.2). Burton (1954), however, expounded it in a precise and quantitative form in such a way as to clarify our thinking on the subject. Omitting for a moment the behaviour of smooth muscle about which information is rather scanty and which is a minor component of large arteries, we may consider the behaviour of a wall composed of elastin and collagen. Elastin is a very extensible substance and has a Young's modulus of about

3×10^6 dynes/sq. cm/100 per cent elongation. Collagen on the other hand is much less extensible and has a modulus of about 1×10^9 dynes/sq. cm (values from Burton 1954). If both are plotted on a stress-strain diagram they will be represented respectively by straight lines but of very different slopes. The behaviour of each is assumed to conform approximately to Hooke's law. If the two materials were stretched in parallel the elastic diagram would, of course, be dominated by the less extensible component, i.e. the collagen, and if this conformed to Hooke's law then so would the mixture. To explain a non-linear elastic diagram it is postulated that at small extensions the collagen fibres have not been pulled out "straight" and that the stress-strain behaviour is entirely determined by the elastin which is being stretched. As the extension increases the collagen is also stretched and the modulus of the wall increases rapidly. The simplest analogy to this is the familiar one of a rubber bulb surrounded by a loose net of string. This distends easily until the string is taut and then becomes very difficult to inflate. In its simplest form the stress-strain diagram would be a straight line of low slope and then have a fairly sharp discontinuity and continue as one of a very high slope. Burton illustrated a curve of this type derived from a vein. I have derived similar curves from the behaviour of the smaller peripheral arteries on longitudinal stretching (Fig. 8.3 shows a femoral and a saphenous artery). In these it is interesting to note that the region of most rapid change occurs at a length very close to that of the excised specimen *in situ*. The usual curves for the circumferential stretch of arteries, and also longitudinal stretch in the aorta, are the smooth curves such as that shown in Fig. 8.1. To explain this type of curve one has to postulate that the degree of "slack" in the collagen fibres varies greatly and that, with increasing length, more and more fibres are progressively stretched. There is no direct histological evidence for this but it is possible to imagine such a situation in a tissue with a very variable orientation of the fibrous components.

From this hypothesis we should anticipate that at small extensions the effective modulus of the arterial wall was the same as that of elastin. The accompanying table shows this is approximately true although the lowest values for the arterial wall appears to be appreciably lower than those for the ligament. As the "modulus" here is calculated from the cross-section of the tissue, while the elastic behaviour will depend on the cross-section of the material, such as elastin or collagen, that is put under stress, such differences in the values may easily be due to different tissue structure.

Equally from the hypothesis we should expect that at the upper limit of the physiological range of extensions the elastic modulus should approximate to that of collagen (1×10^9 dynes/cm²). It can be seen from the table that only in the case of some peripheral arteries extended longitudinally do we get values even approaching this order of magnitude. In the tangential moduli which have been recorded in my laboratory a value of 5×10^7 dynes/cm² in the femoral artery represents the upper limit, and usually it is considerably less. This is less than the value for tendon by a factor of 20. To account for this either we must assume that only a small fraction of the collagen is being involved (for as we have seen

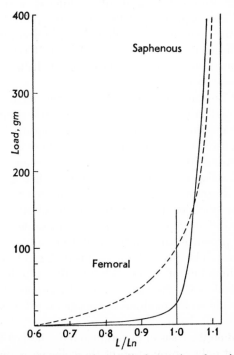

FIG. 8.3. Elastic diagrams for longitudinal extension of specimens of femoral and saphenous arteries of the dog. Ordinate—load in grams; Abscissa—ratio of length to that of the specimen *in the body*. It will be observed that at this length the extensibility of the artery is rapidly increasing (see Table III for values of modulus).

30 per cent of the peripheral arterial wall is collagen), or that the collagen of arterial wall has a much lower elastic modulus than that in tendon.

Similar results have been derived from attempts to separate the two components of the wall artificially. Hass (1942a) extracted the collagen from the thoracic aorta with concentrated formic acid. As seen in the table the remaining elastin had a modulus of the same order of magnitude as the whole arterial wall at small extensions. It should be noted, however, that his data are calculated on the basis of the cross-section of *dried* tissue. As Harkness *et al.* (1957) have shown (p. 162 above) that the normal water content is about 70 per cent of the wall, values on dried specimens can be up to three times too large. If this is so Hass's corrected values would be about $1\cdot0 \times 10^6$ dynes/cm² which is considerably lower than the corresponding values for ligamentum nuchae and for intact arterial wall. This suggests that the somewhat powerful chemical treatment of the tissue may have altered its physical properties. In the case of collagen it is well known (e.g. Wood, 1954) that chemical treatment which causes no visible histological change may greatly reduce its tensile properties.

Roach and Burton (1957) have extended this technique. Hass's method for extracting collagen was used and compared with similar specimens digested with commercial trypsin. This enzyme preparation normally contains elastase but will not digest collagen. They demonstrated that the two preparations, one of "elastin" and the other of "collagen" from the arterial wall, had approximately linear elastic diagrams. The slope of the collagen preparation, as expected, was much steeper than that of the elastin. The results show that the difference in slope (which in the same specimen will represent the proportionality of the moduli) is only of the order of 10 times at most. This fits with the results deduced from the limits of the values found in intact vessels but hardly, as indicated above, fits quantitatively with the values originally proposed by Burton (1954), where the elastic modulus of collagen is given as 300 times greater than that of elastin.

To proceed on the basis of the original hypothesis it is necessary to assume that only a proportion of the collagen is implicated in the situations where stress is being applied. Further it suggests that the orientation of the fibres is an important factor affecting the proportion involved. Experimentally this can be tested by measuring the elastic behaviour under the influence of simultaneous longitudinal and circumferential stresses. Preliminary experiments of this type were made by applying pressure to segments of arteries and loading them longitudinally at the same time. The results showed that, although increasing the length by loading tended to increase the modulus in the tangential direction, the change was usually small. The largest increase observed was about an 80 per cent increase in tangential modulus for a 100 per cent increase in length. Over the whole series, as stated, the effect was much smaller. Clearly this requires a much fuller investigation with more refined techniques but the results make it difficult to apply the "elastin-collagen mixture" hypothesis of Burton with any quantitative precision. Lawton (personal communication) has tested the hypothesis in a different way. He has measured the elastic modulus of strips of thoracic aorta cut in various directions— longitudinally, transversely and with varying degrees of obliquity. No significant difference was found. As a result he considers that the arterial wall should be considered as a homogeneous and isotropic structure, albeit of somewhat unusual elastic properties.

The arterial wall as a homogeneous elastomeric structure

The analysis of the elastic behaviour of the arterial wall in terms of elastomeric (or "rubber") theory is, unfortunately, very incomplete at present. This is discussed at some length in the "Proceedings of the Symposium on Tissue Elasticity" (Remington, 1957), to which reference should be made. Unlike the hypothesis of Burton discussed above we cannot utilize data from previous papers on the arterial wall because, without measurements of the dynamic behaviour it is impossible to deduce the elastomeric constants. Lawton's pioneer experimental work in this field has already been quoted, and this has stressed the qualitative similarity between the behaviour of elastomers like rubber and the arterial wall. In terms of thoracic aorta, which has the most linear behaviour of arterial specimens studied, we can see from the table that the modulus may increase by a factor of 10 over the physiological range of blood-pressure, although it is usually less than this, especially in Bergel's recent experiments (see footnote to Table III). This represents an extension of 70–80 per cent in length and seems to be quantitatively much more non-linear than rubber. Lawton has, however, said (personal communication) that it is quite possible to synthesize a rubber tube of exactly the same characteristics as the dog thoracic aorta.

From the measurement of pulse-wave velocity and the limited information on elastic moduli available (see Table III) it seems that the arterial tree gets less extensible as one moves peripherally. This appeared in my own earlier investigations as a more rapid rise in modulus with increasing pressures from values that were similar below 40 mm Hg from thoracic aorta to femoral; Bergel's results, however, indicate that the increase is mainly in dynamic elastic modulus. As Harkness *et al.* (1957) have shown that these effects are not due to progressive changes in composition, it suggests that there is a structural change. Lawton (personal communication) has made a preliminary comparison of strips of thoracic and abdominal aorta and found that the principal change was in the damping factor.

The experiments using a complete arterial segment (Bergel, 1958) have already been mentioned. Curves illustrating the

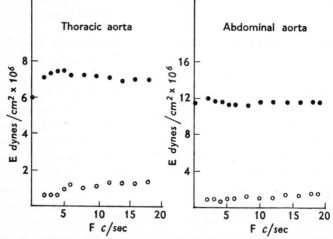

FIG. 8.4. The dynamic elastic constants of whole arterial segments (thoracic and abdominal aorta) measured by the method of Bergel (1958). The relevant equations (8.12–8.14) are explained in the text. The upper (solid) points in each case are the values of the "elastic" term E_{dyn} and the lower points (open circles) the "viscous" term $\eta \omega$. The ordinate is in the units of Young's modulus (dynes/cm^2); abscissa—frequency of oscillation. The mean pressure in each case was 100 mm Hg; the imposed oscillation about ± 5 mm Hg. The Young's modulus measured under static conditions is that of the solid circle at zero frequency; in this case the "tangential" modulus at 100 mm Hg is shown so that the values are higher than some of those in Table III. (From unpublished results of Dr. D. H. Bergel.)

dynamic behaviour of segments of thoracic and abdominal aorta are shown in Fig. 8.4. It can be seen that the damping (which is a function of the lower curve, representing $\eta\omega$—see eqn. 8.12 to14) is indeed somewhat higher in the abdominal aorta. These measurements were performed at a mean pressure of 100 mm Hg and it can also be seen that the static modulus is higher in the abdominal than in the thoracic aorta. The elastic component of the dynamic modulus (*E dyn*—upper curve) is also higher in the abdominal than in the thoracic aorta at all frequencies from 1–20 c/sec. At present we are far from making any interpretation of these results (if confirmed by later experiments) in terms of structure.

The main evidence on the progressive change in elastic properties in the peripheral regions of the arterial tree is derived from the progressive increase in pulse-wave velocity. Taylor (1957*b*) has shown that proximity to a reflecting point will cause an increase in apparent wave velocity, a condition likely to be found, for example, in the femoral artery. Thus it is important that we should be able to differentiate changes in wave velocity due to changes in arterial wall structure from those due to reflection. Until this is resolved calculations of moduli based on wave velocity (Table III) should be treated with suspicion. (See also Ch. 10).

To summarize the present position it is fair to say that the consideration of the arterial wall as a moderately homogeneous viscoelastic substance offers the most comprehensive yet simple description of all aspects of its behaviour, but it may yet be more specifically described in terms of elastomeric theory. When the extension of the arterial wall approaches its physiological limits it does seem, as Burton has postulated, that some of the collagen functions as a restraining fibrous network and that this accounts for the marked rise in elastic modulus under these conditions. In the body, however, the artery is "tethered", that is subject to considerable longitudinal restraint by its attachments to the surrounding tissues. The effects of this, as is seen in the next chapter, probably modify the viscoelastic properties that have been studied in the isolated specimen.

The effect of the smooth muscle in the arterial wall

The contribution of smooth muscle to the functional behaviour of the larger arteries is obscure. This is due to the fact that the tensile force produced by muscle appears to be small compared with the wall tension in a large artery. Burton (1954) considered that the probable value for the Young's modulus for contracted smooth muscle was $1·0 \times 10^5$ dynes/cm^2. The actual tensile force it could exert would obviously be much less than this. The modulus for elastin, as we have seen, is about $2–3 \times 10^6$ dynes/cm^2. The tangential tension in the wall of, for example, the dog's thoracic aorta is about 6×10^5 dynes/cm for a wall of unit thickness at 100 mm Hg pressure. Even if we allowed for 10 per cent of the wall to be muscle this would give a force per unit area of muscle fibre of 6×10^6 dynes. If the quoted value for the Young's modulus is correct the contractile force of the muscle would be utterly ineffective at this tension. This led Burton (1954) to postulate that the muscle fibres were connected to the elastin-collagen matrix in such a way as to exert a mechanical advantage, of say 100 to 1, so that they could contribute to the elastic behaviour of the wall. This postulate had the disadvantages that (1) there was no histological evidence for it, and (2) while the tensile effect could be created, equally, by the law of the lever, it meant that the dimensions of the artery could only be altered by 1/100th of the shortening of the muscle fibres. This latter point meant that contraction of the muscle merely meant the addition, in parallel, of an element similar in elastic modulus to the elastin; functionally this would not seem to serve any purpose, and would be impossible to detect.

Investigation of the experimental evidence suggests that the value of Young's modulus for smooth muscle is grossly inaccurate. Burton's figure was derived from one of the few papers available, that measured on the retractor penis of the dog (Winton, 1926). It is very difficult to maintain adequate oxygenation in a relatively thick muscle of this nature and probably only the outer layers of fibres were contracting effectively. Bozler (1957) suggests that the correct value for the Young's modulus of striated muscle is at least 500 times greater—he quotes a value of $6·2 \times 10^7$ dynes/cm^2 "on a water-free basis".* This would certainly seem to be more reasonable physiologically in terms of the tensions in the walls of arteries of various sizes without the necessity of postulating elaborate fibre attachments within the wall. In vessels the size of the thoracic aorta it is known that procedures such as nerve stimulation that cause smooth muscle contraction do not cause measurable changes

*Abbot and Lowy (1958, *J. Physiol*, **141**, 385–397) measured a maximum tension of $3.5–8 \times 10^6$ dyn/cm^2 in molluscan smooth muscle which suggests a value for the modulus of the same value for this muscle as that quoted from Bozler.

in calibre at normal arterial pressures. The tension on the muscle fibres here is of the same order of magnitude as the Young's modulus (which it will be remembered is the force which will cause 100 per cent elongation). When we get down to vessels of one-tenth the diameter (1 mm) active muscular alteration of the calibre begins to be feasible. With vessels of 200–100μ in diameter the contractile force of the muscle fibres will be greater than the wall tensions—and these are, of course, the arterioles where we know that smooth muscular control is all important. The relation of wall tension to the radius also explains why one may see active closure of, say, a femoral artery in a rabbit but not in a dog or a human. Wehn (1957) has produced evidence that the femoral artery of the rabbit actually gets narrower with each pulse, which he attributes to rhythmic contraction of the arterial smooth muscle in time with the heart beat. As he has subsequently found the same effect in the femoral arteries of the dog and one human subject (Wehn—personal communication) this cannot be dismissed as an effect only seen in small arteries. However, very simple procedures such as cannulating a side-branch to record the arterial pressure apparently paralyses the smooth muscle so that his records then show an orthodox dilatation with each pulse. This effect, and, indeed, the speed of contraction of the muscle required for his hypothesis, are difficult to reconcile with the known physiological behaviour of smooth muscle. The hypothesis is virtually a revival of the old concept of an active contraction of the arteries contributing to the propulsion of the blood and hence forming a "peripheral heart". As this concept was abandoned by the early 1920's there seems at present insufficient evidence to revive it.

In summary, contraction of the muscle fibres scattered in the walls of large arteries in the bigger mammalian species may produce a slight modification of their elastic properties. For physical reasons the effect is likely to be small. In the present analysis, therefore, this factor is neglected until there is definite experimental evidence to the contrary.

Determination of pulse-wave velocity from the elastic constants of the arterial wall

In the investigation of the dynamics of the circulation the determination of the pulse-wave velocity is of great importance. It will be shown in the succeeding chapters that while the velocity

TABLE III. *Elastic moduli of arteries*

Tissue	Method of measurement	Young's modulus dynes/cm² × 10⁶	Author	Comments
Ligamentum Nuchae	Longitudinal strip	4·6	Krafka (1939)	Calculated by Burton (1954)
,,	,,	40	Reuterwall (1921)	Small extensions
Thoracic aorta	Longitudinal strip (dog)	1·24	Lawton (1955 Fig. 3)	70% extension, i.e. "natural" length
,,	,, (static)	3	,,	Range from 10–70% extensions
,,	,, (dynamic)	2–18	,,	Extensions up to 40%
,,	(dog, cow)	1·4	Krafka (1939)	Calculated by Burton (1954)
,,	Whole vessel with collagen extracted	3	Hass (1942a, b, 1943)	
,,	Tangential modulus from p.w.v. (dog)	2·5	Personal	Calculated from pulse-wave velocity of c. 500 cm/sec found by Dow & Hamilton, 1939; Laszt & Müller, 1952a
,,	Whole vessel (longitudinal) (dog)	2·0–3·0	,,	Extensions from excised length up to 10% greater than "natural" length
,,	Whole vessel (tangential) (static)	3·0	,,	Pressures 20 mm Hg – 100 mm Hg (Fig. 8.1)
,,	,,	20·0	,,	Maximal value found in any specimen at 200 mm Hg
,,	,,	1·2	Bergel (1960)	At 40 mm Hg (mean of 10 specimens)
,,	,,	4·4	,,	At 100 mm Hg (mean of 10 specimens)
,,	,,	16·1	,,	At 200 mm Hg (mean of 10 specimens)
,,	(tangential) (dynamic)	4·7	,,	2·0 c/sec 100 mm Hg (mean of 10 specimens)
,,	,,	5·3	,,	18·0 c/sec 100 mm Hg (mean of 4 specimens)

Abdominal aorta	From pulse-wave velocity	5·0	Personal	Calculated from values of Dow & Hamilton 1939; Hale *et al.* 1955
,,	Longitudinal	3·4	,,	Small extensions
,,	,,	53	,,	Maximal value at 10% above "natural" length
,,	Tangential (static)	1·2	Bergel (1960)	At 40 mm Hg (mean of 7)
,,	,,	9·2	,,	At 100 mm Hg ,,
,,	,,	13·1	,,	At 200 mm Hg ,,
,,	Tangential (dynamic)	10·9	,,	2·0 c/sec 100 mm Hg press. (mean of 7)
,,	,,	12·2	,,	18·0 c/sec 100 mm Hg press. (mean of 4)
Femoral	,,	10·0	Personal	Calculated from pulse-wave velocity
,,	Tangential (static)	1·2–16·1	Bergel	Range from 40–200 mm Hg
,,	Whole artery longitudinal	2·0	Personal	Average value up to 90% "natural" length
,,	,,	60	,,	Maximal value at slightly above "natural" length (Fig. 8.3)
Carotid	Tangential (static)	1·0–12·8	Bergel	Range from 40–200 mm Hg
Saphenous	,,	1·0	Personal	Small extensions
,,	,,	200	,,	Above "natural" length (Fig. 8.3)

All "personal" and Bergel results are for the dog and are calculated for each increment of extension (approximately the slope of the tension-length diagram at each point). Bergel also gives values for carotid: 2 c/sec—11·0, 18 c/sec—12·8, static (100 mm Hg)—6·9; femoral, 2 c/sec—12·0, 18 c/sec—12·0, static (100 mm Hg)—9·0 (Bergel, D. H., 1960, *J. Physiol.*, **150**, 34*P*). These dynamic values for arteries show that the only significant rise in modulus is between 0–2 c/sec and thereafter it is not frequency-dependent up to 18 c/sec (the femoral actually shows a slight fall from a maximum of 12·0 at 5 c/sec).

of wave propagation is largely determined by the elastic behaviour of the arteries, it can be substantially modified by the viscosity of the fluid and by the presence of reflected waves. For full experimental analysis it is necessary that we should be able to separate these factors. The inconclusive review of the elastic behaviour of the vessels made above shows clearly that at present we have insufficient information to predict the "ideal" wave velocity of any given artery. The early work correlating wave velocity and elastic constants only aimed at getting average values over large sections of the arterial tree. Hamilton, Remington and Dow (1945) attempted to correlate wave velocities measured in segments of the arterial tree with those predicted from stretching arterial rings. They found considerable discrepancies but the ring technique is open to so many doubts as to its accuracy that it is difficult to interpret the cause of the difference between observed and calculated values.

The measurements of Dow and Hamilton (1939) and Hamilton *et al.* (1945) of the pulse-wave velocity which measured the transmission time of the "foot" of the wave (the foot-to-foot velocity) are the most detailed measurements we have for comparing various regions of the arterial tree. These agree fairly well with the results of Laszt and Müller (1952*a* and *b*). On this basis I am assuming in subsequent discussions that at an average mean arterial pressure in the dog the wave velocity in the thoracic aorta is 400–500 cm/sec, in the abdominal aorta 550–650 cm/sec and in the femoral artery 800–1,000 cm/sec. This makes the assumption that the foot-to-foot velocity is the best measure of the "ideal" or "natural" wave velocity that we have. From the evidence presented in Ch. 10 this appears a reasonable working value, at least for the higher frequencies in the pulse-wave, but it leaves much to be desired in the approximations it involves. In particular it gives no information on the variation of wave velocity with frequency, for as seen above an artery may get "stiffer" at higher frequencies and hence have a higher wave velocity. For many purposes the absolute values are not so important as their ratios, and it can be seen from Table III that these fit reasonably well with available measurements of the effective Young's moduli. The lack of accurate measurements of the elastic constants over the whole arterial tree constitutes a major barrier to the testing of the mathematical analysis, as will be seen in the succeeding sections.

CHAPTER IX

PULSATILE FLOW IN AN ELASTIC TUBE

We have already seen that the hydrodynamic problems of pulsatile flow are considerably more complicated than those of steady flow even in pipes of unvarying diameter. The figures presented in Ch. 5 showed that we can make reasonable approximations while ignoring the movement of the arterial wall, yet it is clearly unsatisfactory to leave the physical analysis at this stage. In this chapter it is proposed to give an account of the hydrodynamic properties of oscillatory flow in an elastic tube system with an indication as to how valid it seems to be when applied to arteries. In view of our relative ignorance of the complex elastic properties of arteries that was shown by the review of existing knowledge in Ch. 8, it is clear that we are inevitably some way from a complete solution.

As always it is necessary to consider what approximations may reasonably be made and what is the most realistic physical model of an artery. The model, that has usually been regarded as the most obvious, is that of a thin-walled tube with walls that are perfectly elastic. This is because we think of arteries as independent pipes running through the body, and the behaviour of such a model must be considered. Anyone who has attempted to define an artery by dissection, however, is aware that it is difficult to define precisely where the adventitia ceases and the surrounding tissue begins. In terms of the intact animal one can make out a very good case for regarding the arteries as tubes drilled through the body mass. The mathematical model for this is a cylindrical hole in an infinite elastic body, and in certain cases has been studied in detail, as in the properties of oil wells. Womersley has used this model in an exploratory way but the analysis has not been pursued because it does not seem the most realistic model for the circulation and because the mathematical forms are rather intractable.

From the consideration of the relation of the arterial wall, which was described as "tethering" in Ch. 8, and in view of the fact that arteries are surrounded by tissue masses, Womersley (1957) has developed a further model. This is essentially that of an elastic tube which is subjected to a longitudinal restraint (the "tethering") with walls that are loaded by additional mass. This appears to be the most realistic model that has been studied fully up to the present time. An extension of this model to include visco-elastic properties of the wall has also been made (Womersley 1958a) and has been tested recently by Taylor (1959b) on a rubber-tube model. He finds that the viscous element in the wall increases the apparent longitudinal "tethering".

In addition to making approximations as to the physical behaviour of the wall we have also to consider the physical properties of the blood. The simplest case is to neglect its viscosity and treat it as a non-viscous fluid. We have seen (Ch. 5) that in large vessels or at the higher frequencies the effects due to viscosity are relatively small and use of this was made in the calculations of Fry *et al.* (1956). Karreman (1952) has given one of the most extensive recent analyses of the oscillatory motion of non-viscous fluid in a thin-walled elastic pipe. From this emerges the classical Moens-Korteweg equation (8.16) for the velocity of the pulse wave

$$c_0 = \sqrt{\frac{Eh}{2R\rho}}$$

and he also points out that the pressure-flow relationship is of the form of the standard water-hammer equation of Allievi (1909). The simplest form of this is

$$P = \rho \bar{V} c \quad \dots\dots\dots\dots\dots\dots\dots \quad 9.1$$

where P is the pressure, ρ the density of the liquid, $\bar{V}$ its average velocity across the pipe and c the wave velocity. In an elastic tube this velocity as shown in the equation above is determined by the properties of the wall for, by comparison, the fluid is incompressible. In the more familiar experience of "water-hammer" as in the domestic water supply with rigid metal tubes the value of c is very high, being of the order of the velocity of sound in water, and it can be seen why very high pressures are developed. The same factors operate in the production of cavitation e.g. around ships' screws.

In spite of the approximation involved in neglecting viscosity this simple formula forms a useful guide to the pressure developed by the rapid injection of fluid into an elastic tube or an artery. Taylor (unpublished) showed for example that the first step in aortic pressure produced by the injection of a rectangular pulse of liquid (Peterson, 1954) can be predicted quite closely by this means. Starr's results with rapid injection of blood into the cadaver fitted this equation better than any other less simple ones (Starr and Schild, 1957). King (1947*a*) has also studied the behaviour of non-viscous fluid in an elastomeric tube.

Nevertheless it is clear from the simple theory set out in Ch. 5 that the effects of viscosity are far from negligible in pulsatile flow in tubes of the calibre of arteries. The mathematical consideration of the oscillatory motion of a viscous fluid in a free elastic tube was first studied by Witzig (1914) and this was extended by Karreman (1952). A fuller analysis, however, was that of Morgan and Kiely (1954) followed a few months later by an independent treatment with essentially the same results by Womersley (1955*c*). As the latter considered the motion of the liquid as well as wave propagation and was more specifically related to the dimensions of the arterial system its conclusions will be described here. Although, as already remarked, the free elastic tube is not entirely satisfactory as an arterial model, it is necessary to consider its physical behaviour to test it against other models and the circulatory system *in situ*. The primary assumptions made in this treatment are (1) that the wall is perfectly elastic and thin in comparison with the radius of the lumen; (2) that the wave-length of the oscillation is long compared with the lumen and (3) that the tube is extended infinitely, i.e. that the motion is established with no entrance effects and no end-effects in the form of reflections of the wave. In terms of arteries the assumption of thinness is reasonable, as noted above (p. 161) $h/2R$ is about 0·08. The condition of long wave-length is also satisfactory; the wave velocity of the arterial system is of the order of 500 cm/sec so that the wave-length of the fundamental component of a human pulse (70/min) is almost 5 metres, and in a dog (2/sec) 250 cm. Even if we consider frequencies up to 20/sec (e.g. the 6th harmonic of a dog with a pulse frequency over 3/sec) the wavelength is still 25 cm compared with an aortic diameter of 1 cm. The assumption (1) of perfect elastic behaviour we have already seen in the previous chapter to be untrue and it is certainly an exaggeration to consider an artery as infinitely extended and, as will be seen in Ch. 10, end-effects in the form of reflections do occur.

The full mathematical analysis given by Womersley (1955*c*) is too complex to be repeated here and it will suffice to describe the physical results. These may be considered under these headings:

(A) Movements of the wall.
    1. The longitudinal movement due to the viscous drag of the liquid.
    2. The radial dilatation.
(B) The change in the pressure-flow relationship compared with that of the simple theory (Ch. 5).
(C) The properties of the propagated wave.
    1. The wave velocity and its dependence on the frequency.
    2. The damping of the wave.
(D) Non-linearity of the equations.

(A) MOVEMENTS OF THE WALL

1. The longitudinal movement

An important effect of the viscosity of the liquid is that the resulting drag pulls the wall in a longitudinal direction. The magnitude of this effect is sensitive to changes in Poisson's ratio and as Womersley has calculated its value for various values of α (eqn. 5.8) it might serve as a means of studying the elastic properties of the arterial wall under dynamic conditions. With parameters analogous to those of the dog's femoral artery ($\alpha = 3 \cdot 34$ and $\sigma = \frac{1}{2}$ or 0.5) the computed value of the velocity of movement of the wall is approx. $0 \cdot 12$ of the average velocity of the liquid, which is surprisingly high. Also this velocity of movement of the wall leads the average velocity in phase; in the example quoted, by 74° (Fig. 9.1). This phase effect may be understood by reference to the diagrams of the velocity profiles (p. 43 and Fig. 3.1) where it can be seen that change in direction of flow begins at the wall of the pipe. This longitudinal movement has not previously received much attention but it can easily be seen when an oscillating flow is created in a rubber tube. I have, however, failed to observe any longitudinal movement of a comparable magnitude (Fig. 9.1 predicts an excursion of almost 1 cm in the femoral artery) in the wall of any arteries studied with high-speed cinematography. This adds further evidence to the suggestions that the outside of an artery is subjected to a longitudinal tethering or constraint and will be discussed further when the behaviour of the tethered tube is considered.

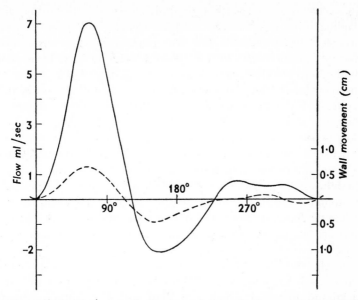

FIG. 9.1. The flow curve for the femoral artery (ordinate on left) with the computed curve of the longitudinal movement that the wall would make if it behaved like a free elastic tube (broken line—ordinate on right). This longitudinal movement is due to the viscous drag of the liquid within it. It can be seen that the total excursion would be of the order of 1 cm whereas in fact none can be observed at all. This is additional evidence that the artery is strongly constrained by its connections with the surrounding tissues.

For the fundamental component the velocity of the wall leads the corresponding flow lag by 74° but the total movement (plotted here) lags by 16°; the higher components lag by rather less. (*Curves computed but not published by J. R. Womersley; data given in Womersley, 1958a.*)

2. The radial movement

The second relation that emerges from this work is of greater practical importance. It is shown that the radial dilatation is related to the velocity of flow and not directly to the pressure. The relation is a very simple one

$$\frac{\overline{V}}{c} = \frac{2\xi}{R} \qquad \dots\dots\dots\dots\dots \quad 9.2$$

where again $\overline{V}$ is the average velocity, c the wave velocity, 2ξ the radial expansion, i.e. $\pm\xi$ about R the "resting" radius, that is the radius at the mean pressure.

At first sight this seems a most surprising conclusion because we are accustomed to regarding the pulse-*pressure* as the prime distending force in an artery. Further thought will make it clear, however, that in pulsatile flow in an elastic tube any short section that we consider will, during the acceleration of flow, have more fluid entering it than there is leaving it and that the distension of the segment is due to the increase in the amount of fluid in this segment. From the equation we see that for a given velocity of flow, the slower the pulse-wave, the greater the dilatation. As a slow pulse-wave means a lower Young's modulus, that is a more distensible arterial wall, we see that this is a perfectly reasonable relation. From the values for pulse-wave velocity and Young's modulus given in Ch. 8 it is therefore explained why the pulsatile dilatation is less in the abdominal than thoracic aorta and smaller still in the femoral artery. The quantitative aspects of this relationship are discussed below after considering the modifications in behaviour of the tethered tube model.

As the velocity of flow is not in phase with the pulse-pressure but leads it in phase (see Fig. 5.1) it is also apparent that the maximum dilatation, which is in phase with V/c, will also *precede* the peak of the pressure pulse. This is not quite so simple as it appears because the value c is a complex number and has a phase component in it (see p. 185 below), and in the "tethered" tube this is further modified. Precise recording of the dilatation of an artery and of the pulse-wave velocity would, theoretically, be a method of deriving the phasic flow in an artery. Unfortunately the expansion of an artery and the pulse-wave transmission time are very small and without a great refinement of technical methods the results would be very inaccurate.

Rushmer (1955*b*) has made simultaneous recordings of aortic circumference with a mercury-in-rubber strain gauge, and of aortic pressure. He found that in the living animal the maximum dilatation *preceded* the pressure peak. In the excised aorta that was distended, on the other hand, and also in a rubber tube, he found that the dilatation either moved with the pressure (as in the rubber) or lagged slightly behind in the case of the aorta (which was to be expected from the hysteresis phenomenon in a visco-elastic tube discussed above p. 153, Ch. 8). The difference between the living animal and excised aorta fits the prediction that the dilatation is following the changes in velocity of flow. The quantitative aspects of this are discussed below (p. 194).

(B) THE PRESSURE-FLOW RELATIONSHIPS IN THE FREE
ELASTIC TUBE

Expressing the pressure-flow equation for the elastic tube in terms comparable with those used for the simple tube we can write down the following relations. For the mathematical derivations and the full definition of the functions reference should be made to Womersley (1955c).

If we take a sinusoidal pressure gradient of the form

$$\Delta P = A_1 e^{i\omega t} \quad \dots\dots\dots\dots\dots\dots\dots\dots\dots\dots\dots\dots \text{9.3}$$

of which the real part is

$$\Delta P = M \cos(\omega t - \phi) \quad \dots\dots\dots\dots\dots\dots\dots\dots \text{9.4}$$

it will be recalled that, from eqns. 5.7 and 5.14

$$\overline{W} = \frac{MR^2}{\mu} \cdot \frac{M'}{a^2} \sin(\omega t - \phi + \varepsilon) \quad \dots\dots\dots\dots\dots \text{9.5}$$

where $a = R\sqrt{\dfrac{\omega}{\nu}}$ i.e. is a function of the radius (R) of the tube, the frequency of the motion (ω) and the kinematic viscosity of the liquid (ν). M' and ε' are dependent solely on a. $\overline{W}$ is the average velocity in the direction of the Z-axis.

The corresponding equation for the elastic tube may be written

$$\overline{W} = \frac{A'_1 R^2}{\mu} \cdot \frac{M''_{10}}{a^2} \cdot (\sin \omega t - \phi + \varepsilon''_{10}) \quad \dots\dots\dots\dots \text{9.6}$$

In this equation A'_1 is derived from the modulus of the pressure-gradient; M''_{10} and ε''_{10} are, like their analogous factors M' and ε, in eqn. 9.5, dependent on the parameter a, but also on the Poisson's ratio (σ) and on the relative thickness of the tube (h/R). This last ratio is called K which is useful, for the modifications due to tethering and loading of the tube may be all combined into modifications of this factor. The values of M''_{10} and ε''_{10} have been tabulated (Womersley, 1958a). It is found that for most conditions M''_{10} is slightly larger than M', and ε''_{10} slightly smaller than ε at the same a. This means that both amplitude and phase-lag are increased. For example, taking the Poisson's ratio as 0·5 which is a close approximation to that in arteries (see p. 149) and $K = 0·1$ (which is a little low for arteries; $K = 0·16$ is more generally correct, p. 161) we find over a typical range for the femoral artery

a	M''_{10}	M'	ε''_{10}	ε
3·34	0·7373	0·6551	29·26°	30·98°
6·67	0·8471	0·8096	11·59°	13·49°

With lower values for σ the effect is decreased until when $\sigma=0$ it is reversed and M''_{10} is actually smaller than M' and ε''_{10} is larger than ε.

In calculating a flow curve accurately it is also necessary to introduce an allowance for the pulsatile variation in diameter—this in effect means substituting $(R+\xi)$ for R into the equations where the dilatation (ξ) is defined by the relation in eqn. 9.2 above. The effect of these corrections is shown in Fig. 9.2 applied to one set of

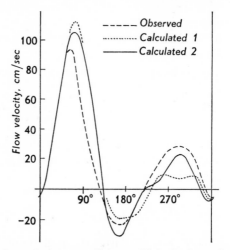

FIG. 9.2. A flow velocity curve ("observed") in the femoral artery measured by high-speed cinematography compared with two calculated curves. "Calculated 2" is computed from the equations of motion of liquid in a free perfectly elastic tube (see text) compared with "calculated 1", computed from eqn. 5.2 in which it is assumed there is no movement of the wall.

It can be seen that the corrections do not alter the pattern very much but do tend to improve to fit with the observed curve—especially in the period of diastolic forward flow. (*Redrawn from Fig.* 5, *Womersley,* 1955.)

data in the femoral artery reported by McDonald (1955a). It will be seen that the modifications of the original calculated curve are small but, in this case, alter the curve in the right direction in relation to the observed curve. The peak systolic flow rate is slightly decreased and the diastolic flow increased. In other cases the curves calculated from the simple theory are the better fit. The differences in these parameters are small compared with the probable errors in the flow measurement so that the exact form of the flow curve is not a critical test of minor variations in the physical relationships.

For ease of mathematical manipulation the equations expressed above are better kept in their complex form. A travelling pressure-wave (P) which at the origin is $A\ e^{i\omega t}$ will be represented in general as

$$P = e^{i\omega(t-z/c)} \quad \dots\dots\dots\dots\dots\dots\dots\dots\dots \text{ 9.7}$$

at any point distance z along the tube.

The velocity of flow (cp. eqn. 9.6) is then

$$\overline{W} = \frac{A}{\rho c} \cdot e^{i\omega(t-z/c)}\ M''_{10}\ e^{i\varepsilon''_{10}} \quad \dots\dots\dots\dots\dots \text{ 9.8}$$

and as the rate of flow, $Q = \pi R^2 \overline{W}$, the corresponding equation for flow may easily be written.

The presence of the factor $1/c$ recalls that the pressure-gradient along the tube (eqn. 5.11) for a sinusoidal oscillation

$$-\frac{\partial P}{\partial z} = \frac{1}{c} \cdot \frac{\partial P}{\partial t}$$

This emphasizes once more that in the hydrodynamics of elastic tubes, of whatever properties, the wave velocity is one of the most important parameters.

(C) THE PROPERTIES OF THE PROPAGATED WAVE

1. The wave velocity. 2. Damping

When a wave is propagated in a viscous medium it will be progressively damped, that is, its amplitude will decrease exponentially as it travels. This is apparent from the very nature of viscosity as discussed at the beginning of Ch. 2. In mathematical terms this means that the actual velocity, c is a complex quantity so we write

$$c_0/c = X - iY \quad \dots\dots\dots\dots\dots\dots\dots\dots \text{ 9.9}$$

where the velocity of the wave in a perfect fluid, c_0, is $(Eh/2R\rho_0)^{\frac{1}{2}}$ as before (eqn. 8.16).

This means that the phase velocity, c_1, is given by

$$c_1/c_0 = 1/X \quad \dots\dots\dots\dots\dots\dots\dots\dots \text{ 9.10}$$

and the percentage damping over one wave length, D, is given by

$$D = (1 - e^{-2\pi y/x})100 \quad \dots\dots\dots\dots\dots \text{ 9.11}$$

Thus as the velocity comes close to that of the perfect fluid, the damping becomes small.

The values of c_1/c_0 are illustrated graphically in Fig. 9.3 and they vary with the value of the parameter a. a, it will be recalled, is $R\sqrt{\dfrac{\omega}{\nu}}$ that is, it increases directly with the calibre of the tube and the square root of the frequency. With values of a about 3 which represents a vessel of the size of the femoral artery, c_1 is about 90 per cent of the ideal velocity and in larger vessels or at higher frequencies it gradually increases to a value of about 95 per cent. In the large vessels the slowing effect of viscosity, therefore, is

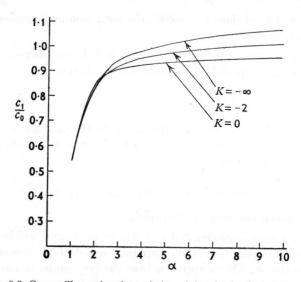

Fig. 9.3. Curves illustrating the variation of the phase velocity of a wave in a perfectly elastic tube filled with viscous liquid as the value of $a(=R\sqrt{\omega/\nu})$ varies. Ordinate—ratio of phase velocity, c_1, to the wave velocity, c_0, of the same tube filled with a liquid of zero viscosity (eqn. 8.16); abscissa—value of a. The term K is defined by eqn. 9.14. The curve for $K=0$ represents the behaviour of the free elastic tube; $K=-\infty$ is a tube rigidly constrained in the longitudinal direction (see section on the tethered tube). $K=-0\cdot2$ is a tube with a partial constraint.

The fall in velocity where $a<2$, i.e. in small arteries, is marked in all cases. In the femoral artery a is app. $2\cdot5$ for the fundamental, so that it can be seen that in a free tube of this and larger size that the viscosity of the liquid has little effect on the wave velocity; the ratio is within 10 per cent of the limiting value of $1\cdot0$. Longitudinal tethering increases the limiting value to $1\cdot16$ but even so the effect of size or frequency is not very great for $a>3$.

In a tube with a visco-elastic wall the rise in wave-velocity with frequency might be expected to be more marked than in a purely elastic tube. The results of Taylor (1959b), however, show that in a rubber tube the wave-velocity for values of a up to 90 fits very well with the curve for limiting longitudinal restraint ($K=-\infty$). (*Womersley*, 1957.)

relatively small. It is of interest that Moens (1878) added this value of 0·9 as an experimental constant to the formula for the wave velocity in an ildea fluid. The part of the curve that is highly significant in circulatory physiology is the steep fall of actual velocity at values of α less than 3. With an α of 1·0 it is only half the ideal value and at smaller values becomes uncomputable.

This slowing of the pulse-wave velocity must be associated with increased damping. In Fig. 9.4 the value of $\exp -2\pi Y/X$ is shown also in relation to α. The ordinate here represents the transmission, i.e. the fraction of the wave remaining after travelling over one wave-length. This damping increases markedly as α decreases from 10 until it is very nearly 100 per cent when α=1·0. For the larger mammals such values will be found for the fundamental in such vessels as the saphenous artery (in the dog α=0·8 to 1·0) and indicates the precise physical basis for explaining the disappearance of the pulse-wave in the arterioles even though their length is a small fraction of a wave-length.

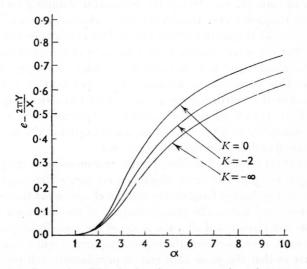

Fig. 9.4. Curves describing the damping, or attenuation, of a wave travelling in an elastic tube under the same conditions as in Fig. 9.3. Ordinate here is the proportion of the wave remaining after travelling over one wave-length, i.e. damping is virtually 100 per cent when α< 1·0. Tethering the tube (e.g. $K = -\infty$) increases damping. When the increase is due to an increase of frequency the damping *per unit length* increases because the wave-length becomes shorter. When the wall has visco-elastic properties the damping is dependent on the frequency alone as well as on the value of α and may be considerably greater than these values for the purely elastic tube (Taylor, 1959b). (*Womersley*, 1957.)

The relation of damping to the size of the vessel involved is therefore very important. The importance of the frequency of the wave is of equal significance and slightly more complicated. Considering a tube of constant size the effects of increasing a are then due to increase of frequency of the oscillation. The curve in Fig. 9.3 thus shows that, in a viscous fluid, velocity of propagation rises with frequency. From Fig. 9.4 it can be seen that the damping *per wave-length* also decreases, but with increasing frequency the wave-length becomes shorter. As the wave velocity is the product of the frequency and the wave-length this is not quite so simple as, for example, the calculation of the wave-length of radio waves, because the velocity also changes with the frequency. The net effect is, however, that the wave-length always decreases with frequency. (The wavelength also is shorter in large arteries such as the thoracic aorta, which have a lower wave-velocity because the wall has a lower elastic modulus.) As damping in practical terms needs to be considered in terms of distance the result is that over a length of tube of, say, 10 cm the percentage damping increases with the frequency even though the wave velocity increases. Thus for an $a=3\cdot34$ Womersley (1955c) in the free elastic tube has computed that the wave velocity is 91·4 per cent of the ideal and the amplitude is damped to 27 per cent of its initial value in one wavelength. This represents a damping of 5·4 per cent in a 10 cm length. For the fourth harmonic, i.e. at four times the frequency ($a=6\cdot67$) c_1 is 94·2 per cent of c_0, and the amplitude of the wave is only reduced to 63·6 per cent *in one wave-length* but the damping per 10 cm length is increased to 7·5 per cent.

This effect must be considered in the transmission of the pulse-wave generated by the heart which is a mixture of harmonic frequencies. The higher frequencies will travel somewhat faster than the lower, and hence the phase relations of the harmonic components will change and alter the shape of the wave by dispersion. At the same time, however, the higher frequencies will be damped out first so that the pulse as it travels peripherally will lose high frequency components, for example, the incisura of the central aortic pulse becomes damped out rapidly.

With a complex wave, which clearly still has a corporate existence even though it alters in shape, the term *group-velocity* is used to express the modal velocity of the group of components which have velocity dispersion. The velocity of individual harmonic waves is referred to as their *phase-velocity*. It is difficult to make a measurement of the group-velocity of a wave like the pulse-wave that would satisfy a mathematician and it is doubtful what value this concept has in the presence of reflections.

Müller (1951) has measured the phase-velocity, and what he calls the group-velocity, of sinusoidal waves in a rubber tube using both water and a glycerine solution. Group-velocity was here measured from the foot of the first wave he generated, but this is more probably the velocity of the highest frequencies because at such a discontinuity there would be, theoretically, a complete spectrum of frequencies. It is, in fact, seen from his results that the phase-velocity, which increases with frequency, becomes virtually the same as the "group-velocity" at 20 c/s. The phase-velocity was measured from the waves when they had settled down to a steady state oscillation. His illustrations show vividly the change in wave velocity and damping with frequency qualitatively similar to those predicted by Womersley. Womersley has calculated that in arteries with $a > 3$ the difference between phase- and group-velocity would not be more than 2 to $2\frac{1}{2}$ per cent.

(D) NON-LINEARITY IN THE EQUATIONS

It has been assumed throughout the previous discussion that there is a simple relation between individual harmonic components of the pressure and flow waves. Thus the Fourier series for the pressure-gradient can be transformed into flow, term by term. This is the principle of superposition, and for the simple theory in the "rigid" tube this is true. In the elastic tube, however, this is no longer strictly accurate and the harmonics will show an interaction. The mathematical reason for this is that the non-linear terms of the full equations are no longer negligible. The physical basis of this is that (1) as a result of the changes in radius there is a radial component of flow, and (2) the inertia terms. In addition (3) the interaction between the oscillatory and the steady flow term (taken in Ch. 5 as simply additive) has to be considered. (1) This was computed in the paper dealing with the free elastic tube (Womersley, 1955c) and found to be small as also are the inertia terms (Womersley, 1958a). At greatest they are only a few per cent. (3) The interaction between steady and oscillatory flow was also studied in Womersley (1955c) but much more fully by Womersley (1958a). An earlier treatment of a small oscillatory motion in a large steady flow was investigated by Morgan and Ferrante (1955). Womersley concluded that in a situation such as the femoral artery the oscillatory terms might alter the steady flow by as much as 14 per cent, which is far from negligible. In terms of a phasic flow curve the steady flow is very small compared with the oscillating components and it is difficult to detect whether this amount of alteration occurs. The "steady" pressure-gradient is, as observed in the discussion of the calculation of the flow curve (p. 86) so small that it cannot be measured accurately. The presence of the interaction means that Poiseuille's law cannot strictly be applied even to the steady pressure-gradient and flow in the presence of oscillatory terms.

The presence of a steady flow also modifies the wave velocity. This has been studied mathematically by Morgan and Ferrante (1955) and Womersley (1958a). It may be taken that the wave velocity in the presence of a steady flow is the algebraic sum of the normal wave velocity and the steady flow velocity. Some experiments of Müller (1950) appeared to show that there was a slightly different effect when the wave was "with" or "against" the stream but there seems to be no physical reason for this and the observation is slightly suspect because he used transient waves and did not allow for dispersion which alters the wave form as it travels. The *steady* flow component in arteries is so slow in comparison with the pulse-wave velocity that these effects are of little practical importance at present. The presence of a steady stream has in addition a slight effect on the damping. Womersley (1958a) predicts a very small increase in damping. Morgan and Ferrante (1955) predict a decrease in damping when the wave is running *with* the stream and an increase when against the stream. The relative magnitude of the steady flows considered relative to the oscillatory amplitude were so different that both calculations may be correct.

The presence of non-linearity of the kind discussed at the beginning of this section may most easily be seen by generating a pure sinusoidal wave in a system. In a non-linear system this will generate other harmonics and the sinusoidal form of the wave will appear distorted. The small magnitude of such non-linearity has been shown in our laboratory by the use of the pump designed by Taylor (1957b) which in a rubber tube showing comparable radial dilatation to that of the aorta, only generates about 3 per cent of second harmonic and no measurable amount of any other harmonic. Mathematically and experimentally one can be confident that this type of non-linearity, generated within the liquid, is very small and may be neglected. This is indeed fortunate, for any major departure from linearity would make the physical treatment of the problem unmanageably complex. Some theoretical and experimental investigations of this subject have been made by Taylor (unpublished). These appear to show that the non-linearity due to the wall will be small compared with those due to the motion of the liquid, so that they may be regarded as unimportant.

THE EFFECT OF EXTERNAL RESTRAINT. THE TETHERED AND LOADED TUBE

In the discussion above of the most realistic mathematical model of an artery it was pointed out that the anatomical attachment of the arterial wall to its surroundings suggested that the wall was "tethered", i.e. subject to an external restraint. Some evidence was put forward for this in Ch. 8. Further it was observed that a free tube would have a longitudinal movement due to the viscous drag of the liquid. This is not, in fact, observed in arteries *in situ* again indicating that they are not free to move longitudinally.

Womersley (1957*b*) has treated this mathematically by introducing a factor into the constant K, which in the free tube represented the relative thickness of the wall. The constraint is assumed to act purely in the longitudinal direction and has a natural frequency, m. The factor he introduces is

$$\left(1-\frac{m^2}{n^2}\right) \dots\dots\dots\dots\dots 9.12$$

where n is the circular frequency of the oscillation (equivalent to ω in other equations).

The "loading" of the tube adds to the wall a mass that takes no part in the elastic deformation. This increases its inertia. The factor used in this case is the same as that introduced by Morgan and Kiely (1954) as a mathematical means of describing the effects of surrounding tissue masses on the artery. The thickness of the wall of the tube, h, in the original equations is replaced by a term H' such that

$$\frac{H'}{h}=\left(1+\frac{h_1.\rho_1.R_1}{h.\rho.R}\right) \dots\dots\dots\dots 9.13$$

where h_1, ρ_1 and R_1 are the thickness, density and radius of the added mass and h, ρ, and R that of the tube wall.

Combining these two factors Womersley (1957*b*) defines K as

$$K = \left(1 + \frac{h_1 . \rho_1 . R_1}{h . \rho . R}\right)\left(1 - \frac{m^2}{n^2}\right) \dots \dots \dots \dots 9.14$$

From this it can be seen that with a fairly stiff constraint, $m > n$, then K will be negative. With a very stiff constraint, $m \gg n$, $K \to -\infty$. If $m = n$ then $K = 0$ and the wall behaves as though it has no mass.

With this alteration in the definition of K the mathematical equations are of exactly the same form as those for the free elastic tube discussed above (eqns. 9.6, 9.8). The values of M''_{10} and ε''_{10} are dependent, as before, on the parameter a, the Poisson's ratio and on K. These have been tabulated (Womersley 1958*a*) for values of K from $0 \cdot 4$ to -10. There is no direct way of evaluating K at the present time, that is, the dimensions of the "added mass" and the natural frequency cannot be measured directly.

From the evidence of the tethering effect it would appear to be stiff and hence we should expect K to have a fairly large negative value. The most interesting fact that emerges from the tables is that when $K \to -\infty$ then $M''_{10} \to M'$ and $\varepsilon''_{10} \to \varepsilon$, i.e. the values used in the simple theory (Ch. 5) and given in Table VI in Appendix 1. These values are very nearly the same with negative values of K of -10 or greater.

We may consider briefly the physical behaviour of oscillatory flow in such a tethered and loaded elastic tube under the same headings as for the free elastic tube.

MOVEMENTS OF THE WALL

1. Longitudinal

The condition of external constraint that has been postulated naturally tends to prevent any longitudinal movement. It was my own observations that virtually no such movements occur that led to the suggestion that such a longitudinal constraint existed. Hosie (personal communication) has made the same observation but full details are not yet available. Lawton and Greene (1956) have reported small variations in length but they appear to be in the opposite direction to that which might be anticipated, i.e. there is a contraction of length in systole. The movement is, however, very small. Evans (1956) has suggested that this must be due to aniso-tropism in the wall, but this may be regarded as a special case of constraint in the longitudinal direction.

The presence of a longitudinal constraint must be conceived physiologically as due largely to the connective tissue attachments on the outside of the artery. The viscous drag on the inside of the wall will still tend to move it and so will create a shearing stress in the wall. In such a thin wall it is unlikely that the inner side would be able to move more than a fraction in excess of the permitted movement of the outer side. Nevertheless there must be a continuous oscillating shear in the wall with each heart beat. As some present-day investigators of arteriosclerosis, such as Duguid (e.g. Duguid and Robertson, 1957) are stressing the role of mechanical factors in its causation, this shearing force is probably one of the most important. Its magnitude is mainly dependent on the degree of pulsatile variation in flow velocity and the degree of tethering. It would, therefore, be interesting to seek for a correlation between regions of the arterial tree where these are maximal and the commonest sites of arteriosclerotic degeneration.

2. The radial movement

From the equation relating dilatation to flow velocity (eqn. 9.2) and the equation (9.8) relating the velocity to the pressure, it is easy to relate the pressure to the flow, thus

$$\frac{2\xi}{R} = \frac{P}{\rho c_1^2} . M_{10}'' e^{i\varepsilon_{10}''} \quad \dots \dots \dots \dots \dots 9.15$$

$$= \frac{P}{\rho c_0^2} \left(\frac{c_0}{c_1}\right)^2 M_{10}'' e^{i\varepsilon_{10}''} \quad \dots \dots \dots \dots 9.16$$

where $\frac{c_0}{c_1}$ is the reciprocal of the velocity ratio plotted in Fig. 9.3. For all finite values of K this means that the expansion always leads the pressure in phase but the lead becomes progressively smaller with increasing negative values of K. When $K \to -\infty$ the limiting form is

$$\frac{2\xi}{R} = (1-\sigma^2)\frac{P}{\rho c_0^2} \quad \dots \dots \dots \dots \dots \dots 9.17$$

or for $\qquad\qquad\qquad \sigma = 0 \cdot 5$

$$= \frac{3}{4} . \frac{P}{\rho c_0^2}$$

and pressure and frequency are in phase at all frequencies.

B.F.A.–O

Womersley (1957) applied this form of analysis to the measurements of expansion and pressure measured simultaneously in the abdominal aorta by Lawton and Green some of which are illustrated in their (1956) paper. Potentially this provides a good method of testing the theory. In the present case there were inconsistencies in the results but it appeared that the phase lead of expansion over pressure was small, certainly less than 10°. It is, therefore, suggested that on present evidence the mathematical theory of stiff constraint, which also has the simplest form, is the best description of the situation.

The measurements of pulsatile dilatation of Lawton and Greene (1956) were made from cinematograph film. This method has also been used by Hosie and I know from personal experience that it is both laborious and subject to error. Rushmer (1955b) used a mercury-in-rubber strain gauge and reported a larger phase lead of dilatation over pressure. It is possible that this gauge introduced some instrumental error to account for the discrepancy with the results analysed above but it may be a more accurate record. Although the pulsatile dilatation of arteries is small an accurate experimental method for measuring it should not be impossible to devise and would be of great value.

The radial expansion of arteries with the pulse is so obvious to the eye that it is suprising to find that it is difficult to measure because it is so small. The femoral artery of a large dog may be 5 mm in diameter, but even with a large pulse pressure it will not expand by more than 0·2 mm. It appears greater because we see light reflected from the curved surface which changes, and the movement of the light beam magnifies the apparent movement. Bends in vessels also tend to straighten out with an increase of pressure and this is the cause of the apparent pulsatile dilatation of small arteries such as in the mesentery or on the surface of the brain. From cineradiographic studies Reynolds *et al.* (1952) denied that arteries dilated at all, but their illustrations showed it in the aorta of a similar degree to my own observation as measured by cinematography. In the umbilical artery, with which they were mainly concerned, it is virtually immeasurable. Their further contention that the volume of arteries increased in systole only by lengthening did not seem to be proved by their own evidence, and, as stated above, my own experience is that very little longitudinal extension can be demonstrated.

Wehn (1957) has also expressed the opinion that arteries do not expand with the pulse and quotes many earlier workers of the same persuasion. His own results using a photo-electric method on the femoral artery of the rabbit sometimes show a small increase and sometimes a decrease at each pulse. These are of the order of 1.5 per cent (which is only a few microns in this vessel).

In the dog the maximum radial dilatation I have observed by measuring the projected image of individual frames of a cine film has been 10 per cent in the thoracic aorta under the influence of noradrenaline. The normal values in my records are 5–7 per cent and this is similar to that measured by Rushmer. In the abdominal aorta I usually record 4–5 per cent (Lawton and Greene, 1946, recorded only about 3 per cent expansion), and in the femoral artery 3–4 per cent. In the rabbit a dilatation of up to 15 per cent has been observed in the thoracic aorta after dissection of the adventitia (McDonald, 1952*c*) and in the abdominal aorta about 5 per cent.

If eqn. 9.2 relating expansion to the flow and the wave velocity is applied it will be found that these measured arterial expansions are considerably smaller than would be predicted. For example, in one case in the femoral artery where both flow and film records were available in the same artery the foot-to-foot wave velocity was 850 cm/sec and the peak systolic flow 88 cm/sec. $\overline{W}/c$ is therefore a little over 10 per cent while the measured expansion was about 4 per cent. This discrepancy may be due to visco-elastic effects in the wall, but it must be repeated that until the magnitude of the effects of wave reflection have been estimated we cannot directly apply the description of the physical behaviour of a propagated wave in a very long tube to that of the arterial tree.

THE PRESSURE-FLOW RELATIONSHIP IN THE CONSTRAINED TUBE

The essence of the modification into the flow equations have already been discussed in the discussion of the radial dilatation. If the constraint is such that K has a large negative value it was shown that the form of the equation became identical with that for the simple theory (eqn. 5.2). The curves calculated using this formula and illustrated in Ch. 5 must stand as evidence that this physical model is a reasonable one.

The wave-velocity and the damping

The addition of a longitudinal constraint has, as we might expect, a stiffening effect on the wall and this results in a relatively greater wave velocity compared with the free elastic tube. This is shown in the upper curve of Fig. 9.3 which represents the limiting curve for a stiff constraint ($K = -\infty$). It will be seen that the form of the curve is similar to that of the free elastic tube. The limiting value of c_1/c_0 in this case, however, is not unity as in the case of the free tube, but is

$$\text{Limit } \frac{c_1}{c_0} = \frac{(M^1)^{\frac{1}{2}}}{\sqrt{1-\sigma^2}} \sec \frac{\varepsilon'}{2} = 2/\sqrt{3} \text{ (if } \sigma = 0{\cdot}5) \ldots \ldots 9.18$$

$$= 1{\cdot}16$$

If the data on the elastic constants of arteries were accurate enough to predict c_0, the fact that a stiff longitudinal restraint leads to wave velocity values up to 16 per cent greater could be used as a test of the model.

Stiffening the tube also has the effect of increasing the damping. This is also illustrated in comparison with the free elastic tube in Fig. 9.4. The degree of damping this appears to predict may seem high, but it must be appreciated that the arterial system is a fairly short one in terms of wave-length and the diminution of the pulse-wave by damping is more than offset by the presence of reflections due to the effects of changing calibre and wall behaviour in the arteries. This is discussed more fully in Ch. 12, where an attempt is made to synthesize all the effects to explain the actual behaviour of the pulse-wave as observed in the arterial system.

Recent experiments by Taylor (1959*b*) with an hydraulic model consisting of a long rubber tube filled with liquids of different viscosity appear to agree very reasonably as regards wave velocity with values predicted in Fig. 9.3 where $K = -\infty$, i.e. where the tube is "tethered". The tube in Taylor's experiments was not externally restrained other than by its attachment to the pump at the origin and by its supports. The close agreement that was found with the "tethered tube" equation therefore suggests that an important effect of a viscous element in the wall is to restrain the longitudinal movement in it that would otherwise result from the motion of the viscous liquid. By contrast, the damping is considerably greater in a visco-elastic rubber tube than it would be for a perfectly elastic tube. Earlier work by Müller (1951) seemed to

suggest that the wave velocity would go on increasing with frequency to a greater degree than Womersley's equation would
suggest. As the viscous element in rubber tubes appears to be of
the same order of magnitude as that in the arterial wall (Hardung,
1952, 1953; Bergel—personal communication) these results seem
to give further support to the idea that the equations for the
"tethered" tube, which closely approximate to the "simple"
theory set out in Ch. 5, are the best representations of pressure-
flow relations in an artery.

Landowne (1953, 1954, 1957a and personal communication
1956) has made observations on the velocity of artificially generated
impulses in arteries. He created sinusoidal oscillations in the
brachial artery of human subjects by means of an externally applied
mechanical oscillator and recorded the wave velocities between the
brachial artery and the radial artery at the wrist. From frequencies
of 6/sec up to 50/sec, or even to 100/sec the wave velocity continued to rise. He attributed this to an effective increase in stiffness
of the wall with frequency and this is, in a sense correct, but
Taylor's experiments indicate that this will mainly be effective in
limiting the longitudinal movements and so prove difficult to
separate from the restraint that the artery is normally subject to
in the body. The same effect would account for the high velocity
of propagation of single spikes imposed on the arterial pulse by
Landowne (1957b) and which have been discussed by McDonald
and Taylor (1959). Over the range of frequencies that have an
appreciable amplitude in the pulse-wave, say from 2/sec to 12/sec
in the dog, the change in wave velocity is not large in comparison
with other factors causing a change in shape of the pulse wave as
will be seen in Ch. 12, but there appears to be little doubt as to the
presence of the effect.

A subsidiary observation from his experiments is of some
interest. The non-linear elastic behaviour of the arterial wall which
was described in Ch. 8 might be expected to cause the generation
of higher harmonics (see p. 189 above). In Landowne's ingenious
experiments with sinusoidal waves no visible distortion was seen
although a detailed analysis was not made to look for it.

Now we have seen that the amount of dilatation of arteries due
to the pulse-pressure is also smaller (p. 195) than that obtained by
applying a similar pressure slowly to isolated segments. The
elastic diagram of the arterial wall indicates that the modulus

increases with increasing tension. It is, however, the change in length of the wall that determines the change in modulus, and not the change in tension. Thus as the dilatation of the artery in vivo is smaller than would appear from the elastic diagram, over the full range of the pulse-pressure, then the elastic behaviour of the artery will probably be more linear in the living animal than it is with slowly applied pressures in the isolated arterial segment. Although the magnitude of the oscillations Landowne used were relatively small his observations provide some support for this optimism.

CHAPTER X

WAVE REFLECTION

So far we have considered pulsatile flow in arteries as though they were long tubes with a remote end. The actual situation with the repeated occurrence of branches ending in the capillary bed makes it necessary to consider what effect, if any, changes in the vessel beyond the point of observation will have on the pressure and flow. Any such effect will be due to the creation of reflected waves and it is generally agreed that such waves occur. The only point of dispute is "how important is wave reflection in arterial dynamics?"

A travelling wave such as the pulse-wave will be reflected to some extent wherever there is a discontinuity in the system. The extreme cases are where a tube is either completely blocked or opens into a large reservoir, either of which cause total wave-reflection though in the latter case it is in the opposite sense, i.e. 180° out of phase with the former. In the circulation we are obviously dealing with intermediate conditions causing only partial reflection but the terms "closed" or "open" are convenient to describe their character. The discontinuity may be a change in calibre, as at a point of branching, or merely a change in the elastic properties of the wall. It might, therefore, seem obvious that the arterial tree which has many discontinuities of this sort would create large reflections and that there are no grounds for argument. The case for the contrary is probably best summed up by the remark that Womersley made when he was first confronted with the problem—"If you wanted to design a perfect sound-absorber you could hardly do better than a set of tapering and branching tubes with considerable internal damping such as the arterial tree." The experiments of Peterson and Shephard (1955) further-more appear to bear this out because they showed that a large pressure-wave created by a rapid injection pulse of blood retro-gradely into a femoral artery caused no detectable effect in the pressure-curve recorded at the root of the aorta. Their interpreta-tion was that any reflected waves created in the periphery, which would undoubtedly be very much smaller than their experimental ones, would be very rapidly damped out. This bore out the earlier findings of Peterson (1954) that the pressure curve due to an injection pulse in the arch of the aorta contained no components which could be attributed to discrete reflected waves. Wehn (1957) quotes several earlier authorities who have questioned the importance of reflections. On the other hand the fact that the pulse-wave normally develops secondary humps such as the dicrotic wave as it travels peripherally is usually ascribed to the presence of reflected waves. Indeed much of the analysis of arterial dynamics is based on the assumption that not only are there centripetal reflected waves but that these are in turn reflected at the aortic valves and re-traverse the system, setting up a condition of "resonance"; this is an integral idea in the development of the Windkessel hypothesis and is used as a basis for estimating the length of the Windkessel (Wezler and Böger, 1939; Wetterer, 1956). Allied to this is the description of "a standing wave" in the arterial system (Hamilton and Dow, 1939).

There have been so many conflicting opinions of these points that it is desirable that the elementary properties of reflected waves should first be recapitulated. To keep this consistent with the previous chapters we will first consider the behaviour of a system in steady-state oscillation. Then we can attempt to correlate this with the other hypotheses that have been put forward based on the idea that the pulse is a transient response, a distinction that has been discussed in Ch. 1.

REFLECTED WAVES IN A STEADY-STATE OSCILLATION

If the wave we are considering is in the form of a simple harmonic oscillation which is not being damped and is completely reflected at a closed end, then there are two components, the incident and the reflected waves which are equal in size, but travelling in opposite directions. At the point of reflection they are in phase and the oscillation of the two waves sums together. Moving away from the reflecting point they will progressively cancel each other out until at a distance of one-quarter wave-length there will be no oscillation at all. This point is called a node while the points of maximal oscillation are antinodes, and the two are spaced alternately at quarter wave-length intervals (Fig. 10.1). If the whole tube is, say, one wave-length long then the reflection phenomenon will be repeated exactly at the origin, the summation of waves will

build up and the tube will be in resonance. There will be a very
large oscillation at both ends and in the middle of the tube—the
antinodes—and two nodes at intermediate points where there is
no oscillation at all. The demonstration of this is familiar in the
standard classroom demonstration in physics of Kundt's tube. The
oscillations at the antinodes will be exactly synchronous and so the
whole is called a stationary, or standing, wave. If the far end is
closed, resonance occurs at a half wave-length and its integral

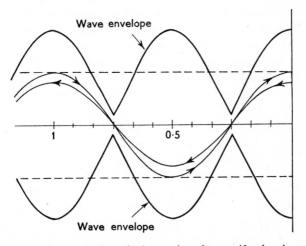

FIG. 10.1. A diagram to show the interaction of a centrifugal and a reflected
wave at a closed end (vertical line on right). For clarity it is assumed that only
80 per cent of the wave is reflected (i.e. reflection coefficient=0·8). The individual components are shown at one instant of time with arrows to identify them.
The abscissa is marked in fractions of a wave-length. At the point of reflection
both waves are in phase and sum together. With reference to a point one-quarter
wave-length away the incident wave is 90° earlier, and the reflected wave 90°
later, so that they are always 180° out of phase and almost cancel. This point is a
node and the only oscillation is the difference between their maximum amplitudes. At one half wave-length they are separated by a full cycle (360°) and so in
phase again and the waves sum together for another maximum—an antinode.

The total excursion throughout the cycle is represented by the wave envelope
(heavy outer lines). If there were no reflections and no damping, as we have here,
this would be a straight line (broken lines). In all subsequent figures only half the
envelope is shown as "the amplitude (or modulus) of the oscillation".

If reflection was complete the nodes would be at zero and the anti-nodes twice
the amplitude of the incident wave. Repeated reflection from the origin, as
shown here, would not increase this. If, however, the origin were one-half, or
one, wave-length from the end, summation would occur here as well and then be
repeated again at the far end. Thus, theoretically, the antinodes could become
infinitely large for this is the condition of resonance.

In the presence of damping the incident wave would be larger nearer the
origin and the reflected wave would be growing smaller towards the origin and
mutual interaction would be progressively smaller—as shown in Fig. 10.2.

multiples; if it is open, at a quarter wave-length and its integral multiples. In terms of pressure this means that in resonance the origin is always an antinode but is a node of flow.

When dealing with liquids, however, damping must be taken into account. This was studied in detail by Taylor (1957a) in a mathematical analysis based on the analogy of an electrical transmission line and the conclusions were verified by testing on a simple hydraulic model (Taylor, 1957b). This consisted of a long water-filled rubber tube which was attached to a pump with a sinusoidal output. The first point that he showed was that in such a system true standing-waves cannot occur because there are no points where no oscillation occurs, and so no true nodes. This is because, in the presence of damping, the reflected wave is smaller than the incident wave and so cancellation cannot occur. Points of maximum and minimum oscillation however, do occur which may

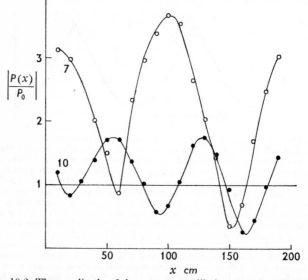

Fig. 10.2. The amplitude of the pressure oscillation at various points along a tube closed at 200 cm from the pump. The ordinate, $P(x)/Po$ is the ratio of the pressure amplitude (modulus) to that in the tube without reflections; abscissa—distance from the pump. Open circles—7 c/sec; full circles—10 c/sec.

The wave-velocity was app. 1,400 cm/sec. At 7 c/sec this section of tube was one wave-length and the tube is resonating. There are antinodes of pressure at both ends, with another at the half wave-length position—all of large amplitude. At 10 c/sec the tube represents 1·43 wave-lengths and there is no resonance. There are still marked antinodes and nodes at quarter wave-length intervals but the variation in amplitude is much less. (*Taylor*, 1957b.)

be called relative antinodes and nodes (Fig. 10.2) and are spaced at approximately quarter wave-length intervals. The discrepancy in size of the incident and reflected components increases as the distance from the reflecting point increases and so the maxima decrease in amplitude while the minima increase. The oscillations also are no longer synchronous but will appear to travel away from the origin, although this apparent phase velocity will vary greatly, being at a maximum at a relative antinode and at a minimum at a relative node (Fig. 10.7); this is discussed in a later section.

It will be simpler to consider first a tube with a closed end (as in Figs. 10.2 and 10.7), and compare it with that of an open end later. The amplitude of the pressure oscillations are always at a maximum at the end because the incident and reflected waves are exactly in phase. The position of the other maxima and minima are determined by the distance away from this point and independent of the total length of the tube, that is to say they will occur whether, or not, the tube is resonating. Their locations do not, therefore, depend on successive reflections from the beginning of the tube and the occurrence of maxima and minima does not, necessarily, indicate a condition of resonance. As we are driving the system with a pump we have a condition of *forced oscillation* at the frequency of the pump, and only that frequency will appear in a system whose behaviour obeys linear equations. If it is non-linear, as the arterial system certainly is, then some oscillation at the frequencies of the harmonic overtones may be generated. This point is of some importance when discussing the problem of "natural" frequencies of the system which are postulated in the theories which consider the pulse as a transient phenomenon.

The physical analysis of the arterial system which we are considering makes the fundamental assumption that the regularly repeated heart-beat creates a steady-state oscillation. It is, therefore, similar to the rubber tube with a sinusoidal pump. The arterial flow is thus in a condition of forced oscillation at frequencies determined by the pulse-rate. To look for evidence of reflection it is therefore necessary to separate the harmonic components of the pulse-wave by Fourier analysis and see whether they show maxima and minima. One example is analysed below (Fig. 10.3) and it can be seen that they do occur. From the frequency of the heart beat and the wave-velocity characteristic of the arteries involved (which we assume to be that of the rate of travel of the sharp "foot" at the front of the wave) we can calculate the wave-lengths of each harmonic component, because wave-length is the wave velocity divided by the frequency. The position of the pressure antinodes and nodes, then tells us how far away are the reflecting sites that are causing them.

CHANGES IN PRESSURE AMPLITUDE DUE TO REFLECTIONS

Fig. 10.3 shows the results of Fourier analysis of the pulse-wave forms recorded at six points along the aorta. These were measured

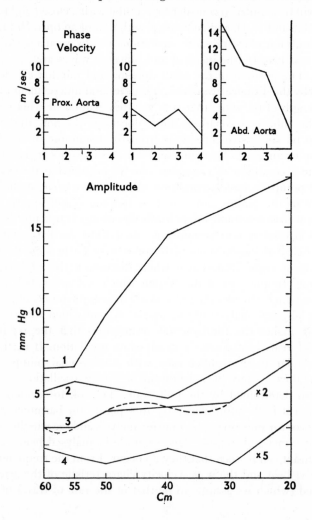

with a capacitance manometer, at successive points in the aorta through a long cardiac catheter introduced into the distal part of the femoral artery. In order to preserve their time relations, in respect to phase-shift, the E.C.G. was also recorded and the QRS complex taken for all curves as the origin of time. Values of the phase-velocity calculated from these phase-shifts are also shown in Fig. 10.3.

The distances are measured from the point of insertion of the catheter. In terms of anatomical position the 20 cm position is a few cm within the iliac artery, the diaphragm was some 40 cm distant and the farther point 60 cm in the arch of the aorta some 3 cm distal to the aortic valves. The pulse-frequency was 2·85 c/sec. The fundamental oscillation at this frequency is seen to be at a minimum close to the heart and to rise steadily as the wave travels peripherally. The fact that the values at 60 and 55 cm are very similar suggests that there is a relative node there but one could not, on the record of this single frequency, predict whether the most peripheral point was an antinode. The higher harmonics all wax and wane but it can be seen that in the interval farthest from the heart the amplitudes are all rising. This immediately suggests that the wave is near a region which is causing a reflection of a closed type.

Turning to the points of least amplitude it is seen that, for the second harmonic, one occurs at 40 cm, for the third harmonic at about 33 cm and again at about 58 cm, and for the fourth harmonic at 30 cm and again at 50 cm. We have already seen that the 60 cm

---

Fig. 10.3. The harmonic analysis (first four components) of a series of pressure pulses measured at six points along the aorta defined in terms of the length of catheter inserted (abscissa); tube 60 cm is close to the aortic valves and 20 cm at the origin of the iliac artery.

Lower curves—amplitude variation (the third harmonic is plotted at double amplitude with dotted line to indicate probable fluctuation between measuring points; the fourth harmonic is plotted at five times actual amplitude). Pulse frequency—2·85 c/sec; fourth harmonic—11·4 c/sec; the corresponding wave-lengths are 160 cm and 40 cm. Between the 30 and 20 cm positions the amplitudes of all the components are increasing together indicating that they are within a quarter wave-length of a region caused by a "closed" reflection. The distribution of the maxima and minima is consistent with this (see text).

Upper curves—the phase shift, expressed as apparent phase velocity for three of the intervals; on left between 60–55 cm; centre, 50–40 cm; on right, 30–20 cm. Abscissae refer to harmonies. The increase in apparent phase velocity where the amplitude is rising is most clearly seen in the first harmonic. (Five of the recorded pulses analysed here—omitting that at 55 cm—are shown in Fig. 12.1; another series is shown in Fig. 12.4 and analysed in Fig. 12.5.)

position probably represents a node of pressure for the fundamental. These minima, or nodes, should occur at a quarter of the wave-length proper to their respective frequencies. This can only fit the findings in all four harmonic components if there is a reflecting site close to the 20 cm position, that is a few centimeters distal to the termination of the aorta. This is the region between the division of the aorta and the arteriolar bed of the pelvic viscera, and it appears from this set of data that the reflected waves in the aorta mainly arise from this site. This may be more marked in the dog than in man because the arterial supply to the pelvic organs commonly arises as a midline single vessel forming a "trifurcation" rather than the bifurcation that we speak of in man.

It can be seen that if the length of the aorta, which is approximately 40 cm in this case, is a quarter wave-length, then the wave-length is 160 cm and the pulse-wave velocity would be 456 cm/sec (160×2.85) which is a very reasonable figure. The second harmonic has a wave-length of 80 cm and shows an antinode at the reflecting site, a relative node in the region of the diaphragm, 20 cm away, and a small antinode near the origin of the aorta. The length of the aorta is about one-half of a wave-length for this frequency. The fourth harmonic at twice this frequency has a wave-length equal to that of the aorta and has two nodes (at 10 and 30 cm distance) with an antinode between them at the level of the diaphragm, and another antinode at the root of the aorta. The third harmonic is intermediate in wave-length between these two and has a node in the proximal abdominal aorta (about 13 cm away) and another near the origin with an antinode in the thoracic aorta.

The positions of these relative nodes and antinodes will, of course, vary with the pulse-frequency and so one cannot generalize, except within wide limits, as to where they will occur. Even assuming that the reflecting conditions, which are modified greatly by changes in vasomotor activity, remained the same, the pulse-frequency might be only one-third of that in this experiment. The distances of the nodes would, correspondingly, be about 3 times farther away as all the wave-lengths would be increased. Then only the third and fourth harmonics would show a node, the former at the origin and the latter about 10 cm away from it.

With the particular example that we have been discussing we have seen that the distance from the heart to the main reflecting point is almost exactly a half wave-length for the second harmonic, and a wave-length for the fourth harmonic, and so at lengths at which resonance might be expected to occur. Nevertheless the variation in amplitude of these two components is not very marked. This emphasizes that even in conditions of frequency and wave velocity that might, theoretically, be expected to cause resonance, and hence great amplification of the oscillation at the antinodes, this does not occur. This must be attributed to the fact that the arterial system is highly damped, and reflections are incomplete.

So far a somewhat artificial simplicity has been created by neglecting the vascular systems of the two hind-limbs. This has been necessary in part because with measurements made with a catheter in the way that we did here, an occlusion of the femoral artery is involved. Therefore in withdrawing the catheter along the external iliac artery we are recording in a "blind end" with complete reflection where the catheter is held by a ligature. This means there is total wave-reflection 20 cm beyond the last point recorded. In addition the catheter is causing a relatively greater obstruction in these smaller arteries. Laszt and Müller (1952a) have already criticized this method of recording aortic-pulse waves as it was used by Hamilton and Dow (1939). Occlusion of one femoral artery caused an increase of amplitude of some 50 per cent in the 4 c/sec component in the pulse-wave recorded near the terminal division of the aorta (see Fig. 10 of McDonald and Taylor, 1959), but was barely perceptible 12·5 cm away in the proximal abdominal aorta or in the thoracic aorta. A similar effect is probably contributing to the unusually large increase in the modulus of the fundamental oscillation seen in Fig. 10.3. This emphasizes that when we talk of reflections occurring in the region of the pelvis these are not only due to anatomical subdivision of branches there, but also due to the added effects of reflections along both external iliac-femoral arteries.

It is more difficult to measure the pulse-wave at a similar number of points along the femoral artery without seriously distorting the flow. From Fig. 12.5 and the evidence from the arterial impedance discussed in the following sections it is clear that the reflections in the femoral bed arise from a closed end. The interactions of reflections arising there with those arising in the aorta from the pelvic region will again be dependent on wave-length relationships and so will differ for each frequency component.

Furthermore just as we have to consider a second reflection of reflected waves at the root of the aorta, so will reflected waves from the femoral bed tend to be reflected in turn as they arrive at the distal side of the aortic division. There is the added complication that, if that division is "closed" when looked at from the aortic aspect, it will be "open" when looked at from the iliac aspect.

In fact it is unusual to see clear node and antinode formation, such as we have been discussing in Fig. 10.3, beyond the first node at a quarter wave-length from a reflecting region. This again is to be attributed to the fact that reflection is only partial and the damping is very marked. Hence it is possible to arrive at a surprisingly simple interpretation of the reflection pattern because only the primary reflection is of any significant size.

The phase velocity distribution with frequency is also shown in Fig. 10.3 for three of the intervals between recording points. It has been seen in Ch. 9 that in a visco-elastic tube filled with liquid the wave-velocity would be expected to rise slightly with frequency. In the presence of reflections, however, the apparent rate of travel increases or decreases in a similar way to the distribution of antinodes and nodes of pressure. Thus it can be seen that the phase-velocity of the first harmonic at the root of the aorta rises from 360 cm/sec in the first interval to 460 cm/sec in the second, and at the end of the aorta is enormously increased to 1,500 cm/sec, as it approaches the antinode at the end of the aorta. The second harmonic which initially has almost the same velocity falls to 280 cm/sec in the second interval (which is close to its node) and then rises sharply to 1,000 cm/sec at the end of the aorta. Although it is generally agreed that the abdominal aorta has a higher elastic modulus than the thoracic aorta, this clearly cannot account for these wave velocity changes. In the first place the changes are far too great and even more strikingly, the frequency distribution is quite incompatible with any explanation based on changes in the wall.

THE EFFECT OF REFLECTIONS ON ARTERIAL IMPEDANCE

Hitherto we have only concerned ourselves with the pressure oscillations, but it is physiologically important to consider the flow. The pattern here is the reverse of that of pressure, that is an antinode of pressure corresponds to a node of flow and vice versa. In a tube with a closed end it is obvious that there can be no oscillatory flow at the dead end while we have seen that the pressure oscillation will be at a maximum. At a quarter wave-length distance the pressure oscillations will be at a minimum while the flow will be at a maximum oscillation. The easiest way to relate this behaviour of pressure and flow is in terms of the *fluid impedance*. As was pointed out in Ch. 5 this is, by analogy with alternating electric current, the term for oscillatory flow corresponding to the *fluid resistance* that is commonly used for steady flow. As

$$\text{Impedance} = \frac{\text{Pressure oscillation}}{\text{Flow oscillation}}$$

it can be seen, qualitatively, that near the closed end where the pressure oscillation is great and the flow very small the impedance is very high. Farther away, at a node, the pressure oscillation is at a minimum and the flow at a maximum, so that the impedance will also be at a minimum. The impedance measured at different points along the tube will therefore rise and fall in the same way as the pressure oscillations. This is illustrated by Fig. 10.4, which is a

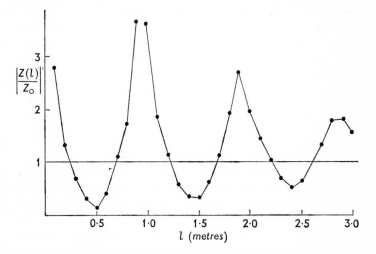

Fig. 10.4. The input impedance, as a ratio of the characteristic impedance (i.e. without reflections) in a rubber tube clamped at various distances from the pump. The model is the same as that used in Fig. 10.2; the frequency here is 7 c/sec throughout so that one wave-length is app. 2·0 metres. Ordinate—ratio of the moduli of the input impedance ($|Zl/Zo|$); abscissa—the distance, from the origin at which the pipe was clamped. The maxima and minima of impedance occur alternately at quarter wave-length intervals in a similar way to the pressure variations in Fig. 2. The effect of damping is shown by the progressively small deviations from the value of 1·0. (*Taylor*, 1957b.)

B.F.A.–P

plot of the modulus of the input impedance due to clamping off a length of rubber tube at different distances from a pump which is creating a known flow.

If the end is open there is a similar pattern of impedance changes but in this case the flow oscillations are at a maximum at the end and the impedance is at a minimum. At a quarter wave-length distance it has increased to a maximum and falls to a minimum again at the half wave-length position.

It is therefore clear that the effects of wave-reflection on measurements made at any single point depend not only on the nature of the ending but also on the distance from that end at which the measurements are made. At first it appears paradoxical when we think of impedance in similar terms to resistance, that a marked narrowing of the end, which will always increase the resistance, can reduce the impedance at certain regions of the pipe. The same applies to the amplitude of the oscillatory pressure and to the phase shift of the resultant wave motion (which is usually expressed as the apparent phase velocity). To interpret such observations it is necessary to record at more than one point to observe the direction of change of these parameters. In the rubber tube model the easiest way to do this is to make measurements at various points along the pipe. In the arterial system this is not usually easy for anatomical reasons, but we can make use of the fact that the distances with which we are concerned are fractions of wave-lengths and that wave-length varies approximately inversely with frequency. The reason this relation is not exact is that the wave-velocity increases with frequency (Ch. 9). An increase in frequency at a fixed point is, therefore, equivalent to making an observation at a greater fraction of a wave-length from the reflecting point. Such changes of frequency may be observed by attaching a pump through a cannula into the arterial system as has been done in preliminary experiments by McDonald and Taylor (1956). A simpler way involving less interference with physiological function is to use the natural pulse-wave and analyse the behaviour of each of its harmonic components independently.

The record of one set of measurements of the arterial input impedance in the femoral artery of a dog has been calculated in this way from the curves shown in Fig. 5.7. The impedance values are shown in Fig. 10.9 for the first eight harmonic components. It can be seen that the value is at a minimum for the frequency of

13·5 c/sec. By analogy with the evidence from Fig. 10.3, discussed in a previous section, we expect the termination of the femoral bed to act as a closed end. The frequency at which the minimum occurs will then indicate that the point of observation is about one-quarter wave-length from the main reflecting region. If this wave-velocity is 800 cm/sec, then the wave-length at 13·5 c/sec is approximately 60 cm. The main reflecting region was therefore 15 cm distant from the point of observation in mid-thigh. In this dog that distance placed the averaging reflecting region a few centimetres proximal to the ankle. If the ending had been open the distance would need to be 30 cm. This would be further than the total length of the leg and so again confirms that the ending must be of a closed type.

The overall change in the phasic flow patterns in different arteries which were discussed in Ch. 7 also emphasize that the ending is closed. The oscillatory component is progressively smaller in the more peripheral arteries (Fig. 12.5). The oscillatory pressure, however, is increasing so that the arterial impedance is increasing in all the major components (which are the low frequency ones—see Table IV).

THE REFLECTION AT A SINGLE ARTERIAL JUNCTION

The evidence that has been discussed seems to indicate that the major sites of wave-reflection are related to the fine arterial termination in a given vascular bed. In the case of the aorta, however, the reflecting-site may well be the actual branching of the aorta itself and indeed this has usually been assumed to be an important site of wave-reflection. In the arterial system we are always dealing with successive reflections which sum together. We can, however, predict theoretically what reflection may be expected at different types of junction, because reflection at a discontinuity is due to the difference of impedance on either side of it.

If an advancing wave of amplitude A_1 is partially reflected at a discontinuity so that a wave of amplitude A_2 is transmitted past it and a wave of amplitude A_3 is reflected, then at the junction

$$A_1 = A_2 + A_3 \dots\dots\dots\dots\dots 10.1$$

and the reflection-coefficient is the ratio of reflected to incident wave i.e. A_3/A_1. Similarly the ratio A_2/A_1 may be termed the transmission coefficient. These waves are, however, not separable but by analogy with electrical theory may be defined by the characteristic impedances on either side of the junction so that

$$A_3/A_1 = \text{Reflection coefficient } (R_f) = \frac{Z_T - Z_0}{Z_T + Z_0} = \frac{1 - Z_0/Z_T}{1 + Z_0/Z_T} \quad .. \ 10.2$$

where Z_0 is the characteristic impedance of the proximal tube and Z_T that of the terminal one; the ratio Z_0/Z_T is often indicated by λ. When the end is completely closed $Z_T = \infty$ and $R_f = +1$; conversely when the end is fully open $R_f = -1$. Partial reflections are often given as the equivalent percentages (as in Fig. 10.5).

In the simplest case we may ignore the effect of viscosity, as was done by Karreman (1952), then the value of λ (i.e. Z_0/Z_T) for a tube of radius r_1 and wave velocity c_1, making a junction with a tube of radius r_2 and wave velocity c_2, is such that

$$\lambda = (r_2{}^2/r_1{}^2)(c_1/c_2) \quad \ldots\ldots\ldots\ldots\ldots \ 10.3$$

or in the case of a bifurcation into two equal branches

$$\lambda = 2(r_2{}^2/r_1{}^2)(c_1/c_2) \quad \ldots\ldots\ldots\ldots\ldots \ 01.4$$

or for n equal branches $\quad \lambda = n(r_2{}^2/r_1{}^2)(c_1/c_2)$

Now if $c_1 = c_2$, i.e. the elastic properties of the vessel wall do not change, it can be seen that λ is the ratio of the cross-sectional areas of the vessels on either side of the junction. As when $\lambda = 1$ the reflection-coefficient is zero and no reflection occurs then, in the simplest case, partial reflection of a closed type will occur when the cross-sectional area of the bed decreases and of an open type when the cross-sectional area increases. In practice, however, the wave velocity in arteries always appears to increase as arteries pass peripherally, i.e. $c_2 > c_1$ so that the condition of zero reflection is at a bifurcation with an area-ratio greater than 1. Karreman (1952) calculated this assuming that the wall thickness remained unchanged, so that from the Moens equation (8.16)

$$c_1/c_2 = (r_2/r_1)^{1/2}$$

and then the point of zero-reflection is at an area-ratio, for a bifurcation, of approximately 1·15.

Womersley (1958b) extended this analysis by incorporating the full equation (5.22) of the impedance for a viscous liquid when, for the tethered elastic tube, he showed that

$$\lambda = 2\left(\frac{r_2}{r_1}\right)^2 \cdot \frac{c_1}{c_2} \left\{\frac{M'(a_2)}{M'(a_1)}\right\}^{1/2} e^{i \cdot 1/2(\varepsilon(\alpha_2) - \varepsilon(\alpha_1))} \quad \ldots\ldots\ldots \ 10.5$$

where $M'(a_2)$ is the appropriate value of M' for the value of a of the branch and correspondingly for the other values $M'(a_1)$, $\varepsilon(a_1)$ and $\varepsilon(a_2)$. The expression can be seen to be similar to that of Karreman with the additional factor to the right of c_1/c_2 which represents the effects of viscosity. Fig. 10.5 shows the resultant curves for values of a from 5 to 10 in the parent branch, values that are appropriate to the abdominal aorta of the dog or man. The assumption made again is that $c_1/c_2 = \left(\dfrac{r_2}{r_1}\right)^{1/2}$ as in Karreman's (1952) paper, and the latter author's curve ($a = \infty$) is also included for comparison. The general impression is that for relatively large values of a e.g. $a = 10$, the reflection conditions for blood are not very different from those of a non-viscous fluid, but the effect of viscosity is to shift the curves to the right. Points of considerable interest are:

(1) With a viscous fluid modulus and phase change in such a way that there is never exact matching of the systems although the minimum reflection at the point of "impedance matching" is only a few per cent.

(2) The area-ratios of branches that are found in the body which are about 1·15 to 1·25 (see Ch. 1) represent very small reflection coefficients in vessels of the calibre of those at the aortic bifurcation.

(3) The phase change from a 0° to a lag of 180° occurs more gradually in vessels containing a viscous liquid, so that in the vicinity of the minimal reflection conditions of intermediate phase shift can occur.

(4) If we regard a as a function of frequency it can be seen that the amount of reflection is not markedly frequency-dependent. There are marked proportional differences in the region of the minimum but the amplitude is so small here that this is of doubtful physiological significance.

It should be emphasized once more that this calculation is an abstraction concerned only with a single junction, with the assumption that the branches are themselves infinitely long tubes. It does, however, emphasize that in large elastic tubes very little reflection will occur unless the change in cross-sectional area is very considerably different from those found in the body. With smaller tubes the effect of viscosity becomes much more apparent and

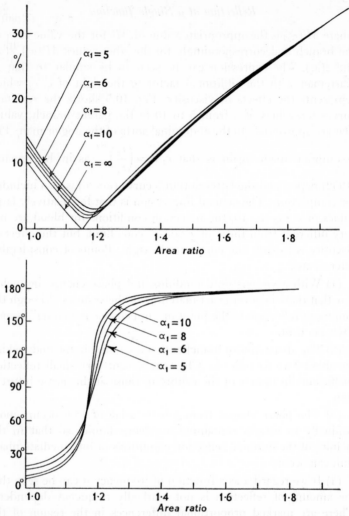

FIG. 10.5. The magnitude of reflections at the point of division of a tube into two equal branches. The radius of the single trunk is R and that of the branches is r. The corresponding wave-velocities (c_1 and c_2) are taken in this case as varying inversely with the square root of the radius, i.e. $c_1/c_2 = (r/R)^{1/2}$. Curves are drawn for four values of α_1 in the incident tube ($\alpha_1 = 5$, 6, 8 and 10) for tubes with limiting longitudinal constraint filled with a viscous fluid, and also for a non-viscous fluid ($\alpha_1 = \infty$). The abscissa is the ratio of the cross sectional area of the two branches to that of the incident tube, i.e. $2r^2/R^2$.

A. The amplitude of the reflected wave expressed as a percentage of the incident wave.

B. The phase-lag of the reflected wave. For the non-viscous fluid this changes from 0° to 180° at the point where the amplitude ratio is zero in A. A phase lag of 0° is a "closed" type of reflection and 180° is an "open" type. (*Womersley*, 1958*b*.)

Fig. 10.6 shows corresponding curves for bifurcations in which the parent branch has an $a=0.5$ (in the dog this represents the fundamental frequency of an artery of the order of the saphenous artery) and $a=2.0$. The same ratio for c_1/c_2 has been taken arbitrarily, in the absence of an exact knowledge, because this approximately offsets the retarding effect on wave velocity that viscosity has in small tubes (Fig. 9.3). The point of minimal reflection is shifted once more towards larger area-ratios; for $a=0.5$ this is now approximately 1·35 and any change in area at a junction smaller than this will cause a closed type of reflection. This value, it will be seen, is approaching that of the area-ratio for identical fluid resistance of steady flow across a bifurcation which is 1·414 (see Ch. 2). Just as it was shown that the resistance changes increase with the number of branches, so will the impedance change increase. This effect is much less with larger branches and if viscosity is neglected as in eqn. 10·5 the reflection is determined by the area ratio irrespective of the number of branches. This is to be expected as the oscillatory flow in small vessels has a pressure-flow relation very close to that of Poiseuille's equation, i.e. is largely determined by the viscosity whereas in large vessels it is mostly determined by the inertia of the liquid. This is also illustrated by the fact that the phase lag changes from 0° to 180° very rapidly at both small and large values of a but is much more gradual at intermediate values, e.g. $a=2.0$, 5·0.

Although it must be recognized that at still smaller vessels prediction of the amount of reflection at individual functions must be highly speculative, nevertheless, unless dramatic and unforeseen changes in the elastic behaviour of the wall occur, it may be expected that reflection will always be of the closed type. If the average area ratio change at each branching is 1·15 then the reflection coefficient in vessels of 1 mm diameter or less will probably be about 13 per cent. The total reflection from an arterial termination will be the summation of a succession of such branches very close together (close, that is, in terms of wave-length) but this will be offset to some extent by the increased viscous damping that occurs as the vessels diminish in size. Compared with this the effects of the origins of the major arterial branches would seem to be very small, for from Fig. 10.5 it can be seen that for an area-ratio of 1·15 the reflection coefficient for $a=5$ is about 4 per cent and for $a=10$ only about 2 per cent. However, calculations based on experimental

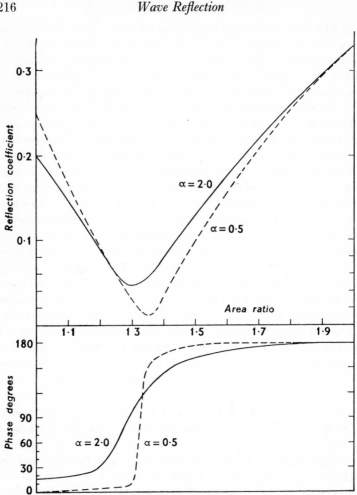

FIG. 10.6. Theoretical curves of the reflection conditions at a bifurcation calculated in the same way as those of Womersley in Fig. 10.5 but for smaller vessels. One curve is for $a=2\cdot0$ in the main artery and one for $a=0\cdot5$; the same wave-velocity assumptions are made. Ordinate—modulus of reflection-coefficient above; phase of reflection below. Abscissa—as in Fig. 10.5 the ratio of total cross-sectional areas of branches to that of main artery.

In the small artery it can be seen that the point of minimum reflection (or closest matching of impedance) is at an area ratio of 1.35 and the reflection is only 1 per cent. The limiting case as the vessels get smaller will be at the area ratio for matched resistance, i.e. 1·414 (see Ch. 2). The phase also changes rapidly from 0° to nearly 180°. The larger artery shows a more imperfect matching of impedance at the minimum although reflection is still only 4·3 per cent at this point; the reversal of phase is, however, much more gradual (cp. curve for $a=5$ in Fig. 10.5).

estimations in this laboratory (Womersley, 1958*b*) suggested a reflection coefficient of 14 per cent (phase shift 40°) at the terminal division of the aorta and about 7 per cent amplitude (phase app. 90°) at the coeliac axis. It should be noted that the simple description above, of "open" and "closed" end reflection effects, cannot be applied to discontinuities where the phase shift is markedly different from 0° or 180°.

The actual reflection-coefficient in the femoral vascular bed of the dog under normal experimental conditions was calculated from the measured phase velocities by the formula of Taylor (1957*a*) and found to be about 50 per cent (using the distance from the reflecting-point estimated from the impedance measurements— see Fig. 10·8). Taylor's paper gives elegant formulae for calculation of the reflection coefficient from the phase-velocities, and he has derived a similar one for the input impedances, but they require the knowledge of the true values of the phase-velocity and the characteristic impedance, i.e. their values in the absence of reflections. These can only be derived indirectly in the arterial tree so that this estimation must only be regarded as very approximate; calculations from the input impedances suggest normal values of the reflection coefficient not higher than 30–40 per cent in the hind-limb.

THE EFFECT OF WAVE-REFLECTION ON PHASE-VELOCITY

When considering the wave-velocity of a single sinusoidal oscillation it must be expressed as the rate of travel of points of identical phase. It is thus dependent on the rate of change of phase in respect to distance, i.e. $d\phi/dz$, and if the circular frequency is ω then the wave velocity is given by

$$c = \omega/d\phi/dz \quad \dots\dots\dots\dots\dots \quad 10.6$$

As the phase-shift has to be measured over a finite interval then the equation used is

$$c = \frac{2\pi f \cdot \Delta z}{\Delta \phi} \quad \dots\dots\dots\dots\dots \quad 10.7$$

When there is no reflection of the wave then the wave velocity is determined by elastic properties of the pipe, but as was seen in Chs. 8 and 9, will vary with frequency owing to the viscous properties of the wall and the viscosity of the fluid within it.

If there is a reflected wave component, however, we have already seen that this interacts with the incident wave and the resultant wave shows waxing and waning of amplitude at different regions of the pipe. Similarly the rate-of-change of phase also varies and hence the *apparent* phase-velocity. This is termed the apparent phase-velocity to distinguish it from the *true* phase-velocity, which is determined by the physical properties of the wall and the contained liquid. The appreciation of the modification of phase shift due to reflections is not easy to see intuitively but may be determined mathematically (Taylor, 1957a). As has been noted above, we find that the apparent phase-velocity in the presence of reflections varies in the same way as the amplitude of the pressure oscillations, with the exception that close to an open-end it continues to rise when the pressure oscillation would be falling. This difference may for the present be ignored as we appear to be concerned in the circulation with reflections of the closed type. Fig. 10.7 shows the variations in apparent phase-velocity in a long rubber pipe that was completely shut off at one end. Measurements over a finite distance will, of course, represent an average of the phase-velocities over that interval. The longer the interval, as a fraction of the wave-length, the more will this average tend to represent the true wave velocity. This is the probable explanation

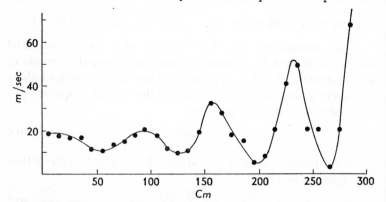

FIG. 10.7. The apparent phase velocity measured in a rubber pipe occluded at 300 cm from the end (the same model as in Fig. 10.2 and 10.4). The frequency was 10 c/sec and the true value of the phase velocity in the pipe without reflections was 14·1 m/sec. The apparent phase-velocity, like the input impedance (Fig. 10.4), oscillated about the value found in the absence of reflections with the first minimum approximately one-quarter wave-length from the distal end of the pipe. The diminution in these variations in velocity, as measurements are made further from that end, is due to damping. (*Taylor*, 1957b.)

of the differences between results that have been recorded by various authors.

The first detailed study of phase-velocities was that of Porjé (1946). He recorded the pulse wave in man at the subclavian artery together with that in the abdominal aorta or in the femoral artery. He made a Fourier analysis of the waves, though only of the first three harmonics, and calculated the apparent phase-velocities for each in the way described above. He found that for the fundamental this was always markedly above that of the rate of travel of the "foot" of the wave, and the same was usually true of the second harmonic. The third harmonic, however, usually had a similar velocity to that of the foot of the wave. These findings he attributed to the presence of reflections. Kapal, Martini and Wetterer (1951) repeated his experiments and obtained similar results. In this laboratory (Fig. 10.8) we have measured phase-velocities over shorter intervals of 5–10 cm in the aorta of the dog (McDonald and Taylor, 1957) and also in the femoral artery.

We have already seen that the apparent phase-velocities of the fundamental frequencies measured in the aorta of the dog can

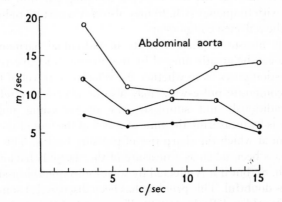

FIG. 10.8. The apparent phase velocities (measured over a 7 cm interval) of the first five harmonic components of the pulse-wave in the abdominal aorta of a dog (●—small full circles). As discussed in the text the rise in these velocities, especially of the lower frequency terms, is considered to be due to the effect of reflections (cp. Fig. 10.7). This is borne out by the fact that the apparent phase velocities are generally increased by artificially increasing the amount of reflection; first, by occluding one external iliac artery (◑—half-full circles), and second by occluding both (○—large open circles). The initial velocities of the first and second harmonics were unusually low for the distal aorta in this experiment (cp. Fig. 10.3 and 12.5). (*Unpublished figure from data of McDonald and Taylor,* 1957.)

change from 380 cm/sec in the root of the aorta to 1,500 cm/sec in the region of the aortic "bifurcation" (Fig. 10.3). The apparent velocity of the second harmonic increased almost as dramatically. Other results are illustrated in Ch. 12. Similar results have been recorded by Landowne (personal communication) in the human subject using a long cardiac catheter. In man he usually found that the apparent phase-velocity was increased above the "pulse-wave velocity" even in the proximal aorta in distinction to the findings in Fig. 10.3. In some cases this is also found in the dog and each example needs to be interpreted in terms of the wave-lengths of the frequencies being considered. This finding in the human agrees with the finding of Porjé (1946) that, even measured over the long interval that he used, the apparent phase-velocity of the low frequency components may be very high. As noted the large interval would tend to average out variations in velocity of the higher frequency components. Using much shorter intervals we have found in the dog (where wave-lengths are shorter owing to the higher pulse-frequency) that only the fifth harmonic shows a relative stability of velocity. This we attribute to the averaging effect of the finite interval, but the fact that the damping per unit length increases with frequency (Ch. 9) may also play a part by reducing the size of the reflected component.

If the measured phase-velocity of individual harmonic components can be greatly altered by the presence of wave-reflection, the question arises as to whether the velocity of travel of the front of the composite pulse-wave may also be affected by reflections. The traditional, and simplest, way of recording pulse-wave velocity is by measuring the time of travel of the foot of the wave—the point at which the sharp rise of pressure begins. This velocity has always been taken as a measure of the elastic behaviour of the wall (Ch. 8), but if it is affected by wave-reflection this assumption becomes doubtful. This problem has been discussed at some length by McDonald and Taylor (1959). They concluded that, the velocity of the "foot", or points near it as used by Kapal *et al.* (1951), was largely determined by the phase-velocities of the higher frequency components. For reasons discussed above these, when measured over a practicable interval, appear to be relatively unaffected by reflections, so that the "foot-to-foot" velocity is the most useful measurement in relation to studying the elastic properties of the wall. This correlation becomes less reliable as the points of observation approach the periphery, when reflection may cause an increase of all the measurable harmonic components and may well give an exaggerated idea of the increase in arterial rigidity in the more peripheral arteries.

THE RELATION OF APPARENT PHASE VELOCITY TO IMPEDANCE

The measurement of phase-velocity like that of the amplitude of the pressure oscillations, can provide information about the presence of reflected waves in a system. Both of these variables require that the pulse form be recorded at at least two points. Equally we have also seen that the measurement of the pressure and the flow at one point gives an estimate of the arterial impedances at the component frequencies of the pulse, and from these one can make deductions concerning the reflection conditions. It is of interest to consider the relations between these different aspects.

The simplest relationship in the consideration of pulsatile flow is that between the pressure-gradient and the oscillatory flow (eqn. 5.2). This is independent of the presence of reflections when a true difference in pressure is recorded, although strictly speaking it only applies to the gradient at a point. Measuring it over a finite interval introduces a small error but this is negligible provided the distance between recording points is reasonably small. Taylor (personal communication) has shown, for instance, that in the femoral artery for an interval of 8 cm between the cannula the error is only about 1·5 per cent for a frequency of 10 c/sec.

The pressure-gradient is related to pressure-wave by the relation (eqn. 5.11)

$$\frac{\partial P}{\partial z} = -\frac{1}{c} \cdot \frac{\partial P}{\partial t}$$

where c has its complex value (eqn. 9.9). In the presence of reflections we can take c as approximately equal to the apparent phase velocity. As the flow is directly related to the amplitude of $\partial P/\partial z$ it can be seen that if the modulus of $\partial P/\partial t$ remains constant but c increases, then the flow decreases. The constant amplitude of $\partial P/\partial t$ implies the constant amplitude of P, hence the impedance, which is pressure divided by flow, also increases. We see, therefore, why it is that in situations where the impedance is increased, the apparent phase velocity is also increased. This explains the apparently paradoxical situation where peripheral vasoconstriction causes an increase in the pulse-pressure but a reduction in the pulsatile flow.

It would appear that either method is equally suitable for studying the effect of changes in peripheral vascular bed upon the oscillatory flow. In practice measurement of the arterial impedance is probably the more direct and potentially more accurate. In view of the criticism offered in Ch. 6 about many flowmeters in use this may seem curious, but that criticism was mainly concerning the distortion of flow that was caused by the meter. Provided that the meters record accurately the flow passing into the vascular bed that is being studied, and provided that the arterial pressure related to that flow is measured, i.e. on the distal side of the meter, then the estimation of input impedance is still correct. The flow recorded may not accurately represent the normal physiological pattern in that vessel; but if it is altered then the arterial pressure wave on the distal side of the meter will also be altered. That pressure and that flow will, however, still be related by the input impedance which is determined by the form of the peripheral bed and its distance from the recording point.

Arterial impedance was apparently first measured by Randall and Stacy (1956*b*). Their electromagnetic flowmeter has a long catheter system which introduces marked damping, and has already been discussed in Ch. 6. Unfortunately they appear to have derived their impedance from the pressure measured at the flowmeter, so that the measured value is that of the vascular bed plus a length of some 15 cm of polythene catheter. This probably accounts for their values of impedance being much higher than those measured in this laboratory, which are discussed below. The method of recording flow in our own experiments have been either the cinematograph method (Ch. 6) or more recently by use of a differential manometer to record the pressure-gradient, and deriving the flow by the use of eqn. 5.6 (Bergel, McDonald and Taylor, 1958). While there is still lack of general agreement about the accuracy of flow recording, it must be recognized that results so far are of a preliminary nature, and the normal range of values will not be established until many more results have been obtained from different laboratories. The discussion above aims, however, to analyse the basis for impedance measurement so that it should be possible at least to sift probable results from those that are manifestly impossible.

By comparison the method of estimating the apparent phase velocity has the advantage that it only requires the use of manometers, and that the characteristics of these instruments have been more closely investigated than have those of flowmeters. Measurement of the phase shift of harmonic components over short distances, however, seems to be very liable to error. Where there is a marked reflection the phase shifts may be very small. As the derivation of velocity involves the reciprocal of this small value, small errors in estimating it can create large variations in the calculated values. The precise matching of manometers with their cannula systems, especially as regards accuracy in phase, is more difficult than is generally assumed. In the present stage of exploratory investigation it is valuable to compare investigations of reflection conditions by both methods, but in my opinion the impedance measurement is easier to interpret and more directly related to the behaviour of the flow with which, as circulatory physiologists, we are primarily concerned.

THE EFFECT OF VASOMOTOR CHANGES ON ARTERIAL IMPEDANCE

The graph of one estimation of arterial impedances has already been discussed (Fig. 10.9) in relation to the expected form of the curve. The impedance here is also quoted in mm Hg/cm³/sec in order that they may be compared with values for the peripheral resistance, which is commonly measured in the physiological literature as Peripheral Resistance Units (P.R.U.) which are mm Hg/cm³/min. In the example in Fig. 10.9 the mean flow was 0·85 cm³/sec (51 cm³/min) and the mean arterial pressure approximately 100 mm Hg, so that the peripheral resistance was about 2 P.R.U. or 120 mm Hg/cm³/sec. The highest impedance (for the fundamental) was less than one-tenth of this, being only 10·4 mm Hg/cm³/sec. This value may be rather low but it indicates that the impedance which is a measure of the "obstruction" to flow of the part of the vascular bed in which pulsatile flow occurs is much less than the resistance which is largely dominated by the fine arterioles and capillaries. Randall and Stacy (1956b) obtained a value of about 1·0 P.R.U. (i.e. 60 mm Hg/cm³/sec) for their fundamental component. This is nearly 6 times as great as that which we record here, but as mentioned above they appear to have included part of the impedance of their flowmeter catheter in this measurement.

Even their higher value is still considerably lower than that of the actual peripheral resistance.

The usual analogy for electrical current in terms of fluid mechanics is that of flow-velocity rather than of volume flow. In Ch. 5 (eqn. 5.22) the impedance was defined in these terms. This

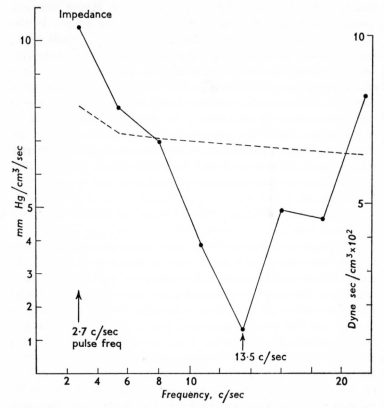

Fig. 10.9. The modulus of the input impedance of the first eight harmonics recorded in the dog femoral artery—full line. This is the same experiment in which the flow curve is displayed in Fig. 5.7. The dotted line represents the characteristic impedance which was used in the calculated flow curve, i.e. assuming that there were no reflections. The differences between the two explain the deviation of the calculated from the observed curves in Fig. 5.7.

The pulse frequency was 2·7 c/sec and there is a minimum of impedance in the fifth harmonic (13·5 c/sec). One quarter wave-length at this frequency is about 15 cm and, as discussed in the text, the graph indicates that the main site of reflections is this distance from the point of observations.

Ordinate—input impedance; scale on left in mm Hg/cm³/sec (i.e. 1/60 of the conventional Peripheral Resistance unit—P.R.U.); scale on right dyne. sec/cm³. These latter units are used for Fig. 10.10 and 10.11 where other impedance values are shown.

has the advantage that the flow-velocity is less dependent on the size of different vessels than is the volume flow. The correct physical units to define fluid impedance would, therefore, appear to be as dynes/cm² (pressure) per cm/sec (flow velocity) or dyne. sec/cm³. This is the standard unit for defining mechanical or acoustic impedances. In the curve already discussed the conversion factor is 94 so that 10·4 mm Hg/cm³/sec is equivalent to $9·8 \times 10^2$ dyne.sec/cm³ (see ordinate scales in Fig. 10.9). The corresponding characteristic impedance is also shown in Fig. 10.9; the curves represent the impedance values taken for the calculated flow curve (Fig. 5.7) which was seen to fit the observed curve fairly well. The differences between the actual impedances as measured and those used in the calculation (which was based on the gradient derived from the time-derivative and pulse-wave velocity (eqn. 5.11) and therefore assumed that the value of c for all components was the same) explains the lack of coincidence in the two curves.

The mean value of the characteristic impedance is rather high relative to the values of the input impedance in Fig. 10.9—one would expect it to be closer to the minimum than it is. As the calculated impedance was based on a wave velocity value of 500 cm/sec whereas a value of 800 cm/sec is more probably correct at least for the higher frequencies, it can be seen (eqn. 5.22) that the characteristic impedance should, in fact, be higher. (The wave velocity of 500 cm/sec was measured by Hale, McDonald, Taylor and Womersley (1955) from peak-to-peak, and it is not clear at present why this value is so different from the usual foot-to-foot velocity, although this point is discussed by McDonald and Taylor, 1959.) Therefore, the measured input impedances are almost certainly too low. The explanation for this is almost certainly due to the tendency for over-estimation of flow-velocity by the bubble method (Ch. 6)—a conclusion which is solely based on these calculations, for it can be seen (Fig. 6.3) that Shipley *et al.* (1943) with the orifice meter recorded flows that are apt to show even greater pulsatile variations than my own.

It is of some interest to try and determine the reflection coefficient from the input impedance. The coefficient can be defined by the terminal impedance (Z_T) and the characteristic impedance (Z_0)—eqn. 10.2. Although we do not know the terminal impedance it is reasonable to suppose that, in a situation like that shown in Fig. 10.9, the input impedance of the lowest frequency is fairly close to the value of the terminal impedance. This assertion is based on the fact that, if the point of observation is one quarter wavelength from the termination for the frequency of the fifth harmonic, then it is only one-twentieth of a wave-length for the fundamental frequency and will not have fallen much in this distance. Calculated on this basis Rf in Fig. 10.9 is only 0·12. This is too low because the impedance values are too low, as indicated above. The value of the reflection coefficient we are currently obtaining in similar conditions is 0·3–0·4.

The changes that are found in the input impedance with changes in vasomotor activity are illustrated in Fig. 10.10. Fig. 10.10*a* shows measurements made in the femoral artery of the same animal under normal conditions and during marked vasoconstriction (intra-arterial nor-adrenaline). They are only analysed to 5 harmonics and a minimum cannot be placed with as much certainty as in Fig. 10.9. It can be seen, however, that the input impedance of the low frequencies is greatly increased, thus indicating a considerable rise in the reflection coefficient. Correspondingly the minimum of the input impedance would be expected to be lower and this seems probable from the graphs shown in Fig. 10.10*a*. In Fig. 10.10*b* we have some impedance values calculated for vasodilatation (from the experiment shown in Fig. 5.8). There is a fall in the input impedance for the low frequencies, but compared with the rise with vasoconstriction it is small (upper curve in Fig. 10.10*b* is measured in the same dog—for flow curve see Fig. 7.7). The "normal" curve is the same as Fig. 10.9. The changes in reflection coefficient these curves represent are normal —0·12; vasodilatation—0·06; vasoconstriction—0·55. If the normal were in fact about 0·35, the other values would be about 0·23 and 0·65—a fall of about 34 per cent, and a rise of some 85 per cent. As the vasomotor changes were here caused by the intra-arterial drugs they must be expected to be maximal. It is clear, from the numerous qualifications made, that I do not regard these values as being at all accurate.

From the fact that the reflection coefficient can be altered so greatly by vasomotor activity, it is clear that a large part of the wave-reflection occurs in the arterioles. It is to be expected that some of the wave-reflection occurs at arterial branches, i.e. vessels that are not altered in size by vasomotor activity. It does not seem possible at present to differentiate this reflection from that in the arteriolar bed because even vasodilatation does not abolish the latter. It merely means that the pulsatile flow penetrates farther, as it were, into the smallest vessels—capillary flow may even become pulsatile. This will move the ultimate site of reflection more peripherally but as the distances involved will be fractions of a millimetre it will be unmeasurable. On the other hand, because

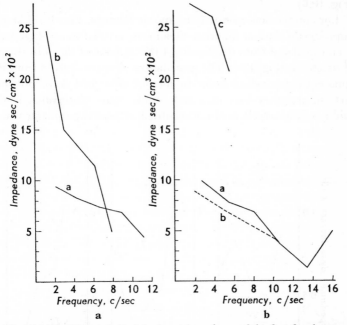

Fig. 10.10. **a.** The moduli of the input impedance of the first five harmonic components measured in the femoral artery of a dog. The flow in these curves was derived from the pressure-gradient recorded with a differential manometer (described in Fig. 11.2) with simultaneous measurement of the arterial pressure (*Bergel, et al.*, 1958).

(*a*) "Normal".

(*b*) After vasoconstriction due to intra-arterial injection of 10 μg noradrenaline. This causes increased wave-reflection with marked increase of impedance in the low frequency components.

b. Some input impedance values showing the effect of vasomotor changes. These are calculated from the pressure and the flow velocity recorded by the high-speed cinematograph method.

(*a*) "Normal" (taken from Fig. 5.7 and 10.9).

(*b*) (broken line) Vasodilatation due to intra-arterial injection of 100 μg acetylcholine (Fig. 5.8).

(*c*) Vasoconstriction with 10 μg i.a. noradrenaline (only three harmonics are shown—Fig. 7.7).

Vasodilatation appears to have a very small effect compared with vasoconstriction but, as discussed in the text, the changes in reflection coefficient are less disparate.

the waves can be thought of as going farther along the minute
vessels, and being more heavily damped, before they are finally
reflected, the reflected waves will be smaller. This would seem to be
the principal cause of the reduction of reflection in vasodilatation
although an increase in the cross-sectional area beyond any given
point of branching will reduce reflection if it is initially "closed"
(Fig. 10.6).

For comparison with the vasomotor changes, Fig. 10.11 shows
impedance values at different sites in the arterial tree. These have
been calculated from the results of the analysis of the pulse-waves
illustrated in Fig. 12.5. The impedances here are derived from the
apparent phase-velocities by the method described in the previous
section, and they vary in a very similar way. Unfortunately the
calibre of the vessels were not recorded in these experiments which

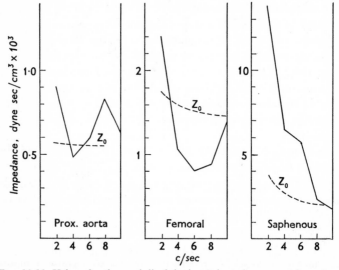

FIG. 10.11. Values for the moduli of the input impedance at various sites in
the arterial tree. These are derived from the pressure and the apparent phase-
velocity using the data displayed in Fig. 12.5 (the analysis of the recorded pressure pulses of Laszt and Muller 1952*a* and *b* and shown in Fig. 12.4). The broken
lines show the characteristic impedance (Z_0) in each situation. Abscissa—frequency in c/sec. Ordinate—input impedance (note that the vertical scale is
different in each graph, and all are one-tenth of that used in Fig. 10.9 and
10.10).

Arbitrary values for the internal diameter of the vessel have been taken as
follows: Prox. aorta—1·0 cm; femoral—0·3 cm; saphenous—0·08 cm. The
significance of the change in the frequency distribution of the impedance is discussed in the text.

are those of Laszt and Müller (1952*a*, *b*) so that arbitrary values
have been used, which are recorded in the legend to the figure, and
the impedance values are only approximate. The impedance distribution in the femoral artery is similar to that shown in Fig. 10.9
which is also recorded in the same vessel although the absolute
values are higher. The minimum here, however, is at a frequency
of 6 c/sec. The animal, however, is clearly a large one and the main
reflecting site at a quarter wave-length is found to be some 10 cm
beyond the point at which the saphenous artery pressure recording
was made, i.e. in the region of the foot. By comparison the impedance pattern in the saphenous artery is seen to be falling
sharply over all the frequencies measured. The difference between
this graph and that for the femoral artery is due to proximity of
the reflecting site. These impedances are measured over a long
interval (25 cm) and so it is more difficult to estimate the distance
from the main reflecting region. If we measure from the centre of
the interval a quarter of a wave-length is 27 cm at the frequency of
the point of lowest impedance, i.e. 14·5 cm beyond the distal
recording-point as compared with 10 cm for the femoral artery
estimation. As there is no indication that the impedance at 10 *c*/sec
is a minimum—in fact, as its value there is close to the calculated
value of the characteristic impedance it is almost certainly not a
minimum—this small discrepancy in estimated distances may be
explained.

In the graph of the impedances in the proximal aorta it can be
seen that there is a well-defined minimum at a frequency of about
4 c/sec. This indicates a reflecting site at a distance of 27 cm which,
taken from the distal point of recording (see Fig. 12.5), is in the
region of the bifurcation of the aorta, a region which was seen in
Fig. 10.3 to cause marked reflection phenomena in the aorta.

The values of the characteristic impedance for each curve are
also shown in Fig. 10.11. It can be seen that the characteristic
impedance at 2 c/sec is 0·56 dyne.sec/cm^3 in the proximal aorta,
1·67 in the femoral artery and 3·75 in the saphenous artery. The
increase in impedance is to be expected as we move into small
vessels by analogy with the resistance to steady-flow. The increase
is, however, surprisingly small when compared with the Poiseuille
resistance which will be larger by a factor of 100 in the saphenous
artery than in the proximal aorta (when recorded in comparable
units, i.e. pressure/average velocity). This increase in impedance

in the smaller vessels shows that all reflections will be of the closed type.

Although the arterial impedance may be derived indirectly there is little doubt that the best way to find it is by direct measurement of pressure and flow. To obtain accurate values requires very careful calibration of both manometer and flowmeter, because for the third and higher harmonics we are dealing with the ratios of components of small amplitude. For practical purposes, once normal values have been established experimentally, the calculation of the first two harmonics will quite likely give most of the information that we need for determining changes in reflection etc. All the discussion above has only been concerned with the modulus of the impedance (see end of Ch. 5); it is possible that the investigation of the accompanying phase changes may add to the information we can derive from this analysis. The work of collecting experimental data on impedance should, in itself, settle many of the disputes about the accuracy of flowmeters which were discussed in Ch. 6. As a quantitative method it is to be hoped that input impedance will be as useful in circulatory physiology as the measurement of the peripheral resistance has been.

THE REFLECTION OF ISOLATED PULSES

The simplest example of wave-reflection that is familiar in everyday life is that of a sound-echo. In a model a similar demonstration can be made by creating a short pressure pulse in a long rubber tube filled with water. If the end of the tube is closed a positive wave returns in the same sense and from an open end it returns inverted as a negative wave. Analysis on this basis would appear to be much simpler than in terms of the sinusoidal oscillations we have been considering, and indeed virtually all previous studies have been along these lines. In the arterial tree, however, difficulties arise in interpretation which have been discussed by McDonald and Taylor (1959) and so will only be outlined here.

In the first place no reflection of a pulse can be observed at the origin of a long rubber tube, until the pulse has travelled to the end and back (e.g. Fig. 2, McDonald and Taylor, 1959). This we may call the "round-trip" time and it will be determined by the wave velocity of the tube and the length of the tube. The height of the pulse will also be reduced by damping and its shape spread out by dispersion, i.e. the difference in wave velocity of the different frequency components of the pulse (Ch. 9). These effects need not concern us at the moment and will be discussed in the next chapter.

If the duration of the pulse is longer than the "round-trip" time the first reflection will be superimposed on it. If the system has many reflecting points this mixture of the original pulse and its reflections may be difficult to interpret. The front of the wave at the origin, however, will always represent the initial disturbance because there is no time for reflections to arrive back and alter it. Theoretically the "round-trip" time for the earliest reflected waves may be very short, for example, if they come from the large branches in the arch of the aorta. In practice, however, the major reflecting sites that have been considered are more remote. The usual ones that have been postulated are in the region of the bifurcation of the aorta (Wezler and Boger, 1939; Sinn, 1956), or in the periphery of the limbs (Frank, 1905; Hamilton and Dow, 1939; Wetterer, 1956). The results presented in the earlier part of this chapter support the location of a closed type of reflection at these sites, although it is directly opposed to the views of Wezler and his colleagues who supposed that the end of the aorta behaves as an open end. The evidence for this was, however, very indirect, for it depended on the so-called period of resonance of the windkessel representing a quarter wave-length.

Considered as a transient response, the first pressure rise of the aortic pulse is determined by the velocity of injection of fluid and the elastic properties of the root of the aorta, and is governed approximately by the "water-hammer" formula (eqn. 9.1). This sharply defined front is especially clear in the response of the aorta to an experimental injection of fluid recorded by Peterson (1954). It is assumed, of course, that the effects of any previous pulse have completely died away, but this is implicit in regarding the pulse as an isolated event.

The requirement that the time of appearance of a reflection is determined by its "round-trip" time has not always been fulfilled in some interpretations of the pulse form that have been advanced in the past. We see that the arteries in any situation cannot respond to a pulse before it arrives, whether it is travelling from the heart or from a peripheral reflecting-point. The introduction of terms such as "resonance" or "standing-waves" to account for apparent synchronous events in different parts of the tree actually leads to additional difficulties. These phenomena must depend on repeated reflections, first from the periphery and then from the heart end and so on. Not until we have sets of centrifugal and centripetal waves interacting can anything of this sort appear, and so it can only occur late in the time-course of the pulse. The round-trip time over the length of the dog's aorta alone is about 0·2 sec, and we cannot consider anything in the nature of resonance until the wave has been over the system at least twice. This immediately raises another problem, in the isolated pulse analysis, for twice the "round-trip" time even for the aorta is close to that of the pulse duration. In Fig. 12.1, for example, the cycle length is only 0·35 sec and so less than twice the time taken to traverse the aorta. Fig. 12.1 can, in fact, be interpreted (with a little imagination) as showing a single reflected wave—the drawn-out pressure rise in the diastolic part of the first (most proximal) curve might be a partial reflection at the end of the aorta of the initial pressure rise due to cardiac ejection. In successive curves one can distinguish a rise in pressure in diastole which is progressively fused with the systolic wave—as one would find if one component was travelling away from the heart and one towards it. The time relations fit in with this interpretation and it can be seen that not only is this first "reflected" wave of small amplitude, but that there is no time in the pulse interval for this process to be repeated.

A certain amount of qualitative information can be derived from descriptive analysis of this sort. In this case the deduction that there is a "positive" or "closed" reflection in the region of the bifurcation of the aorta fits in with the results of the Fourier analysis displayed in Fig. 10.3. The analysis, however, also shows that for a compound wave of this kind it is impossible to speak of "*the* node" of the aorta because the distribution of nodes is different for the various frequency components. The phenomenon of close synchronization of the peaks of pressure and the increase of the amplitude of those peaks can be explained by the interaction of incident and reflected waves without using terms such as "standing waves". When the term is applied to the wave form obtained by measuring the pressure difference between two points in the arterial system (e.g. Hamilton, 1944) it becomes misleading, for it is in fact the form of the pressure-gradient. This is carried to extreme by Spencer and Denison (1956) who measured the difference over 4 cm and then said "this represents the standing-wave in the aorta". Terms such as this have a specific and restricted meaning in physics so that using them in a different sense in physiology can only introduce confusion.

CONCLUSIONS

Referring once again to the doubts expressed by various workers there can be no question as to the existence of reflections. The analogy with a sound absorbing system which was quoted is perhaps a good example of the dangers of neglecting the scale of events in such a comparison. In terms of the wave-lengths we are dealing with, the arterial system is a short one. To eliminate reflections would be comparable with trying to build a perfect sound absorber only about 1 foot long (for the frequency of top C) —so perfect that no distortion could be detected anywhere within it. Nothing approximating to complete reflection occurs anywhere in the arterial tree, and the damping is undoubtedly considerable. At the same time any point of observation is usually less than a quarter wave-length from a major reflecting site, and even small reflections can produce marked local changes in wave-behaviour. These changes, of course, involve both the pressure and the flow and consist of alterations of amplitude and of phase. Both may be used to measure reflection effects although they may be more compactly expressed in terms of the input impedance.

CHAPTER XI

THE DESIGN OF MANOMETERS

Although the main concern of this book has been with the study of pulsatile flow in the circulation this is, of course, intimately connected with the pulsatile pressures. As there is considerable experimental evidence on the pressure wave forms in the arterial tree it is useful to survey this topic. Since the value of this work depends on the fidelity of response of the manometers used it is necessary to discuss the performance of those instruments in common use. The theory on which the design of adequate manometers has been based dates from the work of Frank (1903) and has been greatly extended by his pupils and other workers in subsequent years. As very detailed studies are available, notably those of Hansen (1949) and Hansen and Warburg (1950), the present review will confine itself to the main outlines of the subject. The purposes for which a manometer is used do, however, change our ideas as to its optimum design. Our own quantitative work on the behaviour of the harmonic components of the pressure and flow waves, and especially the complex fluid impedance, emphasizes the importance of both amplitude and phase distortions resulting from manometer performance. The subject of phase distortion, in particular, has tended to be neglected even though Hansen's work has investigated it thoroughly. To be useful in practical terms, however, it is essential first to discuss what frequencies in the pulse-wave we are going to regard as important.

THE FREQUENCY COMPONENTS OF THE PRESSURE PULSE

The main characteristics of a manometer designed to measure oscillating pressure are usually expressed as frequency-response curves, i.e. the graphs of the recorded amplitude and of the phase shift when the manometer is tested with known oscillatory pressures of simple harmonic form (Figs. 11.2 and 11.3). The accuracy to which the various frequency components of the pulse-wave need to be recorded must, therefore, be discussed before the adequacy of any given manometers can be assessed. In addition, as Fourier series have been used extensively throughout the work reviewed in this book, it is desirable to assess the ability of such a

234

series, taken to a relatively small number of terms, to represent the physical events we are recording. The qualification of a small number of terms is necessary, at present, for practical reasons because, otherwise, the method becomes far too laborious.

THE VARIANCE OF A CURVE

To assess the adequacy of a given number of Fourier components to represent a given curve we make use of Parseval's theorem. This states that the variance of a finite set of n harmonic components is given by

$$\text{Variance (series)} = \frac{1}{2} \sum_{n=1}^{n=n} M_n^2 \quad \dots \dots \dots \dots 11.1$$

where M_n is the modulus of the nth component.

The variance of the whole curve is derived from the sum of the squares of the deviation from their mean value. Thus if we measure m ordinates of value y_i (and having a mean value of $\bar{y}$) then

$$\text{Variance} = \frac{1}{m} \sum_{i=1}^{i=m} (y_i - \bar{y})^2 \quad \dots \dots \dots \dots 11.2$$

This is more usually calculated in the following way

$$\text{Variance} = \frac{1}{m} \sum_{i=1}^{i=m} y_i^2 - \left(\frac{1}{m} \sum_{i=1}^{i=m} y_i\right)^2 \quad \dots \dots \dots \dots 11.3$$

The variance of the series that has been calculated from eqn. 11.1 can then be expressed as a fraction, or percentage, of the total variance of the recorded curve. Some values of typical curves are shown in Table IV.

TABLE IV

Recording site		Accumulated sum of the squares of the moduli as percentage of the total variance					
		1	1+2	1+2+3	1+2+3 +4	1+2+3 +4+5	Freq. range
1P	Asc. aorta	56·0	85·3	91·8	94·0	97·6	2·22–11·1
2P	Thor. aorta	63·76	85·4	87·9	90·3	94·8	2·22–11·1
3P	Abd. aorta (prox.)	59·3	90·97	94·25	96·1	97·8	2·22–11·1
4P	Abd. aorta (distal)	56·3	89·2	92·9	94·8	98·0	2·22–11·1
5P	Abd. aorta (distal)	54·9	91·0	96·9	97·8	99·1	2·0–10·0
6P	Femoral	52·45	93·9	99·1	99·41	99·44	2·7–13·5
7P	Saphenous	40·3	84·3	92·0	93·9	98·01	2·0–10·0
8Q	Femoral	37·8	86·46	95·6	97·3	97·8	2·7–13·5
9	Square wave (half-period)	81·1	81·1	90·1	90·1	93·4	—
10	Half rect.: sine wave (1/3 period)	59·6	90·0	98·1	98·6	98·7	—

The accuracy of fit of a Fourier series may be estimated by comparing the variance of the curve with the sum of the squares of the moduli of the harmonic components (eqns. 11.1 and 11.2). The variance of the curve is a measure of its energy content and it can be seen that 5 harmonic terms always give a good measure of the curve and that the first two frequency components account for at least 85 per cent.

The curves marked P are pressure curves; 8Q is a flow curve; the last two are artificial curves (see Fig. 11.1). The total variance is not given in the table: in arbitrary units, where comparable, they were 1—100·37, 2—120·38, 3—187·91, 4—258·75 (all from same animal) 5—552·98, 7—841·03 (same animal). The forms of these curves are reproduced as Fig. 12.5. Curves 6 and 8 are those in Fig. 5.1.

It can be seen that five harmonics will in every case represent the variance of the original curve to within 5 per cent of its true value and in all but one case to within 2·5 per cent. Furthermore, the first two harmonics alone always account for 85 per cent of the variance and the improvement thereafter is progressively much smaller for each additional term. This dominance of the first two harmonics is also marked in the detailed analyses of Randall (1958) where a long series of waves have been analysed by a digital computer. Porjé (1946) also found that over 90 per cent of the variance, of the sum of three harmonics that he measured, was determined by the first two components.

In a pressure-wave the variance represents the energy content and is its most important physical characteristic. Hence we can be assured that the first few terms of a Fourier series give a very good representation, in this respect, of wave forms of this type. It is rather more difficult to generalize about the interpretation of the necessary harmonic components in terms of frequency. Broadly speaking, one needs a rather greater number of harmonics at a low pulse-frequency to obtain the same accuracy as in a pulse-wave with a higher fundamental frequency. It will be seen that, in the femoral artery curve (No. 6 in Table IV) with a pulse-frequency of 2·7/sec, the fourth and fifth harmonic components are considerably smaller than in the other curves. Thus, from the table, one can say that, for the dog, the analysis of frequencies to 8 or 10 c/sec will reproduce, in almost every case, some 98 per cent of the total variance.

THE AMPLITUDE OF THE FREQUENCY COMPONENTS

If the exact form of the wave is the aim of the pressure recording that is made then it is necessary to have an accurate manometer response to far higher frequencies than would be necessary if, for example, only the measurement of the pulse-pressure was needed. This is more difficult to express quantitatively because in analysing a curve one writes it down as a set of ordinates. The number of the ordinates taken limits the accuracy of the analysis. In our laboratory we take 30 ordinates as a routine and such a curve will be fully represented by 15 harmonic terms—no additional ones can be added to it. From the foregoing discussion it can be seen that far less than this number is necessary for reasonable accuracy. Nevertheless a resynthesis will show a considerable "smoothing" of the curve, but to assess the degree to which this is due to omitting terms in the Fourier series the resynthesized curve should be compared with the curve defined by the number of ordinates taken (e.g. Fig. 11.1 C).

Some idea of the contribution to the wave form can be obtained from a consideration of the amplitude of the various components in Table V. For ease of comparison the excursion of each (i.e.

TABLE V

Recording site		Pulse-pressure	Amplitude of harmonics as % of pulse-pressure					Sum %M	Freq. range
			M_1	M_2	M_3	M_4	M_5		
1P	Asc. aorta	33·9	61·1	44·1	20·9	11·9	15·6	153·6	2·22–11·1
2P	Thor. aorta	35·0	69·0	40·2	13·7	13·5	18·3	154·7	2·22–11·1
3P	Abd. aorta (prox.)	40·7	71·5	52·3	16·8	12·6	12·3	165·5	2·22–11·1
4P	Abd. aorta (distal)	49·4	67·5	51·6	17·2	12·4	16·1	164·8	2·22–11·1
5P	Abd. aorta (distal)	52·3	66·7	54·0	21·9	8·4	10·4	161·4	2·0–10·0
6P	Femoral	65·0	63·0	56·0	20·8	5·1	0·9	145·8	2·7–13·5
7P	Saphenous	67·3	54·7	57·2	23·9	12·0	17·4	165·2	2·0–10·0
8Q	Femoral (flow)	—	46·3	52·6	22·8	9·9	5·0	136·6	2·7–13·5
9	Square wave (half-period)	—	127·4	0	42·4	0	25·4	195·2	
10	Half-rect sine wave (1/3 period)	—	76·3	54·5	28·2	7·0	4·2	170·2	

The relative amplitudes of the first five harmonic components of the curves analysed in Table IV. The total excursion of the harmonic is quoted as a percentage of the amplitude of composite curve (i.e. the pulse-pressure for the pressure curves). For curves 6 and 8 further components were calculated thus: 6th Har. P—1·6, Q—2·4 per cent; 7th Har. P—0·94, Q—1·5 per cent; 8th Har. P—0·33, Q—0·3 per cent.

twice the modulus or amplitude in the usual sense) has been recorded, as a percentage of the pulse-pressure, or the total excursion of the composite wave, in the table. The amplitudes of the higher frequency components now appear to make, relatively, a much higher contribution to the wave form than they do to the variance. It should be remembered, however, that in the synthesis of a Fourier series to form the composite wave there is cancellation of the component waves in many parts of the cycle. This is shown by the fact that the sums of the amplitudes of the individual components is always far greater than the total amplitude of the composite wave.

Curves that have sharp deflections or discontinuities in them require high frequency components in a Fourier synthesis if they are to be represented accurately. It is thus of interest to consider two geometric forms that have a rough similarity to pressure-wave forms. The square wave (9 in the tables) is an extreme example of a wave with sharp deflections and the 5th harmonic still has an amplitude of 25 per cent of the total amplitude of the wave, yet

Fig. 11.1 A shows that the resynthesis of these few components (i.e. 1st, 3rd and 5th) gives a not unreasonable representation. (This also shows in a marked way that the addition of higher harmonics often actually reduces the total excursion of the synthesized curve.) Extending the analysis to the 15th harmonic still leaves the oscillations at the discontinuities visible although it considerably reduces them in size. (The values are easy to calculate for they are the corresponding fractions of the amplitude of the first harmonic; i.e. 25·4 is 1/5 of 127·4 for the 5th harmonic, it continues 1/7 for the 7th, 1/9 for the 9th etc.) The proportion of the variance represented by all harmonics up to the 15th is 97·5 per cent which is not a great increase over the value of 93·4 per cent for 5 harmonics. With the half-rectified sine wave (10 in the tables) the synthesis of 5 harmonics gives a good representation

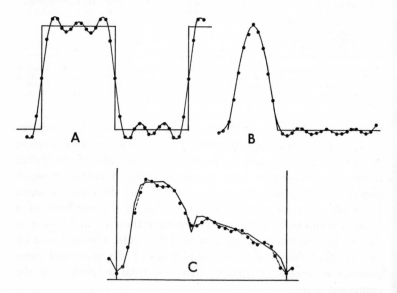

Fig. 11.1. Three representative curves are shown together with the resynthesis of the first five Fourier components. (A) A square-wave. (B) A half-rectified sine-wave, one-third of a cycle in duration. (C) A central aortic pulse-wave (further analytical details are given in Tables IV and V—the pulse-wave used is 1 P). Points on the resynthesis are shown as solid circles. Thirty ordinates were taken and the pulse-curve is drawn using only these thirty points joined by straight lines.

The resynthesized curve shows divergencies at points of sharp inflection, e.g. the incisura in C, but the representation of the total variance by five harmonics is good (93·4 per cent for A; 98·7 per cent for B; 97·6 per cent for C). (*Drawings A and B by courtesy of Dr. M. G. Taylor.*)

(Fig. 11.1 B) in spite of the fact that there are two sharp discontinuities in it. This is reflected in the fact that these 5 harmonics represent 98·7 per cent of the total variance. With a pressure curve the match between the resynthesized and original the main deficiency is once more in representing such sharp deflections as that of the incisura. (Fig. 11.1 C.)

These syntheses of a limited number of frequency components mimic the record that a manometer would make if it responded accurately up to a frequency of about 10/sec and then cut off completely. In fact this is not so in these records, but it could be argued that the small contribution of the higher frequencies in these curves was due to the fact that they were not adequately recorded by the manometer. This is not the situation, however, because in each case the manometer was markedly under-damped with a resonant frequency of 100–200 c/sec; any distortion in the higher frequencies, therefore, would be an exaggeration of their amplitude (see Fig. 11.2). In some records made with manometers having lower resonant frequencies (such as earlier optical models) this probably accounts for the large incisuras that are seen, i.e. they are represented by frequencies which are resonating.

From the comparison of frequency components of the square wave from the 5th harmonic to the 15th mentioned above it would appear that to get real fidelity of recording of wave form it would be necessary to have a manometer without significant amplitude distortion up to frequencies of at least 100 c/sec. This figure is based on the estimate of Broemser (1940) that a true record of the central aortic pulse-wave should include the 40th harmonic (which would mean recording at least 80 ordinates). The tabulated results of Fry, Noble and Mallos (1957) indicate that some modern manometers are capable of accurate recording to such frequencies—provided that short needles are used. This demand can, however, be regarded as unnecessarily stringent. Appreciation of the fact that the amplitudes of the higher frequency components are much smaller than the low frequency terms leads to the acceptance of wider tolerance limits of accuracy. Amplitude distortion up to ±5 per cent is usually regarded as reasonable but at frequencies below 5 c/sec it should be much less than this. In an acceptable manometer we would, therefore, demand that there should be no appreciable distortion below 5 c/sec and that it should not exceed 5 per cent at 15–20 c/sec.

PHASE DISTORTION

In the past the errors in phase introduced by a manometer have not been regarded as very important. They were fully tabulated by Hansen and Warburg (1950) and it can be seen in Fig. 11.3 that phase lag in manometers may be very great under certain conditions. Such phase distortion, which in effect causes a shifting of the harmonic components relative to each other will cause an alteration in form of the recorded wave. An extreme example is shown in Fig. 12.3 where there are two curves composed of a fundamental and 2nd harmonic components; in one curve the 2nd harmonic is shifted by 90° in relation to the other and it can be seen that the combined wave form is drastically altered. On the other hand the total excursion is not greatly changed. Phase distortion will be progressively more marked at the higher frequencies but, as we have seen, these are relatively small so that it is unlikely that the amplitude of the composite wave will be altered appreciably. Equally the qualitative form of the wave is not likely to be noticeably different.

Ideally one would wish to have no phase errors at all. On the other hand when the damping is between 0·6 and 0·8 (see p. 246) the angle of the phase lag increases almost linearly with frequency from zero to resonance, where it is 90°. In a recording with such a manometer all the harmonics will be recorded with the same delay in actual *time* (for the phase angle is referred to the cycle length at each frequency). This will be equivalent to recording the same composite wave undistorted but delayed. If the precise time relations of the wave are not important this is a satisfactory situation; if, however, the transmission time were being related, for example, to the ECG it would introduce an error. It is on account of this lack of distortion, presumably, that Hansen (1949) recommends that a damping value of 0·6–0·8 be used on the grounds that this range is optimal for both amplitude and phase.

While the qualitative form of a pressure curve may not be sensitive to the phase errors introduced by manometers there is no question that for accurate quantitative analysis they are very important. In measuring phase velocities of individual frequency components (as discussed in Ch. 10) an error of 5°, for example, can produce an error of over 100 per cent. Similarly, in the analysis of the dynamic elastic properties of the arterial wall (e.g.

Fig. 8.4) the phase error in even a minimally damped manometer may well be comparable in size with the angle it is desired to measure. When a high degree of precision is required there appears to be no alternative to making calibration curves and correcting the results obtained. As will be seen from the discussion below, this is equally necessary for measurements of amplitude.

THE THEORY OF MANOMETER BEHAVIOUR

Only the main conclusion of the theoretical basis of manometer behaviour will be given here as the outlines of the mathematical analysis are given in Appendix 2.

A manometer may in the first instance be regarded as analogous to a simple oscillating system consisting of a mass attached to a spring. If this is displaced and released it will oscillate in simple harmonic motion and, if the system is ideal, these oscillations will continue unchanged at a constant frequency. This frequency is called its natural frequency (radians/sec). This is described by the equation

$$\omega_0 = \sqrt{\frac{S}{M}} \quad \dots\dots\dots\dots\dots 11.4$$

where S is the stiffness, or elastance, of the spring and M is the mass attached.

If there is a resistance to the movement which is proportional to the velocity of the movement this is called viscous damping, R. If we denote the damping by β_0 then

$$\beta_0 = \frac{R}{2M} \quad \dots\dots\dots\dots\dots 11.5$$

(Damping is usually designated by a e.g. Hansen (1949) and Noble (1953) but in the present work this would lead to confusion with the a introduced by Womersley in relation to oscillatory pressure-flow relationships.)

If the damping factor is equal to the natural frequency, i.e. $\beta_0 = \omega_0$, the mass will not oscillate after being released but will return exponentially to its equilibrium position. This is called the condition of *critical* damping.

If $\beta_0 > \omega_0$ then the rate of return to equilibrium is slower and the condition is called over-damped.

If $\beta_0 < \omega_0$ the mass will oscillate but the amplitude of the oscillation will decay exponentially and the period is longer. This

B.F.A.–R

condition is that of under-damping and is the condition of most manometers unless they are specially modified.

When applying these concepts to a manometer system the term S represents the stiffness of the transducer. Hence increasing this stiffness increases the natural frequency of the manometer. The term M is now the total mass of the liquid in the manometer and the mass of the transducer itself with that of the liquid in the catheter. As it can be shown that by far the greatest role is played by the liquid in the catheter the mass M is given approximately by

$$M = l\pi r^2 \rho \quad \dots\dots\dots\dots\dots \text{ 11.6}$$

where l and r are the length and internal radius of the catheter and ρ is the density of the liquid (which will be taken as $1\cdot0$).

The term S is defined by the pressure-volume relation, E, of the manometer, i.e. $E = \Delta P / \Delta V$, and the linear displacement of the membrane so that we get

$$\omega_0 = \sqrt{\frac{\pi r^2 E}{l}} \quad \dots\dots\dots\dots\dots \text{ 11.7}$$

from which it can be seen that the highest natural frequencies with a given manometer will be obtained with short, wide catheters and that the bore is of greater importance than the length. It also shows that the use of a long narrow catheter will alter the behaviour of a manometer by lowering its natural frequency quite apart from any effect it may have on the damping.

As damping is most easily described as the proportion of critical damping, i.e. when $\beta_0 = \omega_0$ we write from eqns. 11.4 and 11.5

$$\beta = \beta_0 / \omega_0 = \frac{R}{2\sqrt{ME}} \quad \dots\dots\dots\dots\dots \text{11.8}$$

and from Poiseuille's equation (2.6) for the velocity of flow in a pipe it is usual to write an approximate value of the resistance, R,

$$R = \frac{P_1 - P_2}{V} = \frac{8\mu l}{r^2} \quad \dots\dots\dots\dots\dots \text{ 11.9}$$

(Lambossy (1952) was the first to obtain the correct solution for the resistance when the motion of the liquid is oscillatory. This is mathematically the same as that derived by Womersley (Ch. 5) where it can be seen that the fluid resistance rises with frequency (Fig. 5.11). The effects of this are discussed more fully in Appendix 2.)

Substituting for M from eqn. 11.6 we obtain

$$\beta = \frac{4\mu}{r^3}\sqrt{\frac{l}{\pi.E}} \quad \dots\dots\dots\dots 11.10$$

Once again it can be seen that the influence of the bore of the catheter system is far greater than that of length although, with the very long catheters in common use, the effect of increasing length is far from negligible.

FORCED VIBRATIONS

The foregoing discussion describes the behaviour of a manometer when it vibrates freely after a single deflection. It is important to appreciate that critical damping and hence, from common usage, all damping coefficient are defined by behaviour under such conditions. This leads to a standard method of calibrating the characteristics of a manometer which is discussed below (p. 255). The behaviour of the manometer in practice, however, is determined by the fact that it is being continually driven by the force of the arterial pressure. This is the condition of forced oscillation, or forced vibration.

Such a system, with relatively small damping, will respond only at the applied frequency. As this increases the amplitude of the manometer response will increase until it reaches a peak when it is said to resonate. The resonant frequency will be close to but rather less than the natural undamped frequency. The amplitude of response then falls off rapidly (Fig. 11.2). In addition to the amplitude distortion there is also a phase lag in the response. This increases with frequency but the rate of increase varies with the damping. In all cases, however, the phase lag is 90° when the driving frequency equals the natural frequency.

If we call the manometer response x and express it as a fraction of its true value and denote the driving frequency as a fraction, γ, of the natural frequency, ω_0 so that the applied pressure is of the form $\sin \gamma t$ we find that

$$x = \frac{1}{\sqrt{[(1-\gamma^2)^2 + 4\beta^2\gamma^2]}} \sin\left(\gamma t - \tan^{-1}\frac{2\beta\gamma}{1-\gamma^2}\right) \quad \dots 11.11$$

so that the amplitude, A, relative to its true value, is determined by the term

$$A = \frac{1}{\sqrt{[(1-\gamma^2)^2 + 4\beta^2\gamma^2]}} \quad \dots\dots\dots 11.12$$

This is shown graphically in Fig. 11.2, for various values of β.

From eqn. 11.11 it can be seen that when the manometer is driven at the natural frequency, i.e. $\gamma = 1\cdot0$, then

$$A = \frac{1}{2\beta} \quad \dots\dots\dots\dots\dots\dots\dots 11.13$$

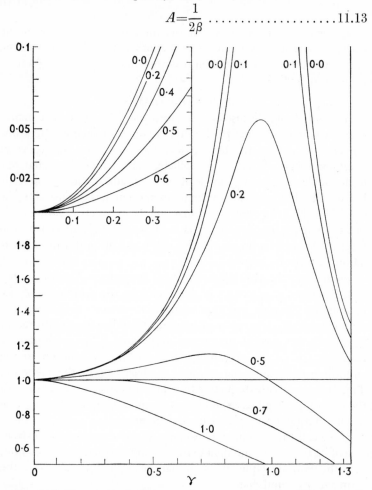

F<small>IG</small>. 11.2. The amplitude response of a manometer, under different conditions of damping, when driven by an oscillatory force of unit amplitude and varying frequency. Abscissa—the ratio of the driving frequency (ω) to the undamped natural frequency (ω_0), denoted by γ, as in the text. Ordinate—amplitude of response. Inset square (top left) is a more detailed display of the behaviour at relatively low driving frequencies. Figures by each curve indicate damping as a fraction of critical damping. The corresponding phase changes are shown in Fig. 11.3. To make recordings that are reasonably accurate with regard to both amplitude and phase it can be seen that one needs a manometer with a natural frequency of the order of ten times the highest frequencies it is wished to record.

With small values of β (e.g. 0·2 or less) this will be very close to its true maximum and the amplitude excursion at resonance will, from this equation, give a good measure of the damping.

The true maximum amplitude occurs when

$$\gamma=\sqrt{1-2\beta^2} \quad\text{.............. 11.14}$$

and it will be seen that, when $\beta=0·707$, γ is zero. At this degree of damping the amplitude never rises above its true value but, as seen in Fig. 11.2, it remains within some 2 per cent of this figure up to about 50 per cent of the natural frequency. This gives a curve which is similar to that at critical damping for free vibrations and is often confused with it when manometer behaviour is discussed. In fact with critical damping the amplitude response falls continuously from zero frequency upwards. Perhaps some term such as "optimal" damping should be used for the 70 per cent damping curve; the common phrase, though it smacks somewhat of jargon, "flat amplitude response to x c/sec" is probably more generally useful. There is nothing of especial practical value in this response curve at 70 per cent damping. Even if only amplitude is considered a curve, which does not deviate by more than 2 per cent, can be obtained with a damping factor of 0·64, up to 67 per cent of the natural frequency.

With manometers in common use, such as capacitance manometers, it is possible to achieve natural frequencies of 200–700 c/sec under working conditions (Fry, Noble and Mallos, 1957). As the Fourier analyses of the pulses-waves in the first section above showed that accurate recording above 15–20 c/sec was not necessary it is clear that we are only concerned in many cases with the part of the curve up to $\gamma=0·1$. In this case the lower the damping, the more accurate the phase recording.

The phase lag ϕ in a record is given in eqn. 11.11 by the angle

$$\phi=\tan^{-1}\frac{2\beta\gamma}{1-\gamma^2} \quad\text{.............. 11.15}$$

This is shown graphically in Fig. 11.3 for various degrees of damping. It can be seen that with low damping the phase lag is small and indeed if accurate phase recording is required then the damping should be less than 0·1. At this value the phase lag is some 2·3° at 0·1 of the natural frequency (i.e. at 20 c/sec if the natural frequency is 200 c/sec). With an increase in damping the phase error at this frequency increases approximately linearly as

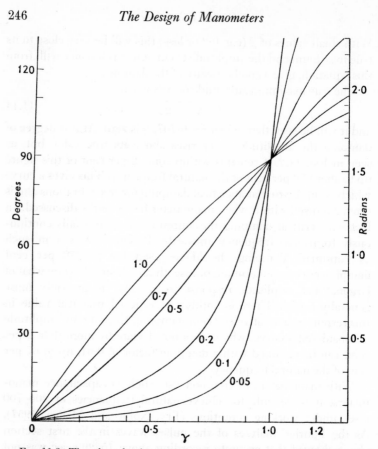

Fig. 11.3. The phase-lag in a manometer driven by an oscillatory force of constant amplitude. With zero damping there is no phase-lag up to the point of resonance and then a sudden change to 180°. Abscissa—ratio of driving frequency to natural frequency (cp. Fig. 11.2); ordinate—phase-lag in degrees (left scale) and radians (right scale). It will be noted that phase distortion is marked unless the damping is kept very low (e.g. less than 0·1 of critical damping).

the damping. As pointed out in a previous section (p. 240) for the purposes of merely recording the form of a wave the phase shifts found with damping of 0·6–0·8 are usually tolerable because the angle increases almost linearly with frequency. As a result the wave is not deformed but is recorded with a uniform time delay.

THE PRACTICAL PROBLEMS OF MANOMETER DESIGN

From the foregoing results it is apparent that it is impossible to construct a manometer that does not distort either the amplitude or the phase of the response if it is necessary to measure a wide band of frequencies. The best approach to simultaneous accuracy for both these characteristics is to have a manometer with a high natural frequency and very small damping. According to the accuracy required one may thus use the lowest 10 per cent or 20 per cent of the frequency curve.

To obtain a very high natural frequency it is necessary to have a very stiff membrane and this reduces the sensitivity so that here it is necessary to effect a compromise. Where it is possible to do so the highest frequencies will be obtained by using short, wide catheters or needles. An even better result is shown by the use of "catheter-tip" inductance type manometers (Ellis, Gauer and Wood, 1951; Wetterer, 1944; Wetterer and Pieper, 1952) which virtually eliminate the hydraulic system of the more conventional manometer and, having a very small effective mass, attain very high natural frequencies (e.g. 980 c/sec for a Gauer type quoted by Fry *et al.*).

Surveying a variety of types of manometer Fry *et al.* (1957) recorded resonant frequencies, when using a No. 18 needle, of between 67 and 740 c/sec. As the damping, estimated from the amplitude recorded at resonance, ranged from 0·03 (with 1,500 per cent increase in amplitude) to 0·14 (360 per cent amplitude) the resonant frequency in these cases will be within 1 per cent of the undamped natural frequency. All of these manometers (with one exception) using a needle of this sort would, therefore, give an amplitude response, accurate to within 5 per cent, up to 50 c/sec and over, i.e. well beyond the 20 c/sec limit suggested above. With this degree of damping the phase error would be small enough to neglect for all but the most precise investigations.

Using a long cardiac catheter, however, the drop in the resonant frequency recorded was very marked and the corresponding range was 10–58 c/sec. The damping was also increased and ranged approximately from 0·2 to 0·12. An amplitude response within 5 per cent of the true value (with the same exception as before) was only obtained up to frequencies of 5–15 c/sec. As the increase in damping and the decreased natural frequency consequent on using such a catheter would, of themselves, introduce a marked phase distortion it would be better in such a case as this to increase the damping to a value of 0·6–0·7. This would give an accurate amplitude response up to some 60 per cent of the natural frequency (although this would be further decreased by increasing the damping). This would be at the expense of increasing the phase distortion but, by making the latter more linearly related to frequency would make it easier to compensate in analysing the records.

The foregoing discussion makes it clear that a "perfect" recording of both amplitude and phase is impossible to achieve. The type of manometer, and extra damping if used, that is preferred for any type of work will always depend on an assessment of the accuracy required and the experimental conditions (e.g. the frequency response requirements would have to be reassessed if one was experimenting on mice where the heart frequency may be 10/sec). In these circumstances the only way to eliminate manometer distortion is to calibrate accurately the amplitude and phase behaviour at various frequencies and correct the results accordingly. We have found this necessary in work on the dynamic elastic properties of the arterial wall (Fig. 8.4 from Bergel), and in the calculation of input impedances etc. in a rubber-tube model (Taylor, 1959*b*). For the calculation of input impedances in the animal if a flowmeter is used such correction of results is even more essential for manometers and flowmeters will have quite different frequency response curves although, as pointed out in Ch. 6, few of them have been rigorously calibrated in the way that manometers have. The need for very precise recording characteristics from manometers is, of course, not felt if records from two similar pieces of apparatus are used. If the behaviour characteristics of both are identical then as far as relative changes in pressure recordings are concerned the frequency response curve is of little interest. The pulse curves analysed in Fig. 10.3 (and shown in Fig. 12.1) are suspect as far as the amplitude of their higher frequency components are concerned. They were, however, all recorded through the same manometer and catheter system—a capacitance manometer and a long cardiac catheter—so that the relative changes seen in the various components at different sites is independent of the manometer characteristics. The same consideration applies to the measurement of phase velocities where the measurement of small phase angles may be involved—but it is important to ensure that the phase distortion of the two manometers used is identical.

Where two pressure transducers are used close together, with a common hydraulic system, coupling will occur. The frequency characteristics of both will then usually be the same in this situation. If one membrane is much less stiff than the other its response will be the dominant one. Thus in the method of measuring arterial impedance used by Bergel *et al.* (1958) a capacitance manometer ($\omega_0 > 100$ c/sec) and a photo-electric differential manometer (see below) which was slightly over-damped but whose amplitude response was within 5 per cent to 8 c/sec. When connected the capacitance manometer, on calibration, had the same calibration curve as the differential manometer. Such situations do not often arise. In this case the two respective records were being used to determine the input impedance and the coupling reduced the error. It does emphasize that calibrations must be carried out under the actual experimental conditions used.

TYPES OF MANOMETER IN USE

The range of available techniques that are suitable for use in manometers has been fully reviewed by Hansen (1949) and more briefly by Noble (1953), so that it need only be briefly summarized here. We have seen that it is desirable that a manometer suitable for recording the arterial pulse-wave in dogs should have an un-damped natural frequency, with its hydraulic system attached, of 200 c/sec. For many purposes 100 c/sec will be sufficient. Any manometer with such a natural frequency will, on its own, necessarily have a very low degree of damping. Hansen (1949) has calculated that the elastance of the membrane used must therefore be of the order of 2×10^{-9} ml/mm Hg pressure. The technical system used will largely devolve on the problem of sensitivity together with the practical needs of stability, simplicity etc.

Optical manometers

The simplest method of recording the bending of a membrane is by the deflection of a beam of light reflected from a mirror mounted on it. Membranes of a suitable stiffness made out of beryllium-copper were introduced by Hamilton (Hamilton, Brewer and Brotman, 1934) and are still in use. The only practical limitation to the optical manometer is that, with a membrane of suitable stiffness one needs a beam of light some 3 or 4 metres long and this entails all the complications of working in a darkened room. If only one or two channels are required this can be circumvented by the use of fixed mirrors causing repeated reflections in a box. In general, these devices are clumsy but this may be reduced to a minimum with technical ingenuity and on the credit side there is the intrinsic simplicity of the method.

Photo-electric recording has been used as a means of increasing the compactness of the optical manometer. A type that we use in this laboratory (manufactured by the Cambridge Scientific Instrument Co.) is based on the design of Müller and Shillingford (1954). In this model a rectangular beam of light is reflected on to two photo-electric cells arranged side by side and a deflection of the beam causes a change in balance of the output of the two cells. This is amplified and recorded. The advantage of this design is that the light beam can operate through water so that the difference in pressure between two points in the arterial system may be measured by applying the pressures simultaneously on either side of the membrane. As these pressure differences are small one can use a sensitive membrane, e.g. with a maximum deflection at 20–30 mm Hg, even though the mean arterial pressure is 100 mm Hg or more. The increase in sensitivity by using a less stiff membrane involves a considerable reduction in natural frequency. In addition the design of this model also makes it necessary to have rather long leads to the experimental animal, and by keeping these wide it has proved possible to record a satisfactory amplitude response up to about 8 c/sec.

Capacitance manometers

This appears to have been introduced into physiology by Lilly in America and is the method used in the manometer designed by Hansen (1949) as a result of his detailed investigation. Of all the electronic methods of recording it combines high sensitivity with high-frequency characteristics and with relative simplicity of manufacture of the transducer.

The principle on which it is based is that the membrane which is moved by the applied pressure forms one side of a condenser. Deflection of the membrane, therefore, alters its capacity. To detect this the condenser is included in an oscillator circuit and the alteration of capacitance is measured by a frequency modulation technique.

The problems encountered in using a capacitance manometer are largely those of any electronic apparatus of moderate complexity. If the amplifiers are well-designed the manometer does not suffer from zero drift but they should be run for 1–2 hours before use to minimize this. The transducer itself is temperature sensitive but sensitivity is not appreciably altered by the usual drifts in room temperature. It should, of course, be calibrated on each working day. Rapid changes of temperature such as those caused by holding it in the hand should, naturally, be avoided but this applies to most pressure transducers. The alignment of the cable connecting the transducer should also be kept as constant as possible because the capacity of this line is, in effect, part of the capacitance of the transducer. In the better commercial models I have never found that cable movements introduce any appreciable errors. In general the capacitance manometer is a very satisfactory instrument and all our arterial pressure recordings are made with instruments of this type. It is, however, difficult to adapt this principle to recording differential pressures.

Strain-gauge manometers

The change in ohmic resistance which occurs in a wire when it is strained has been widely used in a large variety of gauges. The change in resistance is measured by setting the gauge as one arm of a Wheatstone bridge. While the method has all the advantages of stability and simplicity in its electrical circuits, many of these gauges that have been used in manometers have quite unsuitable dynamic properties. Fry *et al.* (1957), for example, state that the Statham P23A has a resonant frequency of 67 c/sec with a needle attached and 10 c/sec with a long cardiac catheter. Even in the former case the amplitude was only accurate (± 5 per cent) up to 5 c/sec. It appears to be difficult to build a strain-gauge manometer with a better frequency response than this for the only model available in this country that I have tested had a rather lower natural frequency than this. In America, however, more recent gauges have been produced which have performances as good as many capacitance manometers, e.g. the Statham P23D, with a needle attached, has a natural frequency of 280 c/sec and very low damping—*c.* 0·03 judging by the results of Fry *et al.* (1959). The technical intricacy of manufacturing the transducer is such that they have to be bought commercially.

Strain-gauge manometers are widely used in clinical practice where a lower frequency response can be accepted (because the heart frequency is slower) and where the most important measurements required are systolic and diastolic pressure rather than the precise wave form. Nevertheless caution should be exercised when they are used with long catheters. The topic of strain-gauge manometers in clinical research has been investigated by Wood, Lensen, Warner and Wright (1954) and they found that it was satisfactory if a flat amplitude response could be achieved to 10 c/sec.

Inductance manometers

The electrical currents induced in a coil when an iron core, or its equivalent, are moved in it have been applied in many ingenious ways to manometer design. Where such a core is actually moved it needs to be made very small if suitably high natural frequencies can be achieved. In other designs the membrane is made to alter the width of an air-gap in a magnetic circuit and as a result the amount and distribution of flux in the magnetic circuit is altered. One advantage of this method is that much lower frequencies of alternating current are required than in the capacitance manometer so that there is very little problem with the electrical properties of the cable. The inductance principle can also be applied more easily to the construction of a differential manometer than can the capacitance technique. The latter is, however, capable of higher sensitivity than an inductance manometer of comparable dynamic properties.

Inductance gauges are of especial interest in that they have been used as very small pressure recording instruments built into the tip of a catheter or sound (Wetterer, 1944; Ellis *et al.*, 1951) and introduced directly into the circulation. They thus eliminate problems associated with the hydraulic system of the catheter in more conventional manometers and, as noted above, the Gauer type has a natural frequency of about 1,000 c/sec. The technical difficulty of manufacture has probably limited their use. In view of the very limited number of papers reporting experiments using this type of manometer it is difficult to assess their potentialities. Their characteristics on calibration seem extremely tempting.

Other types of manometer

A considerable number of physical techniques have been incorporated in manometers at various times, and one is led to assess their practical advantages by the number of workers who have used them.

(*a*) *Conductance*. Pappenheimer (1954) constructed a differential manometer in which applied pressure altered the conductance between two thin glass plates. This appears to be capable of high sensitivities, although as with all manometers this is only at the expense of its frequency characteristics. Of relatively simple construction this apparatus is reported to behave very satisfactorily.

(*b*) *Mechano-electric transducer*. Green (1954) has used the transducer valve RCA 5734, which has a probe attached to the anode, as the basis for a manometer. This valve has been used by several workers as the sensing unit for the bristle flowmeter (Ch. 6). In the same way when a plate is attached to the probe it can be used for pressure measurements. This device is not yet available commercially. The dynamic characteristics seem quite satisfactory but some workers say that this valve is very subject to zero drift.

(*c*) *Piezo-electric effect*. Certain crystals such as quartz develop a difference in potential when they are subjected to mechanical stress. Porjé (1946) used a transducer of this type applied to the exterior of vessels. The crystals have the advantage of having a natural frequency of the order of several kilocycles. Their main disadvantage is that the potential developed during static deformations is very low and, even with good insulation, leaks away so that in practice only the oscillatory pressure terms are recorded. For many purposes this is sufficient but it greatly limits their practical value.

AMPLIFIERS AND RECORDERS

All the discussion of the design of manometers tacitly assumes that there is no subsequent distortion of the recorded pressure. The enormous variety of amplifier circuits and recording devices that have been used makes it impossible to make more than a few general observations here. With mechanical devices such as penwriters the distortions that will be introduced are of the same nature as those in the manometer itself. It is usually arranged so that these are damped to such a degree that there is no resonance (i.e. damping *c*. 0·7 although they are often reported as being critically damped). In this case there will also be a considerable phase lag over frequencies where the amplitude response is undistorted. The natural frequency of penwriters has been greatly improved in recent years. Nevertheless far greater accuracy will be obtained by using a cathode-ray oscilloscope. Our own records are photographed from an oscilloscope on 35 mm film and the curves for analysis are enlarged so that the pulse length is 30 cm on graph paper. Mirror galvanometers are also available which will give a flat response to 600 c/sec and above and, in the frequency range we are concerned with, will give negligible errors.

The errors that may arise from amplifiers are more likely to occur in the low frequency range and so it is more important to control them. A good d.c. amplifier is essential but compensating circuits may introduce other errors. One manometer we have tested was found to have a phase *lead* of some 6° at low frequencies —a minor distortion in most respects but one which caused apparently negative phase velocities of the fundamental components of the pulse-wave measured over short intervals.

In practice it is the behaviour of the whole assembly from catheter to recording apparatus that is of interest. The fact that distortions may be introduced by components other than the pressure transducer only serves to emphasize that the fidelity of a pressure-recording device must always be checked by adequate calibration. The theoretical sections above are only of importance to indicate what distortions one should look for. The mathematical equations are only approximations, albeit close approximations, for they omit such effects as that of secondary resonances in a long catheter and the fact that the resistance term is not independent of frequency.

Where the degree of damping of a manometer needs to be increased it is common practice to do this electrically rather than by modifying the dimensions of the needle or catheter used. The modifications of the frequency response curves by the use of circuits will vary with individual design but will be of the same kind as that caused by hydraulic damping. In particular large phase shifts may be introduced and calibration curves should be made for all such damping circuits that are used.

METHODS OF CALIBRATION

The most direct way of calibrating a manometer for oscillatory pressure is to apply a known forced vibration to it. This can be done by using a device which creates a pressure of constant amplitude and simple harmonic form and which can be run over a wide range of frequencies. Unfortunately such a device is difficult to construct so that one has confidence in the constancy of its amplitude. This necessitates incorporating a manometer into the apparatus and this manometer must itself be calibrated.

Alternatively, the characteristics of the manometer may be measured by applying a transient pressure and studying its free vibrations. This is somewhat less direct, as the behaviour of the manometer is predicted on the basis of the approximations made in the mathematical theory. The method is also rather more difficult to apply if the manometer is critically, or over, damped although Warburg (1950) has described a method of calculation in such a case.

As the free vibrations may be generated very simply this method may be regarded as being the easiest. The transient pressure imposed may be negative as by the sudden withdrawal and release of a syringe plunger. Hansen (1949) uses a syringe with a hole bored through the stem of the plunger which can be closed with a finger. Alternatively a positive pressure may be built up in a small chamber closed by a thin rubber membrane which is suddenly burst (rubber from a surgical glove and a burning cigarette end work very efficiently).

If damping is less than critical there is first an overshoot followed by oscillations dying away exponentially. The period of one complete oscillation is called T_D. If the deflection from the final equilibrium position at the end of one cycle is θ_1 and at the end of the second cycle is θ_2 then

$$\theta_1/\theta_2 = \text{ratio of damping } (\chi) \quad \ldots\ldots\ldots\ldots \quad 11.16$$

and

$$\ln(\theta_1/\theta_2) = \text{logarithmic decrement } (\varLambda) \quad \ldots\ldots \quad 11.17$$

(ln is a natural logarithm i.e. to base e)

i.e.

$$\varLambda = \ln\theta_1 - \ln\theta_2$$

If θ_2 is only a half-period after θ_1 i.e. the next deflection in the opposite direction then

$$\varLambda = 2(\ln\theta_1 - \ln\theta_2) \quad \ldots\ldots\ldots\ldots\ldots \quad 11.18$$

and

$$\varLambda = \frac{2\pi\beta}{\sqrt{1-\beta^2}} \quad \ldots\ldots\ldots\ldots \quad 11.19$$

so that

$$\beta = \frac{\varLambda}{\sqrt{4\pi^2+\varLambda^2}} \quad \ldots\ldots\ldots\ldots \quad 11.20$$

The undamped natural frequency, ω_0, is given by

$$\omega_0 = 2\pi f = \frac{\sqrt{4\pi^2+\varLambda^2}}{T_D} \quad \ldots\ldots\ldots\ldots \quad 11.21$$

where f is frequency in cycles/sec.

Then from the value of ω_0 and β the amplitude and phase response curves of the manometer can be calculated by eqns. 11.12 and 11.15 above.

Calibration by the use of an oscillatory pressure device would appear to be more simple although Hansen and Warburg (1950) give five different methods, in addition to the method using a transient response described above. The simplest way of testing an unknown manometer is that used by Fry *et al.* (1957) where the apparatus under test is compared directly with a manometer that is known to have a much higher natural frequency and so can be assumed to be linear over the test range.

Hansen (1949) has described the somewhat elaborate magnetic pump that he used. A description of the apparatus that Fry *et al.* (1957) or Wood *et al.* (1954) used does not seem to have been published in detail. Linden (1958) has devised a very neat little apparatus which uses a barium titanate strain-gauge to drive a diaphragm. The behaviour of the gauge is dubious below 20 c/sec, however, and requires sinusoidal voltages of the order of ± 200V to produce a reasonable pressure. In general a pressure generator for a closed water-filled system needs a considerable amount of power. It is not easy to arrange such an apparatus so that it is constant in output and pure in form in the low frequency range— which is the range that it is most important to check in relation to arterial pulse-wave investigation.

If air is used in the compression chamber much less power is required. With an oscillatory pump, however, the pressure changes will depend on the frequency because of adiabatic effects. It is, therefore, especially important to measure the actual pressure with a manometer of known characteristics. The amplitude-frequency curve can then be expressed in terms of the ratio with the reference manometer reading. The phase response curve can be recorded in the same way.

It is desirable that apparatus used for calibration should be simple and that checks should be made at each experiment. The presence of even very small bubbles in the manometer system will drastically change the frequency response of a manometer. Fry *et al.* (1957) have stated that they could only get reproducible curves when their manometers were filled with boiled water containing detergent or with 50 per cent alcohol. In addition fibrin deposition inside catheters often occurs during experiments in spite of the administration of heparin but frequently escapes detection if complete blockage does not result. A quick method of checking the frequency response is the most certain way of detecting any recording errors due to this cause, but in practice one cannot keep removing catheters or cannulae during an experiment to do calibration curves. With experience, a marked fall in natural frequency causes an alteration in wave form especially in the disappearance of the small but sharp high-frequency oscillations such as at the incisura. Once again the large safety factor gained by using instruments of high natural frequency is desirable as minor degrees of fibrin deposition will not then cause an appreciable effect. With a sensitive differential manometer or experiments where precise comparison between two manometers is required asymmetry in the cannulae due to this cause is a very real problem. Prevention is then the only real cure and this necessitates frequent flushing with heparinized saline.

CONCLUSIONS

This study of manometer behaviour leads us to the conclusion that accurate recording of arterial pressure-waves is not normally required above about 20 c/sec. To record amplitude and phase reasonably well up to this limit the natural frequency of the manometer should be ten times, or at least five times, this frequency, with damping of not more than $0 \cdot 1$ (of critical damping). If this is impossible, e.g. when using a cardiac catheter, then the optimum damping is $0 \cdot 6 – 0 \cdot 7$ critical, but it is then necessary to make allowance for the phase shift that is introduced. For all very precise work allowance for distortion and phase shift is necessary and this depends on accurate calibration with respect to the frequency range being investigated.

CHAPTER XII

THE SHAPE OF THE PRESSURE PULSE-WAVE

The remarkable change in the shape of the pressure-wave in arteries as it travels from the heart to the periphery has provided a most intriguing problem in circulatory physiology since the first introduction of adequate manometers over fifty years ago. The causes for this change have been discussed at great length in the literature; here it is proposed to discuss the main factors responsible in the light of the analysis of wave propagation that has been put forward in the preceding chapters.

CHANGES IN THE TRAVELLING PRESSURE-WAVE

A set of pulse-waves recorded at intervals along the aorta together with a comparable femoral pulse from another animal are shown in Fig. 12.1 (and others may be seen in Fig. 12.4). The uppermost curve, recorded close to the heart, is fairly typical of the type of curve recorded in this situation. The front of the wave, i.e. the aspect of the left side because time is plotted from left to right, is rising smoothly but not especially rapidly to a rounded summit and then falls to the point of the notch, known as the incisura. This is synchronous with the closing of the aortic valves and hence marks the end of systole. There is thereafter a gradual slow decline throughout the remainder of the curve with small oscillations superimposed on it. Two small humps are seen following the incisura and then a longer, slower one.

In following the curves successively we see the following distinct changes which will be discussed below:

(1) The amplitude of the wave, the pulse-pressure, increases progressively as the wave passes away from the heart—the so-called "peaking" of the pulse.

(2) The rate of rise of the front of the wave increases and becomes steeper.

(3) The sharp inflection at the incisura becomes rounded and then disappears entirely by the time the wave has reached position 5 (in the abdominal aorta at 30 cm distance).

(4) The slight positive wave in the diastolic portion of the first curve is gradually replaced by a slow but marked dip. In the femoral curve we get a marked dip followed by a second hump, often called the dicrotic notch and dicrotic wave respectively.

We may also note that the points of maximum pressure (the peaks) are almost exactly synchronous in curves 4 and 5 which appears to be a similar phenomenon to that shown in the well-known record of Hamilton and Dow (1939) and described as a standing-wave. It may also be commented in passing that, if one is attempting to measure pulse-wave velocity by the transit time of the foot of the wave, then the foot is a very indefinite feature if the pulse is recorded on a reasonably fast time base.

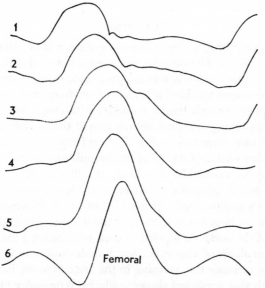

FIG. 12.1. Tracings of the pressure pulses recorded successively at five sites in the aorta with a long catheter. No. 1 is close to the aortic valves and there is a 10 cm interval between each; No. 5 is close to the origin of the iliac artery (see Fig. 10.3). The femoral curve is included for comparison but was recorded from another dog. The "peaking" here is very marked; the pulse pressure in the proximal aorta was app. 110/80 mm Hg, in the distal aorta it was 130/75 mm Hg.

POSSIBLE FACTORS MODIFYING THE WAVE FORM

In a branched system of elastic tubes it might be thought there would be many factors that influence the form of a pressure-wave.

Wiggers (1928) however, needed only four headings for a comprehensive classification (and of these I do not believe it is necessary to invoke the fourth). His classification was:

(1) Damping of waves as they travel.
(2) Various components of the wave travelling at different velocities.
(3) Annihilation or amplification of the components of the pulse by reflected waves.
(4) The occurrence of natural vibrations in various parts of the arterial tree.

To this list might be added "the effects of differences in elastic behaviour and in calibre of arteries", but both these effects cause reflections, as was seen in Ch. 9, and will be discussed under that heading.

DAMPING

Any wave propagated in a viscous system will be attenuated as it travels (Ch. 9). The only simple illustration of this that can be seen in the pulse-wave is the disappearance of the incisura. Any sharp inflection of this kind represents high-frequency components and damping per unit length increases with frequency. The progressive smoothing and final obliteration of the incisura is a result of a progressive attenuation of the highest frequency components.

The other effects of damping on the pulse-wave are not easy to see as they are masked by the effects of reflection. This is seen by reference to a display of the behaviour of the individual harmonic components as illustrated in Figs. 10.3 and 12.5; all frequencies up to 12 c/sec are larger in amplitude at the periphery than they are at the root of the aorta. As a point of personal interest I may say that the first analysis of this type that I undertook was made in an attempt to estimate the damping in the arteries to see how it compared with that predicted theoretically by Womersley (1955c). In fact I am convinced that the actual damping is considerably higher than he predicted, because his theory only considered the attenuation produced by the viscosity of the blood and neglected that due to the viscous element in the elastic wall. The only direct evidence of damping is from experiments such as those of Starr (1957) in which a single impulse is created artificially in a cadaver and dies away very rapidly. Peterson (1954) created an artificial pulse in the living animal, and comparison of the size of the front of such a pulse (which cannot be affected by reflection) recorded in the aorta and the femoral artery shows marked attenuation. More indirectly the rapidity with which the pulse form becomes constant after a sudden change in arterial conditions, such as by releasing an occlusion in an artery (Fig. 12.2), indicates that the arterial tree is highly damped. The main net effect of damping on the form of the pulse-wave is, therefore, the negative one that the changes would be much more marked if the damping were less. From the detailed analysis in Ch. 10 we have seen that reflection effects are relatively small at distances greater than a quarter wave-length from a reflecting site.

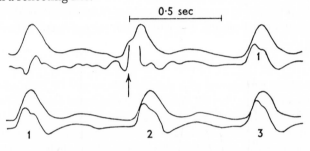

Fig. 12.2. A record of the femoral artery pressure in a dog (upper trace) and the pressure-gradient between that point and another 4 cm distal (lower trace) during and after occlusion of the artery. The artery was clamped 3 cm beyond the distal recording point and released at the point marked by the arrow. The cardiac cycles following the one in which the occlusion was released are shown in the second row (part of cycle 1 is repeated for ease of continuity). It can be seen that these pulse forms are extremely similar in shape as are the pressure-gradients, which are very sensitive to minor variations in wave form. This indicates that the system virtually attains a steady-state in little more than 0·5 sec and must be highly damped.

The arterial pressure in the first cycle illustrated (during occlusion) was 80 mm Hg, end diastolic and 164 mm Hg systolic. The pressure-gradient in the same cycle oscillated from −1·8 to +1·9 mm Hg/cm (i.e. the trace shows a total swing of app. 16 mm Hg). Note the inversion of the form of the gradient during occlusion as compared with that during the hyperaemia following release. The differential pressure was recorded with a Shillingford-Müller type manometer (Cambridge) and the arterial pressure with a capacitance manometer.

DIFFERENCE IN VELOCITY OF VARIOUS WAVE COMPONENTS

It has been seen (Ch. 9) that, in a system with viscous damping, the wave velocity increases with frequency. This causes the effect known as dispersion. It can be most easily seen if a square pulse is generated in a tube. As it travels it becomes rounded and spread out. In the arterial system a similar effect can be seen in the form of the rectangular artificial pulse used by Peterson (1954) when it arrives in the femoral artery. The shape of the cardiac ejection pulse is not known, but it undoubtedly has no sharp discontinuities in it, so that one would not expect to be able to detect this effect over the relatively short distances the pulse-wave has to travel. The main changes in form of the recorded pulse-wave—the peaking effect and steepening of the wave-front—are the opposite of this effect. Dispersion may be regarded as causing only minor effects, although Peterson (1956) has drawn attention to it as a possible cause of "peaking" (see Fig. 12.3).

Another cause of apparent differences in the velocity of components of the pulse-wave, and the only one considered by Wiggers (1928) under this heading, is due to the non-linear elastic behaviour

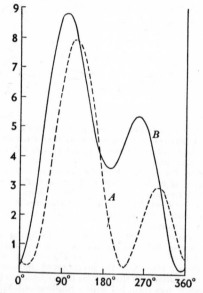

Fig. 12.3. A diagram which demonstrates that it is very unlikely that dispersion can contribute significantly to the peaking of the pulse wave. Both curves A and B are a combination of a first and a second harmonic term of equal magnitude. These have been chosen because they are the largest in the composition of the pulse wave. The second harmonic, however, has been shifted by 45° between the two curves. It can be seen that this produces an increase of some 10 per cent in the total amplitude of A as compared with B. The form of the wave has, however, been altered very greatly and, as plotted, the two curves are no longer oscillating around the same mean value.

The phase shift used here, of one harmonic against the other, is far larger than any ever recorded in the arterial tree—the diagram also omits the effect of damping during travel.

of the arterial wall. It was seen in Ch. 8 that the modulus of elasticity of all arteries increases as they are distended. One result of this is that the pulse-wave velocity increases more or less proportionately to the diastolic pressure (Bramwell and Hill, 1922). By the same reasoning Bramwell and Hill (1923) postulated that the "peak" of the wave would travel faster than the "foot". This, in their opinion, was the cause of the steepening of the wave front. Unfortunately the velocity of travel of the "peak", as represented by the time interval between two points of maximum pressure, is often slower than that of the foot. In a compound wave the point of maximum pressure does not have a separate identity and the simple logic of the argument breaks down on this point. Carried to extremes one would have to argue that each of the points on the wave at each pressure have separate and individual identities and that all travel at different velocities. This is manifestly untrue for points at the same pressure on the rising and falling limbs of the curve.

In terms of steady-state oscillation such as we are considering, the effect of non-linearity has to be expressed in terms of interaction between the harmonic components. A sinusoidal wave propagated in a non-linear elastic tube will become distorted in form due to the generation of higher harmonics. Little is known at present of the magnitude of this effect, which (like the damping), is difficult to detect in the arterial system in the presence of reflections which are altering the magnitude of the harmonic components. This has been discussed by McDonald and Taylor (1959) and has been analysed theoretically and tested on a model by Taylor (unpublished). It probably does contribute in some degree to the increasing steepness of the wave-front.

Both these causes of different wave velocities are, however, very small compared with the changes in apparent phase-velocities which we have seen (Ch. 10) to be due to the presence of reflections. As such they are more properly considered under that heading. It is worth noting, however, that these changes in phase-shift of the harmonic components relative to one another may accentuate the peaking effect that is being caused by the accompanying increase in amplitude of the components. Fig. 12.3 provides a simple illustration of the way in which the shape of a wave can be altered merely by altering the relative phases of its components without changing their amplitude. In the arterial pulse a well marked peak of pressure nearly always indicates the coincidence of a maximun of the two largest components, the first and second harmonics. When the apparent phase-velocities of these components are also very high, as in the interval 4–5 in Fig. 12.1 (see also Fig. 10.3), we get the phenomenon where the peaks are virtually synchronous. As evidence of such synchronicity of the peaks formed the main basis for the description of "standing waves" by Hamilton and Dow (1939) we may arrive at an explanation of this phenomenon which, although different, is nevertheless of the same kind as theirs. The effect is indeed due to interaction with reflected waves (as in a true "standing wave"). In terms of the analysis that we have made, however, it is a purely local phenomenon independent of the resonance which is implicit in the term "standing wave". This escapes the contradictions in the use of the term when it is coupled with measurements of the rate of propagation as a measure of elastic properties of arteries (Dow and Hamilton, 1939)—for a standing wave is "stationary" and does not travel.

REFLECTION

Although Wiggers (1928) has been quoted as considering four categories of factors influencing the pulse-wave form, the only one that has been considered in detail by subsequent workers is that of reflection. All previous work has been on the basis of looking for the reflection of individual parts of the wave, and some of the difficulties in this method have already been discussed in Ch. 10. In terms of steady-state analysis the effects of wave-reflection have been described in detail and the analysis of experimental results has given rise to the same general conclusion—that reflection is the predominant cause of wave distortion in the arterial system.

So far we have presented experimental results in the aorta and in the hind-limb but have tended to regard them as independent. For technical reasons it is difficult to record pressures in experimental animals over the whole arterial bed simultaneously. Consecutive records from the root of the aorta to the dorsalis pedis have been made in man by Remington and Wood (1956) in one of the most detailed studies ever made. Unfortunately they did not publish the whole of their wave forms so that it is not possible to subject them to Fourier analysis. This has been done as an illustration on the records of two separate dogs made by Laszt and Müller

(1952*a*, *b*). Here there are a total of eight recording points from the heart to the saphenous artery. (Figs. 12.4 and 5). By inspection, the progressive changes in wave form in the dog (Fig. 12.4) appear to be similar to those recorded in the human by Remington and Wood (1956). These results are given in addition to our own (Fig. 12.1) because they are made through laterally placed cannulae and there can be no question of increased reflection in the femoral bed due to the use of a long cannula.

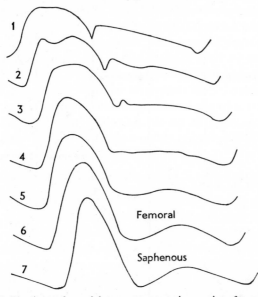

Fig. 12.4. Tracings of arterial pressures at various points from the heart to the saphenous artery. Curves 4–7 are redrawn to the same calibration factor from Fig. 4 of Laszt and Müller (1952*b*). Curves 1–3 are from another dog (Fig. 5 Laszt and Müller, 1952*a*) in which the heart rate was the same but in which the pulse-pressure was lower—the site of curve 4 was common to both. The shape of curve 4 was almost identical in both cases so that the amplitude of the first three curves has been scaled so that they match at this point. The anatomical locations of the recording points are shown in Fig. 12.5.

From Fig. 12.5 it can be seen that the moduli of all the harmonic components shown are larger in the saphenous artery than at the root of the aorta. This phenomenon, which is due to the essentially "closed" nature of the end of the arterial tree, is the principal cause of the increase in total pulse amplitude—the peaking effect that is so marked a feature of the pulse as it travels peripherally. Furthermore there are only two situations where all the harmonics are increasing at the same time. These are at the distal end of the aorta and at the end of the limb (the slight fall in the 2 c/sec component at the saphenous position may reasonably be treated as due to experimental error, and we may regard it as virtually at a maximum throughout the saphenous artery which is close to the termination). As a simple approximation we can regard the arterial tree from the heart to the feet as though it were two chambers in series. The first is the aorta with partial reflection of a closed type

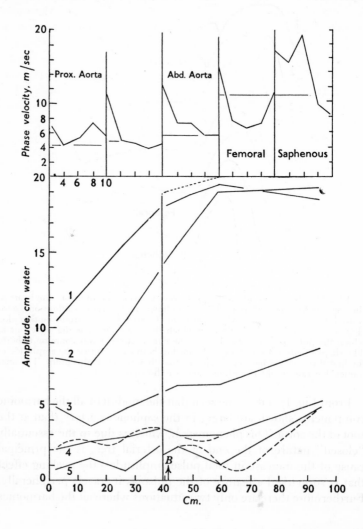

at the region of the bifurcation of the aorta and the pelvic vascular bed; the second is that of the two hind-limbs in parallel with a termination in the region of the feet.

In view of the fact that there are sites of major branches in the coeliac region, and again at the origin of the profounda femoris artery, the picture that emerges from the study of the evidence is curiously simple. The origin of the visceral arteries, in particular, has very reasonably been suggested by previous workers (notably Alexander, 1953) as an important site of reflection. Alexander thought that it acted as an "open" end because the cross-sectional area of all the branches is so much greater than that of the thoracic aorta. If this were so one would expect a tendency for the amplitude of all the harmonics to fall as the wave approaches this region and so far this has never been observed. The only conclusion that can be drawn from present evidence is that the impedance of the total visceral bed is well matched with that of the thoracic aorta. As noted above (Fig. 10.5) Womersley (1958b) has predicted a small reflection at the origins of these vessels with a phase-shift of 90° (i.e. mid-way between "open" and "closed"). This will be modified by the subsequent branching of the visceral arteries; although there is no information at present about their reflection behaviour, by analogy with other terminal beds they will behave as partially "closed". The reflections arising from the arteries to the head and forelimbs have not been studied in detail and as far as the system supplying the rest of the body is concerned can be most easily considered as a part of the reflecting system at the root of the aorta,

---

FIG. 12.5. The results of the harmonic analysis of the curves shown in Fig. 12.4. They represent two different experiments separated by the vertical line. As explained in the legend to Fig. 12.4, the values in the aorta have been scaled up so that the amplitude of the components are the same in the pulse waves recorded at the same location. This is marked by the line just to the left of the point B, which marks the bifurcation of the aorta. All distances are measured from the aortic valves. Dotted lines indicate changes in amplitude that would be consistent with the phase velocities recorded in the upper panels (their abscissae are in c/sec—pulse frequency was 2 c/sec in both animals).

As noted in the text, it can be seen that the amplitudes of all frequencies are rising simultaneously in only two situations—the distal end of the aorta and in the saphenous artery—which indicates that both are close to a major site of reflection. The distribution of nodes and antinodes is not so clearly seen as in Fig. 10.3 but where visible they are consistent with this reflection hypothesis.

The upper panels showing the phase velocities are the values for the first three intervals (in the aorta) and in the femoral (45–60 cm) and saphenous arteries (60–95 cm). The short interval across the bifurcation has been omitted. The horizontal bars represent the foot-to-foot velocities.

because these vessels arise so close to the heart. Reflected waves arising from the hind-end of the body will, of course, be reflected again when they reach the heart. From the point of view of pressure-waves this would appear to be very completely closed—by the aortic valves during diastole and by the wall of the left ventricle during systole. This, however, will be very difficult to separate from the interaction with the impedance represented by the large vessels leading off the arch of the aorta. The analysis of pulse-wave behaviour in the anterior part of the body similar to that presented here for the aorta-femoral systems should help to elucidate this point. By analogy with what is known of the peripheral resistance of these regions it seems at least unlikely that the reflection co-efficients will be higher than in the hind-limb vascular bed, and may be rather less.

The aorta-femoral system can thus be regarded as having at most 50 per cent reflection at the distal end and about the same at the proximal end. Even in the absence of damping any wave travelling over the system will be rapidly attenuated—to at least a half at the first reflection at the periphery, and to a quarter or less after returning to the origin, and so on. When this attenuation is augmented by the viscous damping of the wave as it travels it can be appreciated why there can be very little build-up of pressure-waves in any form of resonance even when (as seen in Fig. 10.3) the wave-length relations in the system might lead one to expect it.

"NATURAL" VIBRATIONS

The concept of natural vibrations occurring in the arterial system has been put forward by many workers. By "natural" is meant a resonant frequency of the system and if an oscillatory force at this frequency is applied there will be a maximum amplitude of response. This phenomenon has to be taken into account and has been discussed in relation to the behaviour of manometers (Ch. 11 and Appendix 2). If we consider the arterial system as being in a steady state oscillation then if it has a resonant frequency this will result in an amplification of any of the component frequencies of the pulse-wave that are close to it. It will be seen from Table V that there is no marked tendency for any harmonic component to dominate the others—the fundamental is the largest and the higher frequencies are all progressively smaller. McDonald and

Taylor (1956) also make a preliminary search for such resonant frequencies by imposing a sinusoidal oscillation from a pump into the aorta (through a cannula in the subclavian artery). The results appeared to show that the amplitude response was flat to 6 c/sec and at frequencies above that declined fairly rapidly. That is, it was a form of curve similar to that of 70 per cent critical or "optimal" damping in a manometer (Fig. 11.2). The response at the higher frequencies was probably inaccurately measured because it appeared that cavitation was occurring proximal to the cannula during the back-stroke of the pump. The method, which is essentially the same as calibrating manometer responses with an oscillator, would appear to be the most direct way of searching for natural frequencies in the arterial tree. In view of all the other evidence on the failure of waves to resonate in the arterial tree (discussed above and in Ch. 10) it seems unlikely that they are of any significance.

CHARACTERISTICS OF THE ARTERIAL TREE

It appears from the evidence that all the changes in wave-form found in the arterial system can be explained by wave-reflection and damping. The special characters of this wave transformation largely arise from the anatomical form of the arterial tree rather than from any peculiar properties of the arterial wall or of the blood. We could probably make a model out of rubber tubes that would show a very similar pattern of wave-propagation.

A most important aspect of the arterial tree that has tended to be overlooked is that it is a short system in terms of the principal wave-lengths involved. When considering wave-transmission the wave-length is a fundamental unit. As the pulse-wave velocity in the aorta is at least 500 cm/sec, and may well be 800–1,000 cm/sec in more peripheral arteries such as the femoral, we can take an average overall wave velocity of 600 cm/sec and still regard it as a conservative estimate. In a human being with a pulse-frequency of 1 c/sec this gives a wave-length of 6 metres. The heart, which generates the waves, is somewhat eccentrically placed in the middle of the arterial tree; the longest distances to the periphery in an average man will be about 1·25 m to the feet, about 0·8 m to the hands and about 0·4 m to the head. Therefore from the heart to the feet is only about a quarter wave-length of the fundamental component of the pulse. The wave-lengths of the higher frequency components will, of course, be proportionately shorter but not until one considers the fourth harmonic will one whole wave-length be reached in this section of the tree. The distance between the heart and the head will similarly be less than one wave-length up to a frequency of 15 c/sec.

Thus although wave reflection is undoubtedly incomplete it can be seen (as was said in Ch. 10) that any point in the arterial tree is always close to a region that will cause reflections. The most remarkable feature of the change in form of the travelling pressure wave is the "peaking" of the wave; that is, the increase in overall amplitude as it travels. This is directly contrary to the expected behaviour of waves propagated in a viscous medium where damping will cause a reduction in amplitude. There are two pieces of evidence especially which emphasize that this must be due to reflections.

In the first place while the pressure pulse is increasing in size the amplitude of the flow pulse is decreasing markedly. This is shown diagrammatically in Fig. 12.6 where some of the flow curves displayed in Ch. 7 are matched against some of the pressure curves discussed in this chapter. As the total amplitude of both of these curves is mainly determined by the size of the first and second harmonic terms, which are of relatively long wave-length, we can simplify the discussion by considering their behaviour alone; that is, we will ignore for the moment the formation of nodes and anti-nodes. The progressive change of amplitude in contrary sense of the pressure and the flow indicates that the peripheral parts of the arterial tree have a much higher impedance than the more central parts. An increased impedance causes wave reflection in a "positive" sense, i.e. as from a partially closed end. In any system without end-effects of this kind the amplitude of the pressure oscillation and of the flow oscillation would be damped by the same amount as they travelled.

The second analysis that makes it evident that there is a reflection of the pressure waves is that when there is "peaking" not only is the amplitude of the wave increased but also its variance. As stated in Ch. 11 the variance is a measure of the energy content of the wave and can only show the apparently paradoxical effect of increasing as it travels if it is summating with a reflected wave. The *variance* of the curve which is derived from the sums of the squares of the ordinates (eqn. 11.2), should not be confused with the *area* under the curve. The area is only a measure of the *mean arterial*

pressure and so will show a small decrease as observations are made more peripherally. The increase in variance is very marked; taking as examples some of the curves analysed in Table IV we find:—
(*a*) from the ascending aorta (1*P*) to the distal abdominal aorta (4*P*) the variance increased from 100·37 to 258·75, i.e. an increase

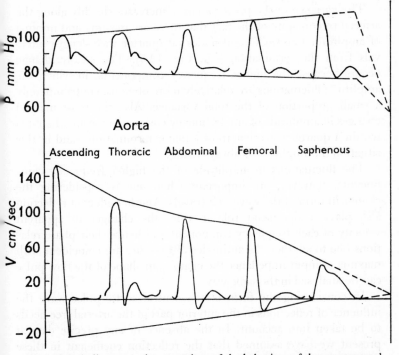

FIG. 12.6. A diagrammatic comparison of the behaviour of the pressure and flow pulses in arteries as they travel away from the heart. Mean pressure falls slowly but the pulsatile pressure variation increases until in the saphenous artery it may be double that at the root of the aorta. The flow oscillation, on the contrary, diminishes markedly. Such behaviour can only be accounted for by the presence of a "closed" type of reflection in the small peripheral vessels. In the absence of reflections damping would cause a parallel fall in pressure and flow oscillations. Ultimately the pressure oscillations must also be damped out—the probable region of this fall is in the smallest arteries and proximal arterioles as indicated by the broken lines.

The increase in ratio of the pulsatile pressure amplitude to that of the flow amplitude is largely determined by the increase in the fluid impedance of the low-frequency components; the change in shape of the pressure wave to that of flow wave depends on the changes in impedance of the various frequency components in terms of their distance from the main reflecting sites, as the impedance is at a minimum at a quarter wave-length distance.

(The pressure curves are redrawn from Fig. 12.4; the flow curves are those of Fig. 7.11.)

of 157·8 per cent; the area of curve 4*P*, however, was only 99·7 per cent that of curve 1*P*. (*b*) The variance from the distal abdominal aorta (5*P*) to the saphenous artery (7*P*) in another animal showed a further rise of 152 per cent. This increase is paralleled by the increase in the impedance of the low-frequency components of the pulse-wave as displayed in Fig. 10.11.

The variance of the pressure curve increases steadily along the arterial tree in spite of the fact that there are maxima and minima of amplitude (antinodes and nodes) at quarter wave-length intervals from the termination (e.g. Fig. 12.5). The steady change occurs because the higher frequency components, in which the amplitude fluctuations are relatively more obvious, contribute only a small proportion of the total variance. Also the most marked changes in amplitude of any frequency component occur when it is within a quarter wave-length of a major termination—and in this situation the amplitude is always rising.

The fluctuations in amplitude of the higher frequency components, however, are important when one is considering the change in form of the wave as it travels. Another effect of reflection also plays a significant role in this—the changes in apparent velocity of each frequency component and hence their phase relations one to another. As antinodes of pressure are coincident with maxima of input impedance the changes in shape of the flow pulse can be analysed in the same way.

In considering the form of the central aortic pulse-wave the influence of reflections in the anterior part of the arterial tree needs to be taken into account. In the absence of any precise data at present we have assumed that the reflection coefficient in these regions is the same as the tentative values we have derived for the pelvic and hind limb vascular beds, i.e. about 40 per cent. The average distance of these terminations from the heart may be taken as approximately half that of the hind-limb terminations. Using a simple mathematical model of this kind Taylor (unpublished) has shown that, assuming the form of the systolic output to be as recorded by Wetterer (Fig. 7.1), one can make a surprisingly good prediction of an average central aortic pulse. This emphasizes that it is quite unrealistic to consider this pulse as being unaffected by reflections as is often assumed when calculations of cardiac output are made (see Ch. 13).

Reflections will always occur at points of subdivision of the arterial tree because one can never get exact impedance matching (as shown in Figs. 10.5 and 10.6). It does seem, however, that in the large arteries this reflection is usually close to the minimum. All the evidence discussed in Ch. 10 points to the fact that reflections mainly arise in the region of the smallest arteries and the arterioles. It is this region that is referred to as the "termination" of the vascular bed.

ARTERIOLES

When considering an artery supplying a specific region, e.g. the superior mesenteric artery, although it appears to be branching constantly the number of subdivisions increases enormously within a few millimetres of the capillary bed. This is well illustrated by the data of Schleier (1918) or Bazett (1941). Again thinking in terms of wave-length this distance is so small that one can think of it as an abrupt end in a large number of small tubes. The total cross-sectional area of these minute branches is, of course, very much larger than that of the parent trunk. This difference in the total size of the vascular bed has often led to the suggestion that reflections should be of the "open" end type; put into other words this means that their fluid impedance must be lower. It is, however, well-known that the vascular resistance increases greatly when the arterioles are reached (the factor being the square of the increase in area divided by the number of branches—eqn. 2.13).

To make precise predictions about the impedance here requires information about the wall elasticity, i.e. velocity of wave propagation, that we do not have but, as shown in Fig. 10.6, there seems no reason to doubt that in very fine tubes the situation for matching fluid impedances will be essentially the same as for matching vascular resistances. It is, in fact, difficult to conceive of any analogous system in which a great increase in resistance is accompanied by a decrease in impedance.

The marked increase in vascular resistance in the small vessels may be attributed to the viscous drag of the blood on the greatly increased vessel wall area. Equally from the properties of wave-propagation in larger tubes (Figs. 9.2 and 9.3) we may anticipate, for the same reason, a very high degree of viscous damping and a reduction of wave velocity. However, the effect on wave velocity of an increased relative thickness of the wall due to the smooth muscle layers is difficult to predict.

In Fig. 12.6 we can see that the pulse pressure increases as far as a small artery such as the saphenous. At some stage of branching beyond this it must start to decrease rapidly because in the capillaries, under normal conditions, there is no pulsation of the wall and the flow is quite steady. From the comparison of the values of the input impedance and that of the vascular resistance that was made in Ch. 10, it was suggested that there is pulsatile flow only in the proximal part of the arterioles. In the example shown in Fig. 10.9 the impedance of the fundamental component was only about 10 per cent of the vascular resistance. Under normal conditions, as discussed in Ch. 2, the arterioles may be reckoned to contribute some 60 per cent of the total vascular resistance. With increasing arteriolar dilatation the pulsatile flow will extend farther through the arterioles and capillary flow itself may become pulsatile. Thus, although reflection in the smallest vessels may be reduced by vasodilatation there will always be an "end" where pulsations are damped out and hence reflected. As, in addition, there is the contribution from the other sites of branching in the larger arteries which do not show vasomotor activity, it will be difficult to separate their "fixed" reflections from the variable contribution from the arterioles. Because the physical effects determining the form of the pulse-wave are so largely centred on the small vessels a more thorough investigation of the patterns of pressure and flow in them should be rewarding.

CHAPTER XIII

ESTIMATION OF THE CARDIAC OUTPUT FROM PRESSURE-RECORDINGS

For its practical value in clinical medicine as well as in physiological research the discovery of a technically simple and non-traumatic way of estimating the output of the heart per beat is something of an Eldorado. Now that the arterial pressure can be relatively easily recorded at the root of the aorta in human beings it is not altogether surprising that many attempts have been made to use this as a measure of the blood flow.

The physical relationships between blood pressure and blood flow that have formed the main theme of this book indicate that the estimation may be approached in one of two ways. The first is to determine the *pressure-gradient* which is associated with the flow, the second is to attempt to discover a formula that will predict the flow from the form of the *pressure*-wave recorded at a single point. It is this second approach which has formed the bulk of the investigations in the past, but an appreciation of the physical problems will make it clear that the first is much more realistic.

PRESSURE-GRADIENT METHODS

The mathematical equations which relate a steady flow in a tube with the concomitant pressure-gradient are well-known in the form of the Poiseuille formula (Ch. 2) and the more general solution which applies to oscillatory laminar flow was given in Ch. 5. Fry *et al.* (1956) have derived a simpler form of this equation and applied it to the measurement of the velocity of flow in the proximal aorta of the dog (Fig. 5.9). This shows clearly that the technique of measuring a pressure-gradient is straightforward and there seems little reason why it should not be applied in the human subject. Owing to the fact that a double lumen catheter must be used it might be preferable to measure the pressure-gradient in the pulmonary trunk. The measurement of the cardiac output of the cat was determined by placing a flowmeter in the pulmonary trunk by Baxter *et al.* (1952) and Brecher and Hubay (1954) similarly

275

used a bristle flowmeter in the dog; this location does have the advantage over using the aorta in that there is no loss of coronary flow. The possible limitations of the method can only be adequately explored by comparing the results of this technique with those obtained using another standard method. The conditions that need to be fulfilled are:

(1) The gradient should be measured over a length of vessel that does not have intervening branches. In this respect the human subject, being larger, is more suitable than a dog in which there is rarely more than 2·5–3 cm between the aortic valves and the origin of the brachio-cephalic artery.

(2) The radius of the vessel must be known, especially if volume flow is to be estimated. The pulsatile variation of radius should also be known but in the aorta it might be neglected as a first approximation. Large pulsatile variations will make any accurate solution very difficult mathematically and so may bar this method from being applied to the pulmonary trunk.

(3) The application, of the equations used, to flow that is turbulent, or has large eddies in it, also needs to be known. Because the pressure-flow under pulsatile conditions in large vessels is largely determined by the inertia rather than the viscosity of the blood this may prove to be unimportant (see Ch. 5). Fig. 5.10 showed the comparison between the curve calculated allowing for viscosity with that if viscosity is zero; the discrepancy is not great and would be smaller in the human adult because the values of α are larger.

These difficulties may seem formidable but I think are far from insurmountable. By comparison any attempt to derive the flow from the recording of a single pulse-wave must be founded on assumptions which are almost certainly untrue. Applying the reasoning of previous chapters, we know that the flow and the arterial pressure run in parallel if the impedance is the same for all the component frequencies. That is to say, the oscillatory flow can be calculated from the pressure curve if there are no reflection effects at the root of the aorta (provided conditions 2 and 3 above can be satisfied). To make this estimation the pulse-wave velocity in the aorta has to be known, and the calculation would be based on the derivation of the pressure-gradient from the time derivative of the pulse (eqn. 5.11). In some cases this approximation is quite close; for example the flow curve for the proximal aorta in Fig. 5.10

which is taken from the pressure-gradient (derived for the first two curves in Fig. 12.1) would be very close to that calculated from the time-derivative, taking a pulse-wave velocity of 400 cm/sec because all the phase-velocities (Fig. 10.3) are close to this value. In a case like that shown in Fig. 12.4 and 5 there would be a considerable error because the apparent phase-velocities (and hence the impedance—Fig. 10.11) are varying considerably. Furthermore the steady flow cannot be derived from a single measurement. The only way these conditions can be checked is by a second pulse recording farther downstream, and if this is done a direct pressure-gradient can be measured.

An ingenious application of the Fry equation (5.12) to the time-derivative of the central aortic pulse has been made by Jones *et al.* (1959). In each experimental animal they "calibrated" the flow obtained by this method against a measurement of the cardiac output by the dye-dilution method. The constant of proportionality will thus include the reciprocal of the wave-velocity (eqn. 5.11) and the cross-sectional area of the aorta (to convert the velocity of flow to volume flow). The added assumption is, as seen above, that the input impedance is the same value for all the major frequency components (which is not necessarily the same as assuming there are no effects of reflection in the proximal aorta— see Fig. 10.3). These authors found by this method a good correlation between the flow calculated from the pressure time-derivative with flows measured by the dye method over a wide range of output and pulse-frequency. The method has thus the advantage of only needing a single lumen catheter together with a reasonable theoretical basis, and appears to be much the best technique, so far proposed, which uses only one pressure record.

PULSE CONTOUR METHODS

The formulae that have been commonly used to calculate the cardiac output are, however, derived from a completely different approach. The basic principle common to them all is that the aortic pulse is treated as though it were the pressure curve of an isolated, but leaking, chamber being filled with liquid. This is, of course, an application of the Windkessel model. The earliest attempt to apply this to estimating the cardiac output was that of Frank (1899), but numerous modifications have been put forward, notably by Broemser and Ranke (1931) and Wezler and Böger

(1939). Apart from the general criticism that this is treating a dynamic system as a static model, the assumptions made in these formulae need to be examined. Firstly, the drainage from the arterial tree is assumed to vary directly with the diastolic pressure or with the diastolic pressure minus 20 mm Hg (Remington, 1954). As this drops considerably from the time of the closure of the aortic valves to the end of the cycle the proportionality can only be true if the flow through the capillaries fluctuates to the same extent. Capillary flow is, however, normally quite free from pulsation. In view of the even larger fluctuations of pressure that occur during the diastolic part of the curve in the more peripheral arteries (Figs. 12.1, 12.4) it is difficult to see how this assumption can seriously be defended. It is much more logical to regard the flow out of the system in relation to the mean pressure throughout the cycle, and it is agreed that this relation is determined by the peripheral resistance, i.e. by vasomotor activity. The second assumption necessary is that the central aortic pulse is not modified by reflected waves, at least, during the systolic part of the cycle. In another form this is an assertion that the pulse-pressure in the proximal aorta is determined entirely by the systolic ejection of the heart, and that it is not affected by vasomotor changes in the periphery. Remington (1954) has actually published a table by which the cardiac index is predicted by the pulse pressure. This is the outcome of detailed studies by the Georgia group, (Remington and Hamilton, 1945, 1947; Remington, Hamilton and Dow, 1945; Remington, 1952) in which the elasticity of the arterial system has been estimated at 10 msec intervals during systolic filling. From the evidence discussed in Ch. 10 it seems impossible to say that reflections play no part in the form of the aortic pulse. They may not be very marked and they may not increase the pulse pressure (as is usually assumed)—in Fig. 10.3 for example, the fundamental component appears to be at a node close to the heart and so is considerably smaller than it would be in the absence of reflections. The predicted ejection curves derived by this group have also been shown by Wetterer (1954) to be quite different from those actually recorded by a flowmeter.* The third assumption involved in

*If the aorta were truly without reflections there would be a pressure pulse at the root very similar in shape to that of the flow velocity curve (Fig. 7.1) and, as the records of Wetterer in 1940 have now been repeated in the almost identical tracings published by Spencer *et al.* (1958) we can

nearly all these derivations is that the elastic behaviour of the Windkessel can be simply determined from the pulse-wave velocity. This is, in essence, reasonable, especially when account is taken of the varying wave-velocities in the more peripheral arteries as in the method of Remington, Hamilton and Dow (1945). In other cases arbitrary values are taken such as by measuring transmission time from the heart to the femoral artery (Warner *et al.*, 1953), and the significance of such a mean value is uncertain.

The values obtained by various methods have been compared with other estimates of the volume of systolic ejection. Hamilton and Remington (1947) compared their calculated results with estimates by the dye-dilution method and found a good correlation. Brotmacher (1957) however, in an independent test of several formulae, found them all unsatisfactory. Starr and Schild (1957) tested the formulae of Broemser and Ranke (1931) and Wezler and Böger (1939), and came to the conclusion that their results did not support the theory on which the formulae were based. One is reminded of the words of Hamilton (1945) himself when he remarked that in the days when Grollman's values for cardiac output were the standards of reference (which are now agreed to be much too low), all the "secondary" methods such as X-ray kymography, ballistocardiography and pulse-pressure methods gave similar results—"These secondary methods are a bit slippery in that they always give results which check with the comparison method, whatever it may be."

A slightly different approach which would appear more promising is that exemplified by Warner *et al.* (1953). They calibrated, as it were, their pulse-pressure estimate in each individual with a direct determination of cardiac output by the dye-dilution method and then used the pressure recording to follow changes in stroke volume under conditions of changing circulatory conditions. This

---

have confidence that it is a common form of the cardiac flow ejection pulse. The pressure pulse is never remotely like this in shape. To talk of a "filling" curve is, strictly speaking, of necessity to invoke reflections because pressure effects from the far end of the chamber (whatever it is) must come into play. Most workers when they write of the absence of reflections merely mean the absence of discrete and recognizable waves, but without any reflections the arterial system would behave as if it were infinite in extent.

emphasizes the potential values of such a method because the standard Fick and the Hamilton dye-dilution methods both require stable conditions, over a considerable period of time, to be valid. Their formula however, is still based on the rather doubtful assumptions that have been discussed above.

An alternative approach would appear to be the application of the water-hammer formula (eqn. 9.1)

$$P = \rho \bar{V} c$$

This would only be an approximation as it assumes a non-viscous fluid, and to convert the velocity into volume flow the cross-sectional area of the aorta would need to be estimated. However, Starr and Schild (1957) in their cadaver experiments found that this simple equation was the best description of their results. More recently Evans (1958) has worked out a formula which is a modification of the water-hammer formula and has applied it to the data of Warner *et al.* (1953) with encouraging results. This suggests that this approach warrants further exploration as it is based on a standard physical formula and is free of the empiricism which surrounds most pulse-pressure formulae. It still leans heavily on assumptions which are hard to justify at present. It requires an absence of reflections, and the estimation of the wave velocity is equally difficult here as in the other formulae. In addition the relation between the phasic flow velocity (which it calculates) and the mean systolic ejection velocity is not known. Evans assumes that the mean velocity is half the peak velocity, which implies that the ejection flow curve is parabolic in form. The curves in Figs. 5.9 and 7.1 indicate that this is a little dubious.

As already indicated, I feel that the work devoted to modifying and justifying these various methods of estimating cardiac output based on a single pressure recording would be far more usefully employed in measuring the pressure-gradient. This is directly related to the flow, although a high degree of technical accuracy is needed to make it reliable. If there is any one single conclusion that emerges from the theoretical analysis and experimental work discussed in the foregoing chapters, it is that one must make a minimum of two simultaneous recordings to derive valid information about a system like the arterial tree. Ideally the phasic flow should be one of these measurements. Failing that, from two pressure measurements one can record the pressure-gradient and the phase velocities, and so describe the conditions of wave-propagation such as the extent to which reflection is occurring. In terms of flow and pressure we can describe the characteristics in terms of the input impedance, which is probably the simplest way that comprises all the factors that are so closely knit together in the arterial circulation.

CHAPTER XIV

SUMMARY AND CONCLUSIONS

It may be useful to survey the overall picture of pulsatile flow in the arterial tree as it emerges from the analysis presented in the preceding chapters.

1. Laminar and turbulent flow (Ch. 2, 3 and 4)

In an hydrodynamic investigation it is first of all necessary to establish whether one is dealing with laminar or turbulent flow. The former can be analysed with precise mathematical methods; the latter is a complex problem. In the circulation we are fortunate in that flow is undoubtedly laminar in all the smaller vessels, although problems of anomalous viscosity are raised by the fact that blood is a suspension of relatively large particles. In the large arteries, however, conditions for turbulence undoubtedly exist during cardiac systole. Nevertheless, even here it is possible to treat the flow as approximately laminar because (a) the periods over which the critical velocities are exceeded are short and it is by no means certain that fully developed turbulence is ever attained, at least in the dog or smaller animals, and (b) turbulence only affects the viscous element in the energetics of flow and in the central arteries, where there are large pulsatile variations in flow velocity, the importance of viscosity is relatively small (e.g. Fig. 5.10 shows that in the proximal aorta the omission of the viscous term makes little difference to the flow curve calculated from the pressure-gradient).

The assumption of laminar flow for the calculation of pressure-flow relations in arteries is thus unlikely to introduce an error detectable with the techniques at present in use. This aspect must be clearly differentiated from the effects of transient turbulence and eddy formation on mixing the blood in the heart and great vessels and in the generation of sounds in the cardiovascular system (Ch. 4). It can be regarded as established that, in the normal heart, mixing is complete by the time the blood leaves either ventricle.

2. The relation of pulsatile pressure-gradient to flow

The simplest type of fluctuating flow to study is one that oscillates sinusoidally. The pressure-flow relationship of such flow, when it is laminar, has been derived by several workers independently but has been explored very thoroughly and the necessary functions tabulated (eqn. 5.2, Fig. 5.3 and Appendix) by Womersley. As might be expected the solution is a general one which reduces to the formula of Poiseuille for steady flow when the frequency of the oscillation tends to zero.

When we remember that the pressure term that we are concerned with in Poiseuille's formula is the pressure-gradient along the tube (the pressure drop per unit length) it is obvious that for oscillatory flow it is also the gradient that must be measured. As the pressure oscillation in this case is travelling away from the heart the difference in pressure between two points will also oscillate (Fig. 5.2). This oscillation will occur in any system with a travelling wave and is no indication of reflected or "standing waves" or resonance in the system (see Ch. 10). If there is no reflection the pressure-gradient (the derivative of pressure with respect to distance) is simply related to the derivative of the pressure with respect to time and the wave velocity (eqn. 5.6). If there are reflected waves this is no longer true. The actual pressure-gradient along the vessel, however, is indissolubly linked to the movement of the fluid within it. This is as true for oscillatory, or pulsatile, flow as it is for the more familiar case of steady flow.

The mathematical equation for oscillatory flow that we use is, strictly speaking, only applicable to a rigid tube, i.e. one in which the walls cannot move. Investigations have shown (Ch. 8) that the connexions between an artery and the tissues around it effectively prevent longitudinal movement. Womersley (Ch. 9) has shown that in this case the equations for the rigid tube apply to arteries very well. The dilatation of arteries is small and although it can be allowed for in the calculations the error due to neglecting it is small and, at present, does not appear to justify the greatly increased complexity of the mathematical working for practical purposes. In fact all Womersley's detailed mathematical investigations indicate that changes in the behaviour and properties of the arterial wall have relatively little effect on the pressure-flow relationships of the blood although they are important with regard to wave propagation.

The solution for a single sinusoidal oscillation may be applied to the pulsatile flow in the arterial system by resolving the pressure-gradient into a set of harmonic components by means of Fourier series (see App. 1). As the heart-beat is regularly repeated this is a standard physical method of analysing a wave such as that of the pulse. It only assumes that the system is in a "steady-state", that is changes due to "starting-up" after any interruption in rhythm have disappeared, and that successive pulses are the same shape. Experience shows that a steady-state is reached in the dog within 0·5–1 sec and in practice this type of analysis is only misleading for the pulses due to single ectopic beats or conditions where the heart rates and force of contraction are markedly irregular.

The rapid attainment of a steady-state is itself evidence for marked damping of pulsations in the arterial tree (see section 4 below) and is the basis for the concept, used by most previous workers, of each pulse being imposed on a system at rest. Technically this would define the arterial pulse as a "transient response". Only at low heart rates is this a reasonable description; even so the proper mode of analysis of a transient response, although set out theoretically by Otto Frank and widely used in other branches of physics, has never been used by physiologists and is far more complex (the usual method is to use the Fourier integral) than the harmonic, or Fourier, series method adopted throughout this book.

It is often overlooked that in addition to the sum of the harmonic terms, the Fourier series has a constant or steady term (eqn. 1.1). This represents the mean value around which the oscillatory components oscillate and sets, as it were, the level of working. When analysing pressure this seems to cause no confusion; in the case of pulsatile flow curves, where the steady flow component is small compared with the magnitude of the oscillatory components, it may decide whether certain special features of the curve (such as backflow at some point of the cycle) are present or absent. The evidence now points strongly to the fact that there is commonly a short period of backflow in the femoral artery in the middle of the cardiac cycle; increasing the steady (or mean) flow as by reactive hyperaemia (Fig. 7.6) or by occluding upstream branches (Fig. 7.9) will cause this backflow to disappear but there will still be a minimum of flow at that point. Equally backflow may disappear if the oscillatory terms are reduced in magnitude, but in this case the total swing between maximal and minimal flow will be reduced. This serves to emphasize that misunderstanding can arise by picking on a single descriptive feature of a record of pulsatile flow, or of pressure.

3. Pressure and flow patterns in arteries. The input impedance

When we consider the changes in the pulsatile pressure and flow that are found as we pass from the heart to the periphery we find that the size of the pressure oscillation, or pulse pressure, usually increases. This has been known for a long time and examples are illustrated in Figs. 12.1, 12.4 and 12.6. The pulsatile flow oscillation on the other hand decreases markedly (Fig. 7.11). Taken by itself the reduction in the fluctuations in flow velocity (as records are made farther away from the heart) might be regarded as caused by the damping due to viscosity. If this were so the pressure oscillation would also decrease in a similar way, as it must in the smallest arteries and arterioles where damping is very high. In the arterial tree it does exactly the opposite. This can only be due to reflections of the travelling wave in the periphery from a "closed" type of termination. The extreme case of such a reflecting system is illustrated by a fluid-filled rubber tube with a pump having a sinusoidal output attached to one end and which is completely closed at the other. Immediately next to the occluded and the pressure oscillation is large but, of course, there can be no flow at a dead end. If on the other hand we move progressively away from the end we find that the pressure oscillation diminishes and the flow oscillation increases until a distance of one quarter wave-length is reached. Here the flow oscillation is at a maximum and the pressure oscillation at a minimum. Moving still farther away changes occur in the reverse direction until, at a half wavelength, pressure is at a maximum and flow at a minimum. The position of these nodes and anti-nodes is determined by their relation to the reflecting site and independent of the position of the pump or the existence of conditions of resonance. If the tube is merely narrowed without being completely closed the same qualitative effects will occur but the relative amplitudes of the maxima and minima will be less for they are determined by the degree of reflection and the viscous damping that is present. Therefore it is called a "closed" type of reflecting site.

The consideration of the distribution of mean pressures in the arterial circulation has clearly shown that the fluid resistance of the peripheral vascular bed is very high compared with that of the central vessels, even though the total cross-sectional area of the vessels has increased enormously. The peripheral resistance of any vascular bed, by analogy with Ohm's law (Ch. 2), is defined as the pressure-drop (potential difference) across it divided by the rate of flow (current). By similar analogy with alternating current theory the ratio of the oscillatory pressure-gradient to the oscillatory flow velocity will define the fluid impedance (Ch. 5). If we are considering the behaviour of a whole vascular bed such as that supplied by the femoral artery we call this the input impedance. As we know that the pulsatile pressure oscillations have disappeared in the capillaries, the pressure-gradient over the whole bed is identical with the pulsatile arterial pressure; put another way this means that by using the arterial pressure and flow we are measuring the input impedance of the vascular bed up to the point (unspecified) where the pulsations disappear.

From the consideration of the simple rubber tube it is easy to see that the input impedance is at a minimum at a quarter wavelength from a closed type of end (pressure—minimal; flow—maximal) and rises steadily towards the termination. The wavelength of each component of the flow gets progressively shorter as the frequency increases. Therefore the distance between any single point of observation in an artery and a reflecting region represents progressively larger fractions of a wave-length as we analyse progressively higher frequencies. Fig. 10.8, for example, shows that at a frequency of 13·5 c/sec there was a minimum of impedance at the femoral artery. The recording point must be approximately one quarter wave-length from the average site of reflections.

The concept of input impedance used in this way is a useful and simple way of describing pressure and flow behaviour in any part of the arterial tree. The use of the term is justified because apart from its most familiar use in electrical theory it is an accepted term, as mechanical, or acoustical, impedance, in other physical sciences. The behaviour of fluid impedance is much more analogous to these latter types of impedance than to the electrical ones and attempts to find simple analogies in an hydraulic system with the components of electrical impedance are almost certainly doomed to failure.

4. Wave reflection

In section 2 of this summary it was stated that the arterial system must be highly damped as it attains a steady-state so rapidly. In section 3, however, large effects due to reflection of waves were mentioned which may appear to conflict with the previous statement. The reason that they are compatible is that, in terms of wave-length, the arterial system is very short. From the heart to the end of the hindlimbs in a dog is normally less than one quarter wave-length of the pulse frequency (e.g. Fig. 12.5), although at fast heart rates this fraction may approximate to the length of the aorta (Fig. 10.3). For the second harmonic the same distances will be about one half wave-length and so on. The present evidence indicates that the pulse-wave undergoes only one major reflection. That is at the periphery and there the reflection coefficient (the ratio of reflected to incident wave) is of the order of 0·3–0·5. Any subsequent reflection at the proximal end of the aorta (aortic valves and the vascular beds supplied by the arch of the aorta) appears to be small. The reason for saying this is summed up in Fig. 10.3 where, by good fortune, we have an animal with a pulse-frequency such that the distance from the heart to the reflecting site near the end of the aorta is close to a half wave-length for the second harmonic and a full wave-length for the fourth harmonic. Both are situations which should resonate, if such a phenomenon occurs, and give rise to marked nodes and antinodes, yet the actual pressure variation is small. This is due both to damping in travel (due to the viscosity of the blood and the viscous element in the arterial wall) and to incomplete reflection at both ends of the aorta.

The study of the arterial system from the heart to the hind-limbs indicates that we can describe the behaviour of reflections as if they were occurring at the pelvic vascular bed and near the extremity of the hind-limbs. Only as we approach these two regions are the amplitudes of all the harmonic components increasing together (Figs. 10.3 and 12.5)—a situation that can only occur if they are all within one quarter wave-length of a closed end. It is also of interest to note that it is only within this distance that any component shows a major change in amplitude; this again points to the fact that the system is, in effect, highly damped.

Now we have seen that for the fundamental frequency a quarter wave-length often includes the whole arterial tree and even for the second harmonic most of the system is included in this interval. A very large proportion of the energy of the pulse is contained in these two harmonics. The energy is proportional to the square of the amplitude and these two components normally account for at least 75 per cent of the total energy—in the femoral artery it is often 85–90 per cent. The behaviour of the low frequency components will, therefore, largely determine the amplitude of the arterial pulse; it is the steady increase of these components of the pressure pulse that is the reason for the progressive "peaking" of pressure that is observed from the heart to the most peripheral arteries; conversely, as the impedance rises towards the periphery it is the resultant reduction in amplitude of the low frequency flow terms that is mainly responsible for the rapid diminution of pulsatile variations in flow velocity.

It is of some interest to consider where reflection of the pulse-wave principally occurs. In a system like this any point of branching, or any region where the elasticity of the arterial wall changes, will mark a change of impedance and give rise to a reflection. From theoretical calculations it appears likely that for the larger branches, like the bifurcation of the aorta, the cross-sectional areas involved are such that reflection is minimal and of the order of 10 per cent at most (Fig. 10.5). In smaller arteries this increases (Fig. 10.6), although we have fewer data as to sizes and wave velocities on which to make predictions. In the small arteries, however, repeated subdivision gets more frequent so that there are good theoretical grounds for supposing that the very small vessels form the major reflecting regions.

Experimentally, there can be little doubt that a large part of the reflection occurs at vessels that are under vasomotor control and, functionally, may therefore be called arterioles. From our own evidence in the femoral artery of the dog it appears that strong vasoconstriction can increase the impedance of the fundamental component by almost three times. With marked vasodilatation the corresponding reduction is much smaller (about 20–25 per cent in our present measurements).

Although these changes in impedance are not so proportionately great as the simultaneous changes in the vascular resistance they can cause large changes in the value of the reflection coefficient.

These quantitative estimates of the size of the reflected components of the pulse-wave are as yet relatively crude because of the dearth of the right sort of experimental data. With the improvement in the accuracy of flowmeters that has been achieved in the last year or so I feel sure that this lack will be remedied; a thorough exploitation of the information that can be obtained from the analyses of pressure-flow relationships in terms of impedance is necessary to test the conclusions that have been put forward here. This is desirable before we can, with any confidence, pass to the practical problems of studying changes in arterial flow in human patients by means of pulse-wave analysis.

APPENDIX 1

THE METHOD OF CALCULATING AN OSCILLATORY FLOW FROM ITS PRESSURE-GRADIENT

The first step necessary in calculating a flow curve is to perform a Fourier analysis of the pressure-gradient. As the oscillatory gradient is a function that repeats periodically this is a valid method of representing it. A Fourier series represents any such curve by a set of sinusoidal oscillations at frequencies which are integral multiples of the repetition frequency; all these components oscillate about the mean value of the function. Mathematically if we have a function $F(t)$ with repetition frequency ω, then we write

$$F(t) = A_0 + A_1 \cos\omega t + A_2 \cos2\omega t + A_3 \cos3\omega t ... A \cos_n n\omega t$$
$$+ B_1 \sin\omega t + B_2 \sin2\omega t + B_3 \sin3\omega t ... B_n \sin n\omega t \quad .... \text{ A.1}$$

where A_0 is the mean value of the function. Each harmonic component is represented by a pair of terms—$A_n \cos n\omega t + B_n \sin n\omega t$. These may also be represented by a single term $M_n \cos(n\omega t - \phi)$. The simplest way of showing this summation of a cosine and sine wave is seen in Fig. A.1. On the left the two components are shown in the conventional way by the rotation of a point around the circumference of a circle. The summation, shown on the right, is that of a point moving on a circle whose radius is the hypotenuse of a right-angled triangle the sides of which represent the amplitudes of the cosine and sine terms. Therefore if

$$A \cos \omega t + B \sin \omega t = M \cos(\omega t - \phi) \quad .... \text{ A.2}$$

then

$$M = \sqrt{A^2 + B^2} \quad .... \text{ A.3}$$

and

$$\tan \phi = B/A \quad .... \text{ A.4}$$

The point P may also be written as a complex number

$$A - iB$$

where $i = \sqrt{-1}$. (Any number which involves the root of minus one is called imaginary; a complex number is so-called because it has real and imaginary parts. When drawn graphically real numbers are represented by distances in the direction of the x-axis and the imaginary numbers by distances in the direction of the y-axis.

The two parts are therefore in essence vectors in two directions at right angles and so are written separately.)

A simple harmonic motion may also be written in exponential form, e^{ix}. The validity of this can be simply shown by expanding the exponential series

$$e^{ix} = 1 + ix - \frac{x^2}{2!} - \frac{ix^3}{3!} + \frac{x^4}{4!} + \frac{ix^5}{5!} \cdots$$

$$= \cos x + i \sin x$$

so that a Fourier term such as in eqn. A.2 may be written as the real part of
$$Me^{i\omega(t-\phi)}$$

i.e.
$$A \cos \omega t + B \sin \omega t$$

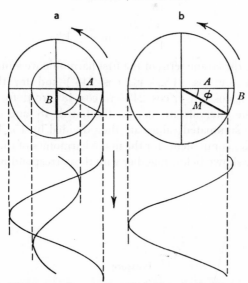

FIG. A.1. Diagrammatic representation of a simple harmonic motion in terms of its Fourier coefficients

(a) A pair of Fourier terms—$A \cos \omega t + B \sin \omega t$; for convenience the sine term is drawn as if it were a cosine projection 90° behind the true cosine component. Thus at $\omega t = 0°$, $\cos \omega t = A$ and $\sin \omega t = 0$; when $\omega t = 90°$ the two vectors A and B have rotated anticlockwise through that angle and $\cos \omega t = 0$ and $\sin \omega t = B$; with $\omega t = 180°$, the cosine is $-A$ and the sine zero. The waves traced out by the points moving around the circles are shown below—the direction of the vertical arrow indicates the values of the two terms as the points move around the circles (curved arrow). The sum of these two curves is shown in the oscillation in the lower part of (b).

(b) The circular diagram shows how the resultant single oscillation described in (a) can be described as a single wave; its initial point is at $-\phi°$ and the amplitude is M. It is thus the curve of $M \cos(\omega t - \phi)$. It can be seen that $M = \sqrt{A^2 + B^2}$ and that $\tan \phi = B/A$ (eqn. A.3 and A.4).

The actual calculation of the Fourier terms of a given curve is best given by an example. In Fig. A.2 is illustrated a pressure-gradient measured by a differential manometer between two points 5 cm apart in the femoral artery. The second curve is the arterial pressure measured at one of these points. The value of the gradient is measured at 30 ordinates throughout the cycle. Each interval therefore represents an angle of $2\pi/30$ radians i.e. $12°$. If the ordinates are y_r where $r=0, 1, 2,...29$ then (referring to eqn. A.1)

$$A_0 = \frac{1}{30} \sum_{r=0}^{r=29} y_r$$

$$A_n = \frac{1}{15} \sum_{r=0}^{r=29} y_r \cos nr \times 12°$$

and
$$B_n = \frac{1}{15} \sum_{r=0}^{r=29} y_r \sin nr \times 12°$$

Thus for the cosine term of the first harmonic we sum $(y_0.\cos 0°+y_1.\cos 12°+y_2.\cos 24°...+y_{29} \cos 348°)$ and for the second harmonic $(y_0 \cos 0°+y_1 \cos 24°+y_2 \cos 48°$ etc.); for the third harmonic the intervals are $36°$, for the fourth $48°$ and $60°$ for the fifth. These summated values are then divided by 15. The values of the Fourier components for the first 5 harmonics of the pressure-gradient are shown below together with the corresponding modulus and phase.

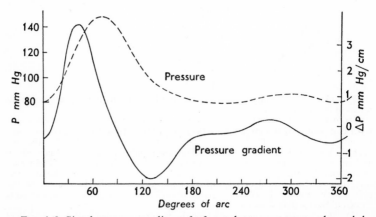

FIG. A.2. Simultaneous recordings of a femoral artery pressure pulse and the pressure-gradient measured between two points 5 cm apart. The gradient curve is subjected to a Fourier analysis and the corresponding flow terms calculated in the text of this appendix.

Fig. A.2. *Fourier analysis of the pressure-gradient* (units mm Hg/cm)

Harmonic	A (cosine)	B (sine)	Modulus (M)	ϕ
1	$+1 \cdot 024$	$+0 \cdot 240$	$1 \cdot 052$	$13 \cdot 2°$
2	$-0 \cdot 126$	$+1 \cdot 346$	$1 \cdot 352$	$95 \cdot 23°$
3	$-0 \cdot 819$	$+0 \cdot 477$	$0 \cdot 948$	$149 \cdot 79°$
4	$-0 \cdot 305$	$+0 \cdot 002$	$0 \cdot 305$	$179 \cdot 62°$
5	$-0 \cdot 260$	$-0 \cdot 144$	$0 \cdot 380$	$209 \cdot 33°$

Mean value $= +0 \cdot 335$ mm Hg/cm.

Note that the angle determined by eqn. A.4 above must be placed in the correct quadrant according to the signs of the cosine and sine terms respectively. (It is a useful practical guide that the phase of each harmonic component of an arterial pressure-wave seems always to get progressively larger with the order of the harmonic; if this is not so we recheck in search of a possible error.)

CALCULATION OF FLOW COMPONENTS

METHOD 1. There are alternative methods of calculating the flow according to which form of the equation is used. The simplest one would appear to be that using eqn. 5.7

$$Q = \frac{\pi R^4}{\mu} \cdot M \cdot \frac{M'}{a^2} \sin(\omega t - \phi + \varepsilon)$$

First the values of a for each harmonic have to be calculated. In the present example $R = 0 \cdot 13$ cm, the pulse-frequency, $f, = 2 \cdot 4$ c/sec; we take $\mu = 0 \cdot 04$ Poise and $\rho = 1 \cdot 055$.

As
$$a_n = R \sqrt{\frac{2\pi n f}{\mu}}$$

for the first harmonic (i.e. $n = 1$) this gives a value of $a_1 = 2 \cdot 60$. The corresponding values for M'/a^2 and ε are then obtained from Table VI. For the second harmonic $n = 2$ and $a_2 = 2 \cdot 60 \times \sqrt{2} = 3 \cdot 67$ and so on for the other harmonics. The "modified modulus" ($M \times M'/a^2$) and the phase ($\varepsilon - \phi$) of the fluid motion is thus established as shown below.

The mean flow is calculated from Poiseuille's equation

$$Q = \frac{\pi R^4 \Delta P}{8 \mu}$$

where ΔP is the mean value of the gradient.

We have seen that

$\Delta P = 0 \cdot 335$ mm Hg/cm $= 0 \cdot 335 \times 1 \cdot 36 \times 980$ dynes/cm³

$$\therefore Q = \frac{3 \cdot 1416 \times (0 \cdot 13)^4 \times 0 \cdot 335 \times 1 \cdot 33 \times 10^3}{8 \times 0 \cdot 04} = 1 \cdot 25 \text{ ml/sec}$$

Harmonic	a	M'/a^2	$\varepsilon°$	$M \times M'/a^2$	$(\varepsilon-\phi)°$
1	2·60	0·0819	42·86	0·0862	$+$ 29·66
2	3·67	0·0508	27·31	0·0687	$-$ 67·92
3	4·49	0·0363	21·17	0·0344	$-128·62$
4	5·20	0·0282	17·83	0·0086	$-151·79$
5	6·80	0·0233	15·76	0·0089	$+166·43$

The factor $\pi R^4/\mu$ is common to all terms and is calculated separately (with the conversion of mm Hg into dynes/cm², i.e. $1·36 \times 980$); here its value is 29·83 so that the total flow (including the mean flow) is given by the equation

$$Q = 1·25 + 2·57 \sin(x + 29·66°) + 2·05 \sin(2x - 67·92°)$$

$$+ 1·03 \sin(3x - 128·62°) + 0·23 \sin(4x - 151·79°) + 0·27 \sin (5x + 166·43°)$$

where x (or ωt) is, as before, successively 0°, 12°, 24° etc. Care has to be taken with regard to the sign of the sine. As the sine is positive from 0° to 180° and thereafter negative, angles between 180° and 360° have been written as negative angles.

This method has the great disadvantage that the sines of every individual term of each harmonic has to be looked up in tables of trigonometrical functions.

METHOD 2. When it is recalled that, in the harmonic terms of the pressure-gradient,

$$A = M \cos \phi \text{ and } B = M \sin \phi \text{ (ref. Fig. A.1)}$$

we can expand eqn. 5.7 into this form, where Q_n is the oscillatory flow of the nth harmonic

$$Q_n = \frac{\pi R^4}{\mu} \cdot \frac{M'_n}{a_n^2}(A_n \sin \varepsilon_n - B \cos \varepsilon_n) \cos nx$$

$$+ \frac{\pi R^4}{\mu} \cdot \frac{M'_n}{a_n^2}(A_n \cos \varepsilon_n + B_n \sin \varepsilon_n) \sin nx \ldots \ldots \text{A.5}$$

This only necessitates looking up the sine and cosine of each value of ε and so, provided a desk calculator is available to do the greater number of multiplications, is much less tedious than the previous method. Not only does it minimize reference to standard tables but it obviates the need to calculate the modulus and phase of the pressure component.

Where $a > 10$ the tables do not apply but simple asymptotic expansions are available to compute M' and ε. Thus

$$M' = 1 - \frac{\sqrt{2}}{a} + \frac{1}{a^2} \quad \dots\dots\dots\dots \text{A.6}$$

and ε (radians) $= \dfrac{\sqrt{2}}{a} + \dfrac{1}{a^2} + \dfrac{19}{24\sqrt{2}a^3} \quad \dots\dots\dots \text{A.7}$

These values are plotted graphically for $10 < a < 20$ in Fig. A.3. When $a > 20$ eqns. A.6 and A.7 may be used but it will rarely be necessary. Even then, when $a = 20$, M' is less than 7 per cent from its limiting value of $1\cdot0$ and ε is only $4\cdot2°$, so that little error will be introduced by taking $M' = 1\cdot0$ and $\varepsilon = 0°$ (cf. Fig. 5.10).

METHOD 3. A further method of calculation is that using the form of the equation for flow given in 5.6. This may be written as

$$Q = \frac{\pi R^4}{i\mu} \cdot \frac{N}{a^2} \left[1 - F_{10} \right] e^{i\omega t} \quad \dots\dots\dots \text{A.8}$$

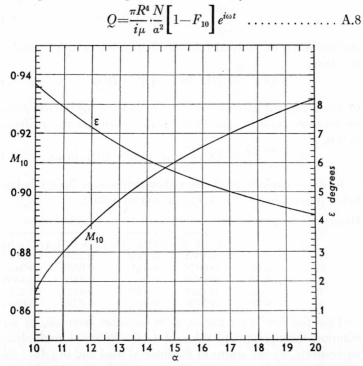

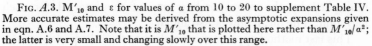

FIG. *A*.3. M'_{10} and ε for values of a from 10 to 20 to supplement Table IV. More accurate estimates may be derived from the asymptotic expansions given in eqn. A.6 and A.7. Note that it is M'_{10} that is plotted here rather than M'_{10}/a^2; the latter is very small and changing slowly over this range.

and expanding a^2 this becomes

$$Q = \frac{\pi R^2 . N}{i\omega\rho}\left[1 - F_{10}\right]e^{i\omega t} \quad \dots\dots\dots\dots \text{A.9}$$

where the pressure-gradient, is the real part of $Ne^{i\omega t}$, that is

$$Re\{Ne^{i\omega t}\} = A\cos\omega t - B\sin\omega t$$

Once again A and B are the Fourier coefficients and the gradient may be written as the complex number $(A-iB)$.

The value of $(1-F_{10})$ in real and imaginary parts is given in Table VII as a function of a and may be written $(C+iD)$.

Therefore to compute eqn. A.9 we write

$$Q = \frac{\pi R^2}{i\omega\rho}\cdot(A-iB)(C+iD)e^{i\omega t} \quad \dots\dots\dots\dots \text{A.10}$$

As dividing by i is equivalent to multiplying by $-i$ we get

$$Q = \frac{\pi R^2}{\omega\rho}(-B-iA)(C+iD)e^{i\omega t} \quad \dots\dots\dots\dots \text{A.11}$$

and following the normal rules of multiplying complex numbers we obtain

$$Q = \frac{\pi R^2}{\omega\rho}(AD-BC)-i(AC+BD)e^{i\omega t} \quad \dots\dots \text{A.12}$$

of which the real part is to be taken, as we are using the real part of the pressure-gradient. Therefore, for each harmonic the oscillatory flow is

$$Q = \frac{\pi R^2}{\omega\rho}(AD-BC)\cos\omega t + (AC+BD)\sin\omega t \dots \text{A.13}$$

In the example worked above these terms have been tabulated below (the values for A and B are set out on p. 293).

Harmonic	a	1–F_{10}		Flow terms	
		C (Real)	D (Imag.)	$(AD-BC)$	$(AC+BD)$
1	2·60	0·4061	0·3738	+0·2884	+0·5063
2	3·67	0·6075	0·3137	−0·8572	+0·3457
3	4·49	0·6835	0·2647	−0·5428	−0·4335
4	5·20	0·7269	0·2337	−0·0727	−0·2212
5	6·80	0·7436	0·2195	−0·2256	+0·0504

Thus the flow is calculated, as in the other methods, by substituting the appropriate value of $(AD-BC)$ and multiplying, successively, by the cosine of the interval used and of $(AC+BD)$ multiplied by the corresponding sine of the interval for each harmonic. The mean flow is also added.

This last method appears more elaborate than the previous ones but is in practice faster because the values of the cosine and sine of the 30 intervals once tabulated for the initial analysis are used throughout. The only additional reference to a table required (which is always the most time-consuming procedure in a computation of this sort) is to read off the value of $(1-F_{10})$. The similarity of eqn. A.13 to eqn. A.5 will be seen to be dependent on the fact that the Real part of $(1-F_{10})$ is $M'\cos\varepsilon$ and the Imaginary part is $M'\sin\varepsilon$.

The steps of the procedure have been written out in full but relatively simple apparatus can be made to carry out much of the work. The model developed by Taylor (1958a)—an improved version of that described by Rymer and Butler (1944)—will perform both Fourier analysis and synthesis. All that is required is the setting of the values of the co-ordinates read from the curve.

For some purposes the resynthesis of the flow curve is unnecessary, for example, in the calculation of the input impedance. In this case it is necessary to divide the pressure components for each harmonic by the corresponding flow terms. If the calculation is in modulus and phase form then the modulus of the impedance is given by

$$|Z_0| = M(Press.)/M\ (Flow)$$

and the phase by the difference

$$Ph\{Z_0\} = \phi(Press.) - \phi(Flow)$$

If the calculation is kept in real and imaginary parts it is necessary to follow the procedure of dividing complex numbers. If the arterial pressure has each harmonic term, $P=(A'-iB')e^{i\omega t}$ and for the flow velocity (following the usage of Ch. 10 in calculating impedance from the average velocity) we set $\bar{V}=(E-iF)e^{i\omega t}$ E and F are $(AD-BC)$ and $(AC+BD)$ in the table above when flow has been calculated from the pressure-gradient.

$$\therefore\ Z_0 = P/\bar{V} = \frac{A'-iB'}{E-iF}.$$

$(1/\omega\rho$ appears when eqn. A.10 is converted to $\bar{V}$ from Q, i.e. dividing by $\pi R^2)$

To divide by a complex number it is necessary to make the denominator real; in this case we multiply the top and bottom of the fraction by $E+iF$ so that

$$Z_0 = \frac{\omega\rho(A'-iB')(E+iF)}{(E-iF)(E+iF)} = \frac{\omega\rho(A'E+B'F)+i(A'F-B'E)}{(E^2+F^2)} \quad ..\text{A.14}$$

To take an example from Fig. A.2—the Fourier coefficients of the fundamental component of the pressure curve were computed (A', B') and the results were as follows.

A'	B'	E	F	$(A'E+B'F)$	$(A'F-B'E)$
$+6·65$	$+23·96$	$+0·2884$	$+0·5063$	$+15·486$	$-3·144$

then multiplying by $\omega\rho/(E^2+F^2)$

$$Z_0=+610·0-i123·8 \quad \text{Modulus,} \quad |Z_0|=6·2\times10^2 \text{ dyne.sec/cm}^3$$
$$\text{Phase} \quad =-11·5°$$

This is the method for calculating the arterial input impedance from the arterial pressure and the pressure-gradient used by Bergel *et al.* (1958).

APPENDIX 2

THE THEORETICAL ANALYSIS OF MANOMETER BEHAVIOUR

Simple harmonic motion is defined in the following way:—If a body moves so that its acceleration is always proportional, and opposite in sign to its displacement from an equilibrium position it is said to execute simple harmonic motion.

If we take as an example a mass (M) hanging on the end of a spring of elastance, S, then if the mass is displaced a distance x from the equilibrium position, the force exerted by the spring will be Sx, which must balance the acceleration; thus

$$M.\frac{d^2x}{dt^2}=-Sx \quad \dots\dots\dots\dots\dots\dots 1$$

If we test for a solution in the form $x=Be^{pt}$, we find

$$p^2=-S/M$$
$$\therefore p=\pm i\sqrt{S/M} \quad \dots\dots\dots\dots\dots\dots 2$$

so that the solution is

$$x=C_1e^{i\sqrt{S/M}.t}+C_2e^{-i\sqrt{S/M}.t} \quad \dots\dots\dots\dots\dots 3$$

where C_1 and C_2 are constants which may be determined from the initial conditions. If, when $t=0$, the body is at the limit of its oscillation then its velocity, $\frac{dx}{dt}=0$ and we set $x=A$.

Then from eqn. 3 we have

$$\left(\frac{dx}{dt}\right)_{t=0}=i\sqrt{S/M}.C_1-i\sqrt{S/M}.C_2=0$$

so that $C_1=C_2$
but $x=C_1+C_2=A$
$\therefore C_1=C_2=A/2$

so that eqn. 3 becomes

$$x=A\frac{(e^{i\sqrt{S/M}\ t}+e^{-i\sqrt{S/M}\ t})}{2}$$
$$=A\cos\left(\sqrt{\frac{S}{M}}t\right) \quad \dots\dots\dots\dots\dots 4$$

299

which is the familiar form of simple harmonic motion described by a cosine wave where the circular frequency (ω_0) is given by

$$\omega_0 = \sqrt{\frac{S}{M}} \quad \dots\dots\dots\dots\dots\dots 5$$

Damped simple harmonic motion is the condition where there is a resistance to the motion that is proportional to the velocity (viscous damping). If we call this resistance factor R the equation of motion corresponding to eqn. 1 is

$$\frac{Md^2x}{dt^2} = -Sx - R\frac{dx}{dt}$$

or

$$M.\frac{d^2x}{dt^2} + R\frac{dx}{dt} + Sx = 0 \quad \dots\dots\dots\dots 6$$

again putting x in the form Be^{pt} we obtain

$$Mp^2 + Rp + S = 0 \quad \dots\dots\dots\dots 7$$

$$\therefore p = -\frac{R}{2M} \pm \sqrt{\frac{R^2}{4M^2} - \frac{S^2}{M^2}} \quad \dots\dots\dots\dots 8$$

for convenience we can write

$$\beta_0 = \frac{R}{2M} \quad \dots\dots\dots\dots\dots\dots 9$$

and as in eqn. 5

$$S/M = \omega_0^2$$

so that

$$x = e^{-\beta_0 t}[C_1 e^{\sqrt{\beta_0^2 - \omega_0^2}.t} + C_2 e^{-\sqrt{\beta_0^2 - \omega_0^2}.t}] \quad \dots\dots\dots\dots 10$$

The behaviour of x in eqn. 10 is determined by the relative values of β_0 and ω_0 and falls into one of three categories (i) $\beta_0 > \omega_0$ (ii) $\beta_0 < \omega_0$ and (iii) $\beta_0 = \omega_0$.

In (i) $\beta_0^2 - \omega_0^2$ is positive, the exponents in eqn. 10 are real and the terms in the square brackets become a hyperbolic function. In terms of the mass-spring analogue we have used, there is now a dashpot in parallel, and the mass, when displaced and released, never oscillates but slowly returns to the equilibrium position. This is often called "dead-beat" motion and the system is spoken of as "over-damped".

(ii) $\beta_0 < \omega_0$, $\beta_0^2 - \omega_0^2$ is negative and its square root is imaginary. Taking the same initial conditions as for eqn. 3 we obtain the solution

$$x = \frac{A\omega_0^2}{\omega_0^2 - \beta_0^2}e^{-\beta_0 t}\cos\left[(\omega_0^2 - \beta_0^2)^{\frac{1}{2}}t - \tan^{-1}\frac{\beta_0}{(\omega_0^2 - \beta_0^2)^{\frac{1}{2}}}\right] \quad \dots\dots 11$$

which represents a sinusoidal oscillation that diminishes exponentially. We note that the "damped natural frequency" is given by $\sqrt{\omega_0{}^2-\beta_0{}^2}$ which is plainly less than ω_0, the natural frequency of the undamped system with the same mass and spring-stiffness.

(iii) In the special case where $\beta_0=\omega_0$ the solution of eqn. 10 becomes

$$x=A\ e^{-\beta_0 t}(1+\beta_0 t)\ \dots\dots\dots\dots\dots 12$$

This resembles dead-beat motion and is the limiting aperiodic case which is called *critical damping*. Damping coefficients are usually expressed as a ratio of this value, i.e. $\beta=\beta_0/\omega_0$. It is important to note that it is defined in terms of free vibrations and that the effect of damping where there are forced vibrations is somewhat different.

When a system that would oscillate naturally in simple harmonic motion is driven by a force that also varies harmonically it is said to be in a state of forced vibration. If there is no damping the resultant motion of the system is compounded of oscillations at both the natural and the driving frequencies. As in any real situation there is some damping the oscillation at the natural frequency dies away and the system only responds to the driving frequency. This is the "steady-state" condition that has been discussed in Ch. 1, i.e. the state after disturbances due to "starting-up" have died away.

If the driving oscillation is $K \sin \omega t$ while the natural frequency of the system is ω_0 as before, then the equation of motion is now (cp eqn. 6)

$$M\frac{dx^2}{dt^2}+R\frac{dx}{dt}+Sx=SK \sin \omega t \ \dots\dots\dots\dots 13$$

and its steady-state solution is, using ω_0 (eqn. 5) and β_0 (eqn. 9)

$$x=\frac{\omega_0{}^2K}{\sqrt{(\omega_0{}^2-\omega^2)^2+4\beta_0{}^2\omega^2}}\ \sin\left[\omega t-\tan^{-1}\frac{2\beta_0\omega}{\omega_0{}^2-\omega^2}\right]\ \dots 14$$

If K and ω_0 are put $=1\cdot0$ and ω is expressed as a fraction, γ, of ω_0 this is identical to eqn. 11.11.

If the damping is so small that $\beta_0{}^2$ can be neglected it can be seen that the amplitude of the response, A, is given approximately by

$$A=\frac{\omega_0{}^2K}{(\omega_0{}^2-\omega^2)}\ \dots\dots\dots\dots\dots 15$$

and will become very large when ω approaches ω_0—the condition of resonance.

Under the same conditions the phase lag is zero for all values except $\omega = \omega_0$ when it becomes indeterminate; in effect the phase lag changes rapidly from $0°$ to $180°$. As the damping increases the phase lag changes progressively with frequency but when $\omega = \omega_0$ it is always $90°$. The changes in phase and in amplitude have already been illustrated in Figs. 11.2 and 11.3.

In applying these equations more precisely to the hydraulic system of the manometer it is necessary to establish the equivalent terms of the generalized oscillatory system that we have considered up to this point. When there is a change in pressure there is movement of a volume of fluid, V, into or out of the system. Under dynamic conditions the effect of such fluid movement can be regarded as determined by its kinetic energy (as Noble, 1953, does) or more rigorously by the analysis of the physical behaviour of oscillations set up by a generator in a fluid-filled system of varying cross-section (as by Hansen, 1950). The velocity of flow with a given change of volume is inversely proportional to the cross-sectional area of the channel. The effective "mass" and the effective "resistance" are thus almost wholly dominated by the dimensions of the narrowest channels—the approximation is of the order of the ratio of the squares of the cross-sectional area of the manometer chamber and that of the needle or cannula. As the ratio of these areas is at least 20:1 it can be seen that the error is about 1/400. The second approximation that is made by Hansen (1950) is that the pressure-flow relationship under oscillatory conditions is that of Poiseuille's equation (2.2). As a result he has re-written the equation of motion (6) for free vibrations in the following form

$$\rho \frac{l}{\pi r^2} \cdot \frac{d^2V}{dt^2} + \frac{8\mu l}{\pi r^4} \cdot \frac{dV}{dt} + \underline{E}V = 0 \dots \dots \dots \dots 16$$

(where V is the volume flow).

In Frank's (1903) original equation the second term (on L.H.S.) was replaced by

$$\frac{k}{\pi r^2} \cdot \frac{dV}{dt}$$

where k was a constant to be determined experimentally. E is the pressure-volume modulus (i.e. $\Delta P / \Delta V$ and not the Young's modulus as in Ch. 8).

Rewriting eqn. 16 so that it is more easily comparable with eqn. 12 (i.e. dividing by $\rho l / \pi r^2$, and putting the density $\rho = 1 \cdot 0$) we

obtain
$$\frac{d^2V}{dt^2}+\frac{8\mu}{r^2}\cdot\frac{dV}{dt}+\frac{E\pi r^2V}{l}=0 \quad\ldots\ldots\ldots\ldots\ldots 17$$

whence we write eqn. 11.7
$$\omega_0=\sqrt{\frac{\pi r^2E}{l}}$$

The damping term β_0 $\left(\text{i.e. } \dfrac{R}{2M}\right)$ is similarly

$$\beta_0=\frac{4\mu}{r^2} \quad\ldots\ldots\ldots\ldots\ldots\ldots\ldots 18$$

As the ratio of the damping to critical damping $(\beta_0=\omega_0)$ is normally used we write (eqn. 11.10)

$$\beta=\frac{4\mu}{r^3}\sqrt{\frac{l}{\pi E}}$$

It is in this term, and in all the other manometer characteristics that involve the damping, e.g. the resonant frequency, that errors due to using the Poiseuille resistance will be apparent. Lambossy (1952b) investigated in detail the changes in predicted manometer characteristics that result from using the pressure-flow relationship of oscillatory flow in place of the approximation used by Hansen. It will be easier here to use the terms derived from Womersley's equations. In Ch. 5 the fluid resistance for oscillatory flow was given (eqn. 5.12) and is illustrated in Fig. 5.11. The new expression for β_0, in place of eqn. 18 becomes

$$\beta_0=\frac{\mu}{2r^2}\cdot\frac{a^2}{M'}\sin\varepsilon \quad\ldots\ldots\ldots\ldots\ldots 19$$

The values of M'/a^2 and ε are tabulated in Table VI and are determined by the term a.

The effect of using the oscillatory fluid resistance in eqn. 19, in place of the Poiseuille resistance (eqn. 18) will be to increase the damping constant as the frequency increases. As a is a function of the radius of the cannula as well as the frequency this effect will vary in degree with the size of tube used and is best illustrated by taking some numerical cases.

In one of Hansen's (1949) examples (that Lambossy, 1952b, also analysed) the characteristics of the manometer were predicted from the dimensions of the apparatus. The calculated value for the damping was 0·22. Now the radius of the needle was 0·0158 cm so that, water-filled, at 6 c/sec the value of $a \doteqdot 0·95$ and the damping calculated from eqn. 19 will be less than 1 per cent greater than that calculated from Hansen's own equation. At the resonant frequency (predicted to be 115 c/sec) the value of $a \doteqdot 4 \cdot 25$ and the damping will be 20 per cent higher than calculated by the Hansen eqn., i.e. $0 \cdot 26$ in place of $0 \cdot 22$.

Lambossy (1952*b*) reached similar conclusions and calculated some of the ancillary effects, e.g. a slightly lower resonant frequency. It is also of interest to note that the frequency-amplitude curve for "optimal" damping, which is that for $\beta = 0 \cdot 707$ (Fig. 11.2) with the simple theory, occurs with $\beta = 0 \cdot 8$ with the modified equation in this example.

This effect must be regarded as being of minor significance. The only situation in which this error might be worth correcting for is that of a manometer calibrated by the free vibration method (Ch. 11). This method, in effect, calculates the damping at the resonant frequency and so, in the working range, it will tend to be too high. Let us take an example from one of our own manometers —with a needle of radius $0 \cdot 02$ cm the resonant frequency was found to be 198 c/sec ($a = 7 \cdot 1$) and the damping at this frequency was $0 \cdot 1$. Applying the correction, this damping is reduced to $0 \cdot 063$ at 30 c/sec ($a = 2 \cdot 75$) and $0 \cdot 06$ at 2 c/sec ($a = 0 \cdot 7$) which is appreciably smaller. The phase error, however, is only *c*. $1 \cdot 5°$ at 30 c/sec with damping of $0 \cdot 1$ and would be actually *c*. $1 \cdot 0°$ if the corrected value were used. The corresponding change in amplitude distortion is to reduce it from 2 per cent to $1 \cdot 9$ per cent. Thus if we use manometers of high natural frequency and low damping so that we can neglect the errors in the low frequency range then we find that the actual errors are in fact smaller than predicted. If the damping is higher through using very fine needles the discrepancy will also be small because the change in fluid resistance is very small when a is small; for example the increase is less than $1 \cdot 4$ per cent for a $0 \cdot 0 - 2 \cdot 0$.

Direct calibration with a generator over the frequency range that it is desired to measure experimentally does not, of course, require any adjustment. It is, in any case, difficult to build a calibration apparatus of sufficient accuracy to detect these deviations from the simple theory of Hansen. The more precise form of the solution, with an estimate of the changes it produces, has been given here in an easily computable form to enable more precise calculation to be made when it is desirable.

TABLE VI

The values of M'_{10}/α^2 and ϵ_{10} for values of α from 0 to 10.

α	M'_{10}/α^2	ϵ_{10}	α	M'_{10}/α^2	ϵ_{10}	α	M'_{10}/α^2	ϵ_{10}	α	M'_{10}/α^2	ϵ_{10}
0.00	0·1250	90·00	2·50	0·0855	44·93	5·00	0·0302	18·65	7·50	0·0147	11·87
0.05	·1250	89·98	2·55	·0837	43·88	5·05	·0297	18·43	7·55	·0146	11·78
0.10	·1250	89·90	2·60	·0819	42·86	5·10	·0292	18·23	7·60	·0144	11·70
0.15	·1250	89·79	2·65	·0802	41·86	5·15	·0287	18·02	7·65	·0142	11·61
0.20	·1250	89·62	2·70	·0784	40·90	5·20	·0282	17·83	7·70	·0140	11·53
0.25	0·1250	89·40	2·75	0·0767	39·96	5·25	0·0278	17·63	7·75	0·0139	11·45
0.30	·1250	89·14	2·80	·0750	39·05	5·30	·0273	17·44	7·80	·0137	11·37
0.35	·1250	88·83	2·85	·0734	38·17	5·35	·0269	17·26	7·85	·0136	11·29
0.40	·1250	88·47	2·90	·0717	37·32	5·40	·0264	17·08	7·90	·0134	11·21
0.45	·1249	88·07	2·95	·0701	36·50	5·45	·0260	16·90	7·95	·0133	11·14
0.50	0·1249	87·61	3·00	0·0685	35·70	5·50	0·0256	16·73	8·00	0·0131	11·06
0.55	·1248	87·11	3·05	·0670	34·93	5·55	·0252	16·56	8·05	·0130	10·98
0.60	·1248	86·57	3·10	·0655	34·18	5·60	·0248	16·39	8·10	·0128	10·91
0.65	·1247	85·97	3·15	·0640	33·46	5·65	·0244	16·23	8·15	·0127	10·84
0.70	·1246	85·33	3·20	·0626	32·77	5·70	·0240	16·07	8·20	·0125	10·77
0.75	0·1244	84·65	3·25	0·0612	32·09	5·75	0·0237	15·91	8·25	0·0124	10·70
0.80	·1243	83·91	3·30	·0598	31·45	5·80	·0233	15·76	8·30	·0122	10·63
0.85	·1240	83·14	3·35	·0585	30·82	5·85	·0230	15·61	8·35	·0121	10·56
0.90	·1238	82·32	3·40	·0572	30·22	5·90	·0226	15·46	8·40	·0120	10·49
0.95	·1235	81·45	3·45	·0559	29·64	5·95	·0223	15·32	8·45	·0119	10·42
1.00	0·1232	80·55	3·50	0·0547	29·08	6·00	0·0220	15·18	8·50	0·0117	10·36
1.05	·1228	79·60	3·55	·0535	28·53	6·05	·0216	15·04	8·55	·0116	10·29
1.10	·1224	78·61	3·60	·0523	28·01	6·10	·0213	14·90	8·60	·0115	10·22
1.15	·1219	77·59	3·65	·0512	27·51	6·15	·0210	14·77	8·65	·0114	10·16
1.20	·1213	76·53	3·70	·0501	27·02	6·20	·0207	14·63	8·70	·0112	10·10
1.25	0·1207	75·44	3·75	0·0490	26·55	6·25	0·0204	14·50	8·75	0·0111	10·04
1.30	·1200	74·31	3·80	·0480	26·10	6·30	·0201	14·38	8·80	·0110	9·97
1.35	·1193	73·16	3·85	·0470	25·66	6·35	·0199	14·25	8·85	·0109	9·91
1.40	·1185	71·98	3·90	·0460	25·24	6·40	·0196	14·13	8·90	·0108	9·85
1.45	·1176	70·77	3·95	·0451	24·83	6·45	·0193	14·01	8·95	·0107	9·79
1.50	0·1166	69·54	4·00	0·0441	24·43	6·50	0·0191	13·89	9·00	0·0106	9·73
1.55	·1156	68·30	4·05	·0432	24·05	6·55	·0188	13·77	9·05	·0104	9·68
1.60	·1144	67·03	4·10	·0424	23·68	6·60	·0185	13·66	9·10	·0103	9·62
1.65	·1133	65·76	4·15	·0415	23·32	6·65	·0183	13·54	9·15	·0102	9·56
1.70	·1120	64·47	4·20	·0407	22·98	6·70	·0181	13·43	9·20	·0101	9·51
1.75	0·1107	63·18	4·25	0·0399	22·64	6·75	0·0178	13·32	9·25	0·0100	9·45
1.80	·1093	61·89	4·30	·0391	22·32	6·80	·0176	13·21	9·30	·0099	9·40
1.85	·1078	60·59	4·35	·0384	22·00	6·85	·0173	13·11	9·35	·0098	9·34
1.90	·1063	59·30	4·40	·0376	21·70	6·90	·0171	13·00	9·40	·0097	9·29
1.95	·1047	58·02	4·45	·0369	21·40	6·95	·0169	12·90	9·45	·0096	9·24
2.00	0·1031	56·74	4·50	0·0362	21·11	7·00	0·0167	12·80	9·50	0·0096	9·18
2.05	·1015	55·47	4·55	·0355	20·84	7·05	·0165	12·70	9·55	·0095	9·13
2.10	·0998	54·22	4·60	·0349	20·56	7·10	·0163	12·60	9·60	·0094	9·08
2.15	·0980	52·98	4·65	·0342	20·30	7·15	·0161	12·50	9·65	·0093	9·03
2.20	·0963	51·77	4·70	·0336	20·05	7·20	·0159	12·41	9·70	·0092	8·98
2.25	0·0945	50·57	4·75	0·0330	19·80	7·25	0·0157	12·31	9·75	0·0091	8·93
2.30	·0927	49·39	4·80	·0324	19·55	7·30	·0155	12·22	9·80	·0090	8·88
2.35	·0909	48·24	4·85	·0319	19·32	7·35	·0153	12·13	9·85	·0089	8·84
2.40	·0891	47·11	4·90	·0313	19·09	7·40	·0151	12·04	9·90	·0088	8·79
2.45	·0873	46·01	4·95	·0308	18·86	7·45	·0149	11·95	9·95	·0088	8·74
2.50	0·0855	44·93	5·00	0·0302	18·65	7·50	0·0147	11·87	10·00	0·0087	8·69

TABLE VII

The function $(1-F_{10})$ for values of α from 0(0·1)10. The function is defined in eqn. 5.6. (Reprinted from Womersley (1958a) by kind permission of the U.S. Air Force.)

	$1-F_{10}(\alpha)$			$1-F_{10}(\alpha)$			$1-F_{10}(\alpha)$			$1-F_{10}(\alpha)$	
α	Real	Imaginary	α	Real	Imaginary	α	Real	Imaginary	α	Real	Imaginary
0·0	0·0000	0·0000	2·5	0·3784	0·3774	5·0	0·7159	0·2416	7·5	0·8109	0·1704
0·1	0·0000	0·0012	2·6	0·4061	0·3768	5·1	0·7215	0·2376	7·6	0·8134	0·1684
0·2	0·0000	0·0050	2·7	0·4322	0·3744	5·2	0·7269	0·2337	7·7	0·8159	0·1664
0·3	0·0002	0·0112	2·8	0·4568	0·3706	5·3	0·7320	0·2300	7·8	0·8182	0·1645
0·4	0·0005	0·0200	2·9	0·4797	0·3657	5·4	0·7369	0·2264	7·9	0·8206	0·1627
0·5	0·0013	0·0312	3·0	0·5010	0·3600	5·5	0·7417	0·2229	8·0	0·8228	0·1608
0·6	0·0027	0·0448	3·1	0·5207	0·3536	5·6	0·7463	0·2195	8·1	0·8250	0·1590
0·7	0·0050	0·0608	3·2	0·5389	0·3468	5·7	0·7508	0·2163	8·2	0·8272	0·1573
0·8	0·0084	0·0791	3·3	0·5557	0·3398	5·8	0·7551	0·2131	8·3	0·8292	0·1556
0·9	0·0134	0·0994	3·4	0·5712	0·3327	5·9	0·7593	0·2100	8·4	0·8313	0·1539
1·0	0·0202	0·1215	3·5	0·5856	0·3256	6·0	0·7633	0·2070	8·5	0·8333	0·1523
1·1	0·0292	0·1452	3·6	0·5988	0·3185	6·1	0·7672	0·2041	8·6	0·8352	0·1507
1·2	0·0407	0·1699	3·7	0·6111	0·3116	6·2	0·7710	0·2013	8·7	0·8371	0·1491
1·3	0·0549	0·1953	3·8	0·6225	0·3049	6·3	0·7746	0·1985	8·8	0·8390	0·1475
1·4	0·0718	0·2208	3·9	0·6331	0·2984	6·4	0·7782	0·1959	8·9	0·8408	0·1460
1·5	0·0917	0·2458	4·0	0·6430	0·2921	6·5	0·7816	0·1932	9·0	0·8426	0·1446
1·6	0·1143	0·2698	4·1	0·6522	0·2860	6·6	0·7849	0·1907	9·1	0·8443	0·1431
1·7	0·1395	0·2921	4·2	0·6609	0·2802	6·7	0·7882	0·1882	9·2	0·8460	0·1417
1·8	0·1668	0·3123	4·3	0·6691	0·2747	6·8	0·7913	0·1858	9·3	0·8477	0·1403
1·9	0·1959	0·3300	4·4	0·6769	0·2693	6·9	0·7943	0·1834	9·4	0·8493	0·1389
2·0	0·2262	0·3449	4·5	0·6842	0·2642	7·0	0·7973	0·1811	9·5	0·8509	0·1376
2·1	0·2572	0·3569	4·6	0·6911	0·2593	7·1	0·8002	0·1789	9·6	0·8525	0·1363
2·2	0·2884	0·3660	4·7	0·6978	0·2546	7·2	0·8030	0·1767	9·7	0·8540	0·1350
2·3	0·3192	0·3723	4·8	0·7041	0·2501	7·3	0·8057	0·1745	9·8	0·8555	0·1337
2·4	0·3494	0·3761	4·9	0·7101	0·2458	7·4	0·8083	0·1724	9·9	0·8569	0·1325
2·5	0·3784	0·3774	5·0	0·7159	0·2416	7·5	0·8109	0·1704	10·0	0·8584	0·1312

REFERENCES

ALBRITTON, E. C. (1952). *Standard values in blood*, pp. 199. Philadelphia: Saunders.

ALEXANDER, R. S. (1953). The genesis of the aortic standing wave. *Circ. Research*, **1**, 145–51.

— (1954). The influence of constrictor drugs on the distensibility of the splanchnic venous system, analysed on the basis of an aortic model. *Circ. Research*, **2**, 140–7.

ALLIEVI (1909). *Allgemeine Theorie über die veränderliche Bewegung des Wassers in Leitungen.* Berlin: Springer. Cited by Karreman, G. (1952).

ANDRES, R., ZIERLER, K. L., ANDERSON, H. M., STAINSBY, W. N., CADER, G., GHRAYYIB, A. S. AND LILIENTHAL, J. L. JR. (1954). Measurement of blood flow and volume in the forearm of man; with notes on the theory of indicator-dilution and on the production of turbulence, hemolysis, and vaso-dilatation by intravascular injection. *J. clin. Invest.*, **33**, 482–504.

APÉRIA, A. (1940). Haemodynamical studies. *Skand. Arch. Physiol.*, **83**, Suppl. 1–230.

ASCHOFF, J. AND WEVER, R. (1956). Die Funktionsweise der Diathermie-Thermostromuhr. *Pflüg. Arch. ges. Physiol.*, **262**, 133–51.

BARCLAY, A. E., FRANKLIN, K. J., AND PRICHARD, M. M. L. (1944). *The foetal circulation and cardiovascular system, and the changes that they undergo at birth.* pp. viii and 275. Oxford: Blackwell.

BARNETT, C. H. AND COCHRANE, W. (1956). Flow of viscous liquids in branched tubes. *Nature, Lond.*, **177**, 740–2.

BARR, G. (1931). *A monograph of viscometry.* Oxford: University Press.

BAXTER, I. G. AND PEARCE, J. W. (1951). Simultaneous measurement of pulmonary arterial flow and pressure using condenser manometers. *J. Physiol.*, **115**, 410–29.

BAXTER, I. G., CUNNINGHAM, D. J. C. AND PEARCE, J. W. (1952). Comparison of cardiac output determinations in the cat by direct Fick and flow-meter methods. *J. Physiol.*, **118**, 299–308.

BAYLISS, L. E. (1952). Rheology of blood and lymph. In *Deformation and flow in biological systems*, ed. Frey-Wyssling, A. Amsterdam: North-Holland Publishing. pp. 355–418.

BAYLISS, L. E. AND ROBERTSON, G. W. (1939). The visco-elastic properties of the lung. *Quart. J. exp. Physiol.*, **29**, 27–47.

BAZETT, H. C. (1941). In *Macleod's physiology in modern medicine*, Ch. 23, p. 408. London: Kimpton.

BERGEL, D. H. (1958). A photo-electric method for the determination of the elasto-viscous behaviour of the arterial wall. *J. Physiol.*, **141**, 22–23P.

BERGEL, D. H., MCDONALD, D. A. AND TAYLOR, M. G. (1958). A method for measuring arterial impedance using a differential manometer. *J. Physiol.*, **141**, 17–18P.

BERGMANN, C. (1937–8). Die "Stromborste", ein elektrischer Geschwindigkeitsmesser für Flüssigkeiten. II. Stromkanüle und elektrische Messanordnung. *Z. Biol.*, **98**, 536–43.

BETTICHER, A., MAILLARD, J. AND MÜLLER, A. (1954). Un manomètre differential à transmission électrique entièrement alimenté sur le réseau alternatif, pour mesurer la vitesse d'écoulement dans des tuyaux et des vaisseaux sanguins. *Helv. physiol. acta*, **12**, 112–22.

BINGHAM AND JACKSON (1918). *Bur. Stand. J. Res., Wash.*, **14**, 75. p. 1993 in *Handbook of chemistry and physics*, 35th Ed., ed. Hodgman, C. D., Weast, R. C. and Wallace, C. W. Cleveland, Ohio: Chemical Rubber Publishing.

BIRCHER, M. E. (1921). Clinical diagnosis by the aid of viscosimetry of the blood with special reference to the viscosimeter of W. R. Hess. *J. Lab. clin. Med.*, **7**, 134–47.

BLUM, E. (1919). Die Querschnittbeziehungen zwischen Stamm und Ästen in Arteriensystem. *Pflüg. Arch. ges. Physiol.*, **175**, 1–19.

BOZLER, E. (1957). Extensibility of contractile elements. In *Tissue Elasticity*, ed. Remington, J. W. Washington: American Physiological Society. pp. 102–9.

BRAMWELL, J. C. AND HILL, A. V. (1922). The velocity of the pulse wave in man. *Proc. Roy. Soc. B*, **93**, 298–306.

— — (1923). The formation of "breakers" in the transmission of the pulse-wave. *J. Physiol.*, **57**, lxxiii–lxxiv.

BRECHER, G. A. (1954). Cardiac variations in venous return studied with a new bristle flowmeter. *Amer. J. Physiol.*, **176**, 423–40.

— (1956). *Venous return*. pp. 148. New York: Grune & Stratton.

BRECHER, G. AND HUBAY, C. A. (1954). A new method for direct recording of the cardiac output. *Proc. Soc. exp. Biol., N.Y.*, **86**, 464–7.

BROEMSER, P. (1928–9). Der Differentialsphygmograph. Eine Methode zur Registrierung der Kurve des Ablaufes der Strömungsgeschwindigkeit des Blutes in uneröffneten Arterien. *Z. Biol.*, **88**, 264–76.

— (1940). Uber die Grundschwingung des arteriellen Pulses. *Z. Biol.*, **100**, 88–96.

BROEMSER, P. AND RANKE, O. F. (1931). Ueber die Messung des Schlagvolumen des Herzens auf unblutigen Weg. *Z. Biol.*, **90**, 467–507.

BROEMSER, P., WETTERER, E., DEPPE, B. AND BAUEREISEN, E. (1943). Haemodynamische Fragen. Zugleich eine Stellungnahme zu den Veröffentlichungen von A. Apéria. *Arch. Kreislaufforsch.*, **12**, 1–47.

BROTMACHER, L. (1957). Evaluation of derivation of cardiac output from blood-pressure measurement. *Circ. Research*, **5**, 589–93.

BRUNER, H. D. (1948). Bubble flow meter. In *Methods in Medical research*, **1**, pp. 80–88. Chicago: Year Book Publishers.

BURTON, A. C. (1951). On the physical equilibrium of small blood vessels. *Amer. J. Physiol.*, **164**, 319–29.

— (1954). Relation of structure to function of the tissues of the walls of blood-vessels. *Physiol. Rev.*, **34**, 619–42.

CATTON, W. T. (1957). *Physical methods in physiology*. pp. ix and 375. London: Pitman.

CLARK, A. J. (1927). *Comparative physiology of the heart*. pp. 157. Cambridge: University Press.

CLARK, J. H. (1933). The elasticity of veins. *Amer. J. Physiol.*, **105**, 418–27.

COPHER, G. H. AND DICK, B. M. (1928). "Stream line" phenomena in the portal vein and the selective distribution of portal blood in the liver. *Arch. Surg., Chicago*, **17**, 408–19.

COULTER, N. A. JR. AND PAPPENHEIMER, J. R. (1949). Development of turbulence in flowing blood. *Amer. J. Physiol.*, **159**, 401–8.

COURNAND, A. F. (1948). Comment on "right heart catheterization". *Methods in medical research*, **1**, p. 231.

DAWES, G. S., MOTT, J. C. AND WIDDICOMBE, J. G. (1955). The cardiac murmur from the patent ductus arteriosus in newborn lambs. *J. Physiol.*, **128**, 344–60.

DAWES, G. S., MOTT, J. C., WIDDICOMBE, J. G. AND WYATT, D. G. (1953). Changes in the lungs of the new-born lamb. *J. Physiol.*, **121**, 141–62.

DENISON, A. B., SPENCER, M. P. AND GREEN, H. D. (1955). A square-wave electromagnetic flowmeter for application to intact blood vessels. *Circ. Research*, **3**, 39–46.

VON DESCHWANDEN, P., MÜLLER, A. AND LASZT, L. (1956). Beitraege zur haemodynamik. *Abstr. Comm. XX Internat. Physiol. Congr. Bruxelles*, pp. 930–1.

DOW, P. (1956). Estimations of cardiac output and central blood volume by dye dilution. *Physiol. Rev.*, **36**, 77–102.

DOW, P. AND HAMILTON, W. F. (1939). An experimental study of the velocity of the pulse wave propagated through the aorta. *Amer. J. Physiol.*, **125**, 60–65.

DREYER, B. (1954). Streamlining in the portal vein. *Quart. J. exp. Physiol.*, **39**, 305–7.

DUGUID, J. B. AND ROBERTSON, W. B. (1957). Mechanical factors in atherosclerosis. *Lancet*, 1957/i, 1205–9.

ELLIS, E. J., GAUER, O. H. AND WOOD, E. H. (1951). An intracardiac manometer: its evaluation and application. *Circulation*, **3**, 390–8.

EVANS, R. L. (1955). On the mechanism of turbulent flow in a liquid. *Proc. 4th Midwestern Conf. on Fluid Mechanics. Res. Bull. Purdue exp. Sta.*, **128**, pp. 235–43.

— (1956). Elasticity of vessel walls. *Amer. J. Physiol.*, **187**, 597.

— (1958). Cardiac output and central pressure data. *Nature*, **181**, 1471–2.

FENN, W. O. (1957). Changes in length of blood vessels on inflation. In *Tissue Elasticity*, ed. Remington, J. pp. 154–67.

FERGUSON, D. J. AND WELLS, H. S. (1959). Frequencies in pulsatile flow and response of magnetic meter. *Circ. Research*, **7**, 336–341.

FOLKOW, B. (1953). A critical study of some methods used in investigations on the blood circulation. *Acta physiol. scand.* **27**, 118–29.

FOLKOW, B. AND LÖFVING, B. (1956). The distensibility of the systemic resistance blood vessels. *Acta physiol. scand.*, **38**, 37–52.

FRANK, O. (1899). Die Grundform des arteriellen Pulses. Erste Abhandlung. Mathematische Analyse. *Z. Biol.*, **37**, 483–526.

— (1903). Kritik der elastischen Membranmanometer. *Z. Biol.*, **45**, 445.

— (1905). Der Puls in den Arterien. *Z. Biol.*, **46**, 441–553.

— (1927). Die Theorie der Pulswellen. *Z. Biol.*, **85**, 91–130.

FRANKLIN, D. L., ELLIS, R. M. AND RUSHMER, R. F. (1959). Aortic blood flow in dogs during treadmill exercise. *J. appl. Physiol.*, **14**, 809–812.

FRANKLIN, K. J. (1937). *A monograph on veins*. pp. 410. Springfield, Ill.: Thomas.

FRY, D. L., MALLOS, A. J. AND CASPER, A. G. T. (1956). A catheter tip method for measurement of the instantaneous aortic blood velocity. *Circ. Research*, **4**, 627–32.

FRY, D. L., NOBLE, F. W. AND MALLOS, A. J. (1957a). An evaluation of modern pressure recording systems. *Circ. Research*, **5**, 40–46.

— — — (1957b). An electric device for instantaneous and continuous computation of aortic blood velocity. *Circ. Research*, **5**, 75–78.

GILMORE, J. P. (1956). Hemodynamic response of the dog to pentobarbital sodium. *Naval med. Field Res. Lab., Proj. No. MNO06.014.04.05,* 9–24.

GOLDMAN, S. (1949). *Transformation calculus and electrical transients.* pp. xiv and 439. London: Constable.

GOLDSTEIN, S. (1938a). *Modern developments in fluid dynamics.* 2 vols. Oxford: Clarendon.

— (1938b). Note on the conditions at the surface of contact of a fluid with a solid body. Appendix to Vol II, *Modern developments in fluid dynamics.* Oxford: Clarendon.

GOMEZ, D. M. (1941). *Hémodynamique et Angiocinétique, étude rationnelle des lois régissant les phénomènes cardio-vasculaire.* pp. xxiii and 731. Paris: Hermann.

GREEN, H. D. (1944). Circulation: physical principles. In *Medical physics,* ed. Glasser, O. New York: Year Book Publishing.

— (1948). Pulsatile flow meters. pp. 101–8 in Vol. I, *Methods in Medical Research,* ed. Potter, V. R. Chicago: Year Book Publishing.

— (1950). Circulatory system: physical principles. In *Medical physics,* vol. II, ed. Glasser, O. Chicago: Year Book Publishing.

GREEN, J. H. (1954). A manometer. *J. Physiol.,* **125**, 4P.

GREGG, D. E. (1950). *Coronary circulation in health and disease.* pp. 227. Philadelphia: Lea & Febiger.

GREGG, D. E. AND GREEN, H. G. (1939). Phasic blood flow in coronary arteries obtained by a new differential manometric method. *Proc. Soc. exp. Biol., N.Y.,* **41**, 597–8.

GREGG, D. E., PRITCHARD, W. H. AND SHIPLEY, R. E. (1948). Changes in arterial inflow in the dog's leg following venous occlusion: evaluation of results obtained with different types of flow recorders. *Amer. J. Physiol.,* **153**, 153–8.

GREGORY, N., STUART, J. L. AND WALKER, W. S. (1955). On the stability of three-dimensional boundary layers with application to the flow due to a rotating disk. *Phil. Trans. A,* **248**, 185–236.

HALE, J. F., McDONALD, D. A. AND WOMERSLEY, J. R. (1955). Velocity profiles of oscillating arterial flow, with some calculations of viscous drag and the Reynolds number. *J. Physiol.,* **128**, 629–40.

HALE, J. F., MCDONALD, D. A., TAYLOR, M. G. AND WOMERSLEY, J. R. (1955). The counter chronometer method for recording pulse-wave velocity. *J. Physiol.,* **129**, 27P.

HAM, A. W. (1950). *Histology.* Ch. 21. Philadelphia: Lippincott.

HAMILTON, W. F. (1944). Arterial pulse. In *Medical Physics,* ed. Glasser, O. Vol. 1, pp. 7–9.

— (1945). Notes on the development of the physiology of cardiac output. *Fed. Proc.,* **4**, 183–95.

HAMILTON, W. F., BREWER, G. AND BROTMAN, I. (1934). Pressure pulse contours in the intact animal. I. Analytical description of a new high-frequency hypodermic manometer with illustrative curves of simultaneous arterial and intracardiac pressure. *Amer. J. Physiol.,* **107**, 427–35.

HAMILTON, W. F. AND DOW, P. (1939). An experimental study of the standing waves in the pulse propagated through the aorta. *Amer. J. Physiol.,* **125**, 48–59.

HAMILTON, W. F. AND REMINGTON, J. W. (1947). The measurement of the stroke volume from the pressure pulse. *Amer. J. Physiol.,* **148**, 14–24.

HAMILTON, W. F., REMINGTON, J. W. AND DOW, P. (1945). The determination of the propagation velocity of the arterial pulse wave. *Amer. J. Physiol.*, **144**, 521–35.

HANSEN, A. T. (1949). Pressure measurement in the human organism. *Acta physiol. scand.*, **19**, Suppl. 68, pp. 227.

— (1950). The theory for elastic liquid-containing membrane mano-meters. Special part. *Acta physiol. scand.*, **19**, 333–43.

HANSEN, A. T. AND WARBURG, E. (1950). A theory for elastic liquid-containing membrane manometers. General part. *Acta physiol. scand.*, **19**, 306–32.

HARDUNG, V. (1952). Über eine Methode zur Messung der dynamischen Elastizität und Viskosität kautschukähnlicher Körper, insbesondere von Blutgefässen und anderen elastischen Gewebteilen. *Helv. physiol. acta*, **10**, 482–98.

— (1953). Vergleichende Messungen der dynamischen Elastizität und Viskosität von Blutgefässen, Kautschuk und synthetischen Elasto-meren. *Helv. physiol. acta*, **11**, 194–211.

— (1957). Zum Gebrauch des Pitot-Rohres bei nichtstationärer Stro-mung. *Arch. Kreislaufforsch.*, **26**, 337–48.

— (1958). Wellenwiderstand und Impedanzen der geraden Schlauch-leitung. *Arch. Kreislaufforsch.*, **29**, 77–88.

HARKNESS, M. L. R., HARKNESS, R. D. AND MCDONALD, D. A. (1957). The collagen and elastin content of the arterial wall in the dog. *Proc. Roy. Soc. B*, **146**, 541–51.

HASS, G. M. (1942a). Elastic tissue. I. A description of a method for the isolation of elastic tissue. *Arch. Path.* (*Lab. Med.*), **34**, 807–19.

— (1942b). Elastic tissue. II. A study of the elasticity and tensile strength of elastic tissue isolated from the human aorta. *Arch. Path.* (*Lab. Med.*), **34**, 971–81.

— (1943). Elastic tissue. III. Relations between the structure of the ageing aorta and the properties of isolated aortic elastic tissue. *Arch. Path.* (*Lab. Med.*), **35**, 29–45.

HATSCHEK, E. (1928). *The viscosity of liquids*. pp. 239. London: Bell.

HAUGEN, M. G., FARRELL, W. R., HERRICK, J. F. AND BALDES, E. J. (1955). An ultrasonic flowmeter. *Proc. Nat. Electronics Conf.*, **11**, 1–11.

HAYNES, R. H. AND BURTON, A. C. (1959). Role of the non-Newtonian be-haviour of blood in hemodynamics. *Amer. J. Physiol.*, **197**, 943–950.

HELPS, E. P. W. AND MCDONALD, D. A. (1954a). Observations on laminar flow in veins. *J. Physiol.*, **124**, 631–9.

— — (1954b). Arterial blood flow calculated from pressure gradients. *J. Physiol.*, **124**, 30–31P.

HERRICK, J. F. (1942). Poiseuille's observations on blood flow lead to a law in hydrodynamics. *Amer. J. Phys.*, **10**, 33–39.

HESS, W. R. (1908). Die Viskosität des Blutes bei Gesunden. *Dtsch. Arch. klin Med.*, **94**, 404–8.

— (1911). Blutviskosität und Blutkörperchen. *Pflüg. Arch. ges. Physiol.*, **140**, 354.

— (1917). Uber die periphere Regulierung der Blutzirkulation. *Pflüg. Arch. ges. Physiol.*, **168**, 439–90.

— (1927). Die Verteilung von Querschnitt, Widerstand, Druckgefälle und Stromungsgeschwindigkeit im Blutkreislauf. *Handb. d. normale u. path. Physiol.* (*Bethe*), Bd. VII, Teil 2, pp. 904–33. Berlin: Springer.

HILL, L. (1900). The mechanism of the circulation of the blood. In *Text-book of physiology*, ed. Schäfer, E. A., vol. II. Edinburgh: Pentland.

HOGBEN, L. (1937). *Mathematics for the million.* pp.686. 2nd Edn. London: Unwin.

HÜRTHLE, K. (1920). Uber die Beziehung zwischen Durchmesser und Wandstärke der Arterien nebst Schätzung des Anteils der einzelnen Gewebe am Aufbau der Wand. *Pflüg. Arch. ges. Physiol.*, **183**, 253–70.

INOUYE, A. AND KOSAKA, H. (1959). A study of flow patterns in carotid and femoral arteries of rabbits and dogs with the electromagnetic flowmeter. *J. Physiol.*, **147**, 209–20.

INOUYE, A., KUGA, H. AND USUI, G. (1955). A new method for recording pressure-flow diagram applicable to peripheral blood vessels of animals and its application. *Jap. J. Physiol.*, **5**, 236–49.

JANSSEN, S., ASCHOFF, J., BAUMGARTNER, G., GRUPP, G., HIERHOLZER, K., HILLE, H., OBERDORF, A., RUMMEL, W. AND WEVER, R. (1957). Vergleich und Kritik verschiedener Durchblutungs-Messmethoden. *Pflüg. Arch. ges. Physiol.*, **264**, 198–216.

JOCHIM, K. E. (1948). Electromagnetic flow meter. pp. 108–15 in Vol. **1**, *Methods in Medical Research*, ed. Potter, V. R. Chicago: Year Book Publishing.

JONES, W. B., HEFNER, L. L., BANCROFT, J. R., AND KLIP, W. (1959). Velocity of blood flow and stroke volume obtained from the pressure pulse. *J. clin. Invest.*, **38**, 2087–2090.

KANI, L. (1910). *Virchows Arch.* (Cited by King, 1947b.)

KAPAL, E., MARTINI, F. AND WETTERER, E. (1951). Ueber die Zuverlässigkeit der bisherigen Bestimmungsart der Pulswellengeschwindigkeit. *Z. Biol.*, **104**, 75–86.

KARREMAN, G. (1952). Some contributions to the mathematical biology of blood circulation. Reflections of pressure waves in the arterial system. *Bull. math. Biophys.*, **14**, 327–50.

KING, A. L. (1947a). Waves in elastic tubes: velocity of the pulse wave in large arteries. *J. appl. Physics*, **18**, 595–600.

— (1947b). Elasticity of the aortic wall. *Science*, **105**, 127.

— (1950). Circulatory system: arterial pulse; wave velocity. In *Medical Physics*, vol. **2**, ed. Glasser, O. Chicago: Year Book Publishers.

KING, A. L. AND LAWTON, R. W. (1950). Elasticity of body tissues. In *Medical Physics*, vol. **2**, ed. Glasser, O. Chicago: Year Book Publishers.

KOLIN, A. (1945). An alternating field induction flow meter of high sensitivity. *Rev. sci. Instrum.*, **16**, 109–16.

KRAFKA, J. (1939). Comparative study of the histophysics of the aorta. *Amer. J. Physiol.*, **125**, 1–14.

KUMIN, K. (1949). *Bestimmung des Zähigkeitskoeffizienten μ' für Rinderblut bei Newton'schen Strömungen in verschieden weiten Röhren und Kapillaren bei physiologischer Temperatur.* pp. 48. Inaug. Diss. Freiburg i.d. Schweiz.

LAMB, H. (1932). *Hydrodynamics*, 5th Edn. (reprinted 1953). Cambridge: University Press.

LAMBOSSY, P. (1950). Aperçu historique et critique sur le problème de la propagation des ondes dans un liquid incompressible enfermé dans un tube élastique. *Helv. physiol. acta*, **8**, 209–77.

References

313

— (1952a). Oscillations forcées d'un liquide incompressible et visqueux dans un tube rigide et horizontal. Calcul de la force de frottement. *Helv. phys. acta*, **25**, 371–86.

— (1952b). Manomètres à l'observation des variations de la pression sanguine. *Helv. physiol. acta*, **10**, 138–60.

LAMPORT, H. (1955). Hemodynamics. pp. 589–611 in *Fulton's Textbook of Physiology*. Philadelphia: Saunders. 17th Edn.

LANDOWNE, M. (1953). Studies of dynamic characteristics of living arteries. p. 540 in *Abstr. Proc. XIX Internat. Congr. Physiol., Montreal*.

— (1954). Wave propagation in human arteries. *Fed. Proc.*, **13**, 83.

— (1957a). Pulse wave velocity as an index of arterial elastic characteristics. pp. 168–76 in *Tissue elasticity*, ed. Remington, J. W. Washington: American Physiological Society.

— (1957b). A method using induced waves to study pressure propagation in human arteries. *Circ. Research*, **5**, 594–601.

— (1958). Characteristics of impact and pulse wave propagation in brachial and radial arteries. *J. appl. Physiol.*, **12**, 91–97.

LANGE, R. L., CARLISLE, R. P. AND HECHT, H. H. (1956). Observations on vascular sounds: the "pistol-shot" sound and the Korotkoff sound. *Circulation*, **13**, 873–83.

LASZT, L. AND MÜLLER, A. (1952a). Über den Druckverlauf im Bereiche der Aorta. *Helv. physiol. acta*, **10**, 1–9.

— — (1952b). Gleichzeitige Druckmessung in der Aorta abdominalis und ihre Hauptästen. *Helv. physiol. acta*, **10**, 259–72.

— — (1957). Über Druck- und Geschwindigkeitsverhältnisse im Coronar Krieslauf des Hundes. *Helv. physiol. acta*, **18**, 38–54.

LAWTON, R. W. (1954). The thermoelastic behaviour of isolated aortic strips of the dog. *Circ. Research*, **2**, 344–53.

— (1955). Measurements on the elasticity and damping of isolated aortic strips of the dog. *Circ. Research*, **3**, 403–8.

LAWTON, R. W. AND GREENE, L. C. (1956). A method for the *in situ* study of aortic elasticity in the dog. *Report No. NADC-MA-5603. A.M.A.L., U.S., Nav. Air Dev. Cent.*

LEUSEN, I., DEMEESTER, G. AND BOUCKAERT, J. J. (1954). Influence des reflexes sino-carotidiens sur le débit cardiaque et la résistance périphérique après hémorragie. *Arch. int. Physiol.*, **62**, 535–9.

LEVY, M. N. (1958). Relative influence of variations in arterial and venous pressures on resistance to flow. *Amer. J. Physiol.*, **192**, 164–70.

LEVY, M. N. AND SHARE, L. (1953). The influence of erythrocyte concentration upon the pressure-flow relationships in the dog's hind limb. *Circ. Research*, **1**, 247–55.

LEVY, M. N., BRIND, S. H., BRANDLIN, F. R. AND PHILLIPS, F. A. (1954). The relationship between pressure and flow in the systemic circulation of the dog. *Circ. Research*, **2**, 372–80.

LINDEN, R. J. (1958). A hydraulic pressure wave generator. *J. Physiol.*, **142**, 44–46P.

MACHELLA, T. E. (1936). The velocity of blood flow in arteries in animals. *Amer. J. Physiol.*, **115**, 632–44.

MCDONALD, D. A. (1952a). The velocity of blood flow in the rabbit aorta studied with high-speed cinematography. *J. Physiol.*, **118**, 328–39.

— (1952b). The occurrence of turbulent flow in the rabbit aorta. *J. Physiol.*, **118**, 340–7.

— (1952c). Lateral pulsatile expansion of arteries. *J. Physiol.*, **119**, 28P.

— (1954). Arterial flow pattern in relation to changes in vascular resistances. *J. Physiol.*, **125**, 36*P*.

— (1955*a*). The relation of pulsatile pressure to flow in arteries. *J. Physiol.*, **127**, 533–52.

— (1955*b*). An apparatus for the analysis of film records. *J. Physiol.*, **127**, 25–26*P*.

MCDONALD, D. A. AND HELPS, E. P. W. (1954). Streamline flow in veins. Film: 16 mm colour sound. Wellcome Film Unit. (Available on loan from Wellcome Foundation.)

MCDONALD, D. A. AND POTTER, J. M. (1951). The distribution of blood to the brain. *J. Physiol.*, **114**, 356–71.

MCDONALD, D. A. AND TAYLOR, M. G. (1956). An investigation of the arterial system using a hydraulic oscillator. *J. Physiol.*, **133**, 74*P*.

— — (1957). The phase velocities of harmonic components of the pulse wave. *J. Physiol.*, **137**, 87–88*P*.

— — (1959). The hydrodynamics of the arterial circulation. In *Progress in Biophysics*, **9**, 107–73. London: Pergamon Press.

MCKUSICK, V. A. (1957). Cardiovascular sound: a clinical survey. *Circulation*, **16**, 424–7.

— (1958). *Cardiovascular sound in health and disease.* pp. 570. Baltimore: Williams & Wilkins.

MCKUSICK, V. A., KLINE, E. W. AND WEBB, G. N. (1955). Spectral phonocardiographic demonstrations of selected varieties of cardiovascular sound. *Amer. Heart J.*, **49**, 911–33.

— — — (1954). Spectral phonocardiography: problems and prospects in the application of the Bell sound spectrograph to phonocardiography. *Johns Hopk. Hosp. Bull.*, **94**, 187–98.

MCKUSICK, V. A., MURRAY, G. E., PEELER, R. G. AND WEBB, G. N. (1955). Musical murmurs. *Johns Hopk. Hosp. Bull.*, **97**, 136–76.

MCKUSICK, V. A., WEBB, G. N., HUMPHRIES, J. O'N. AND READ. J. A. (1955). On cardiovascular sound: further observations by means of spectral phonocardiography. *Circulation*, **11**, 849–70.

MCMILLAN, I. K. R. (1955). Aortic stenosis. A post-mortem cinephotographic study of valve action. *Brit. Heart J.*, **17**, 56–62.

MCMILLAN, I. K. R., DALEY, R. AND MATHEWS, M. B. (1952). The movement of aortic and pulmonary valves studied post-mortem by colour cinematography. *Brit. Heart J.*, **14**, 42–46.

MacWILLIAM, J. A. AND MACKIE, A. H. (1908). Observations on arteries, normal and pathological. *Brit. med. J.*, ii, 1477–81.

MARSHALL, R, J. AND SHEPHERD, J. T. (1959). Effect of injections of hypertonic solutions on blood flow through the femoral artery of the dog. *Amer. J. Physiol.*, **197**, 951–954.

MEIER, P. AND ZIERLER, K. L. (1954). On the theory of the indicator-dilution method for the measurement of blood flow and volume. *J. appl. Physiol.*, **6**, 731–44.

MOENS, A. I. (1878). *Die Pulskurve.* Leiden.

MORGAN, G. W., AND KIELY, J. P. (1954). Wave propagation in a viscous liquid contained in a flexible tube. *J. acoust. Soc. Amer.*, **26**, 323–8.

MORGAN, G. W. AND FERRANTE, W. R. (1955). Wave propagation in elastic tubes filled with streaming liquid. *J. acoust. Soc. Amer.*, **27**, 715–25.

MÜLLER, A. (1948). Uber das Druckgefälle in Blutgefässen, insbesondere in den Kapillaren. *Helv. physiol. acta*, **6**, 181–95.

— (1950). Über die Fortpflanzungsgeschwindigkeit von Druckwellen in dehnbaren Röhren bei ruhender und strömender Flüssigkeit. *Helv. physiol. acta,* **8**, 228–41.

— (1951). Über die Abhängigkeit der Fortplanzungsgeschwindigkeit und der Dämpfung der Druckwellen in dehnbaren Röhren von deren Wellenlänge. *Helv. physiol. acta,* **9**, 162–76.

— (1954a). Über die Verwendung des Pitot-Rohres zur Geschwindigkeitsmessung. *Helv. physiol. acta,* **12**, 98–111.

— (1954b). Über die Verwendung des Castelli-Prinzips zur Geschwindigkeitsmessung. *Helv. physiol. acta,* **12**, 300–15.

MÜLLER, O. AND SHILLINGFORD, J. P. (1954). A manometer for differential and single pressure measurements. *J. Physiol.,* **127**, 2P.

NEWMAN, F. H. AND SEARLE, V. H. L. (1957). *The general properties of matter.* pp. 431. 5th Edn. London: Arnold.

NOBLE, F. W. (1953). *Electrical methods of blood-pressure recording.* pp. 56. Springfield, Ill.: Thomas.

NOORDERGRAAF, A. AND HOREMAN, H. W. (1958). Numerical evaluation of volume pulsations in man. II. Calculated volume pulsations of forearm and calf. *Phys. Med. Biol.,* **3**, 59–70.

NYGAARD, K. K., WILDER, M. AND BERKSON, J. (1935). The relation between the viscosity of the blood and the relative volume of erythrocytes (haematocrit value). *Amer. J. Physiol.,* **114**, 128–31.

PAPPENHEIMER, J. R. (1954). Differential conductance manometer. *Rev. Sci. Instrum.,* **25**, 912–17.

PETERSON, L. H. (1952). Certain physical characteristics of the cardiovascular system and their significance in the problem of calculating stroke volume from the arterial pulse. *Fed. Proc.,* **11**, 762–73.

— (1954). The dynamics of pulsatile blood flow. *Circ. Research,* **2**, 127–39.

— (1956). On the significance of arterial pressure pulse distortion. *Comm. XX Internat. Congr. Physiol. Brussels,* 720–1.

PETERSON, L. H. AND SHEPARD, R. B. (1955). Some relationships of blood pressure to the cardiovascular system. *Surg. Clin. N. Amer.,* **35**, 1613–28.

PHILLIPS, F. A., BRIND, S. H. AND LEVY, M. N. (1955). The immediate influence of increased venous pressure upon resistance to flow in the dog's hind leg. *Circ. Research,* **3**, 357–62.

PIEPER, H. AND WETTERER, E. (1953a). Elektrische Registrierung der Blutströmungsgeschwindigkeit mit neuartigen Strompendeln. *Verh. dtsch. Ges. Kreislaufforsch.,* 19 Tagung, 264–9.

— — (1953b). Strompendel für elektrische Registrierung der Blutströmungsgeschwindigkeit. *Z. Biol.,* **105**, 214–23.

PORJÉ, I. G. (1946). Studies of the arterial pulse wave, particularly in the aorta. *Acta physiol. scand.,* **13**, Suppl. 42, 1–68.

POTTER, J. M. AND MCDONALD, D. A. (1950). Cinematographic recording of the velocity of arterial blood flow. *Nature, Lond.,* **166**, 596–7.

PRANDTL, L. (1952). *Essentials of fluid dynamics.* pp. 452. London: Blackie.

PREC, O., KATZ, L. N., SENNETT, L., ROSEMAN, R. H., FISHMAN, A. P. AND HWANG, W. (1949). Determination of kinetic energy of the heart in man. *Amer. J. Physiol.,* **159**, 483–91.

PRITCHARD, W. H., GREGG, D. E., SHIPLEY, R. E. AND WEISBERGER, A. S. (1943). A study of flow and pattern responses in peripheral arteries to the injection of vasomotor drugs. *Amer. J. Physiol.,* **138**, 731–40.

RALSTON, H. J. AND TAYLOR, A. N. (1945). Streamline flow in the arteries of the dog and cat. *Amer. J. Physiol.,* **144**, 706–10.

RALSTON, J. H., TAYLOR, A. N. AND ELLIOTT, H. W. (1947). Further studies on streamline blood flow in the arteries of the cat. *Amer. J. Physiol.*, **150**, 52–57.

RANDALL, J. E. (1958). Statistical properties of pulsatile pressure and flow in the femoral artery of the dog. *Circ. Research*, **6**, 689–98.

RANDALL, J. E. AND HORVATH, S. (1953). Relationship between duration of ischaemia and reactive hyperaemia in a single vessel. *Amer. J. Physiol.*, **172**, 391–8.

RANDALL, J. E. AND STACY, R. W. (1956a). Pulsatile and steady pressure-flow relations in the vascular bed of the hind leg of the dog. *Amer. J. Physiol.*, **185**, 351–4.

— — (1956b). Mechanical impedance of the dog's hind leg to pulsatile blood flow. *Amer. J. Physiol.*, **187**, 94–98.

READ, R. C., KUIDA, H. AND JOHNSON, J. A. (1958). Venous pressure and total peripheral resistance in the dog. *Amer. J. Physiol.*, **192**, 609–12.

REMINGTON, J. W. (1952). Volume quantitation of the aortic pressure pulse. *Fed. Proc.*, **11**, 750–61.

— (1954). The relation between the stroke volume and the pulse pressure. *Minn. Med.*, **37**, 75–80.

— (1955). Hysteresis loop behaviour of the aorta and other extensible tissues. *Amer. J. Physiol.*, **180**, 83–95.

— (1957). Ed. *Tissue elasticity.* pp. vii and 203. Washington: American Physiological Society.

REMINGTON, J. W. AND HAMILTON, W. F. (1945). The construction of a theoretical cardiac ejection curve from the contour of the aortic pressure pulse. *Amer. J. Physiol.*, **144**, 546–56.

— — (1947). Quantitative calculation of the time course of cardiac ejection from the pressure pulse. *Amer. J. Physiol.*, **148**, 25–34.

REMINGTON, J. W. AND WOOD, E. H. (1956). Formation of peripheral pulse contour in man. *J. appl. Physiol.*, **9**, 433–42.

REMINGTON, J. W., HAMILTON, W. F. AND DOW, P. (1945). Some difficulties involved in the prediction of the stroke volume from the pulse-wave velocity. *Amer. J. Physiol.*, **144**, 536–45.

REUTERWALL, O. P. (1921). Uber die Elastizität des Gefässwände und die Methoden ihrer näheren Prufung. *Acta med. scand.*, **55**, Suppl. 2, 1–175.

REYNOLDS, O. (1883). An experimental investigation of the circumstances which determine whether the motion of water shall be direct or sinuous, and of the law of resistance in parallel channels. *Philos. Trans.*, **174**, 935–82.

REYNOLDS, S. R. M., LIGHT, F. W., ARDRAN, G. M. AND PRICHARD, M. M. L. (1952). The qualitative nature of pulsatile flow in the umbilical blood vessels, with observations on flow in the aorta. *Johns Hopk. Hosp. Bull.*, **91**, 83–104.

RICHARDS, T. G. AND WILLIAMS, T. D. (1953). Velocity changes in the carotid and femoral arteries of dogs during the cardiac cycle. *J. Physiol.*, **120**, 257–66.

RICHARDSON, A. W., DENISON, A. B. JR. AND GREEN, H. D. (1952). A newly modified electromagnetic blood flowmeter capable of high fidelity flow registration. *Circulation*, **5**, 430–6.

ROACH, M. R. AND BURTON, A. C. (1957). The reason for the shape of the distensibility curves of arteries. *Canad. J. Biochem. Physiol.*, **35**, 681–90.

ROBINSON, W. S. (1952). The problem of heart murmurs. *D.S.I.R. Report* (restricted) *Mech. Engineering Res. Lab., East Kilbride, Scotland.*

RODBARD, S. (1957). Transients as a mechanism in the production of heart sounds and murmurs. *Circulation,* 16, 282–3.

ROSSI, H. H., POWERS, S. H. AND DWORK, B. (1953). Measurement of flow in straight tubes by means of the dilution technique. *Amer. J. Physiol.,* 173, 103–8.

RUSHMER, R. F. (1955a). *Cardiac diagnosis: a physiologic approach.* pp. 447. Philadelphia and London: Saunders.

— (1955b). Pressure-circumference relations in the aorta. *Amer. J. Physiol.,* 183, 545–9.

— (1957). Valve mechanics. *Circulation,* 16, 270–2.

RYAN, J. M., STACY, R. W. AND WATMAN, R. N. (1956). Role of abdominal aortic branches in pulse wave contour genesis. *Circ. Research,* 4, 676–9.

RYMER, T. B. AND BUTLER, C. C. (1944). An electrical circuit for harmonic analysis and other calculations. *Phil. Mag.,* 35, 606–16.

SAFFMAN, P. G. (1956). On the motion of small spheroidal particles in a viscous liquid. *J. Fluid Mech.,* 1, 540–53.

SCHER, A. M., WEIGERT, T. H. AND YOUNG, A. C. (1953). Compact flowmeters for use in the unanesthetized animal, an electronic version of Chauveau's hemodrometer. *Science,* 118, 82–84.

SCHLEIER, J. (1918). Der Energieverbrauch in der Blutbahn. *Pflüg. Arch. ges. Physiol.,* 173, 172–204.

SCHONFELD, J. C. (1948). Resistance and inertia of the flow of liquids in a tube or open canal. *Appl. Sci. Res., A,* 1, 169–97.

SHIPLEY, R. E., GREGG, D. E. AND SCHROEDER, E. F. (1943). An experimental study of flow patterns in various peripheral arteries. *Amer. J. Physiol.,* 138, 718–30.

SIMONS, J. R. AND MICHAELIS, A. R. (1953). A cinematographic technique, using ultra-violet illumination for amphibian blood circulation. *Nature, Lond.,* 71, 801.

SINN, W. (1956). Die Elastizität der Arterien und ihre Bedeutung für die Dynamik des arteriellen Systems. *Akad. d. Wiss. u. Lit. Mainz, Jahrgang,* 1956, 647–832.

SMITH, C. A. B. (1954). *Biomathematics: the principles of mathematics for students of biological science.* 3rd Edn. London: Griffin.

SPENCER, M. P. AND DENISON, A. B. (1956). The aortic flow pulse as related to differential pressure. *Circ. Research,* 4, 476–84.

SPENCER, M. P., JOHNSTON, F. R. AND DENISON, A. B. (1958). Dynamics of the normal aorta. "Inertiance" and "compliance" of the arterial system which transforms the cardiac ejection pulse. *Circ. Research,* 6, 491–500.

STACY, R. W., WILLIAMS, D. T., WORDEN, R. E. AND MCMORRIS, R. O. (1955). *Essentials of biological and medical physics.* pp. viii and 586. New York: McGraw-Hill.

STARR, I. (1957). Studies made by simulating systole at necropsy. X. State of peripheral circulation in cadavers. *J. appl. Physiol.,* 11, 174–80.

STARR, I. AND SCHILD, A. (1957). Studies made by simulating systole at necropsy. IX. A test of the aortic compression chamber hypothesis and of two stroke volume methods based upon it. *J. appl. Physiol.,* 11, 169–73.

STARR, I., SCHNABEL, T. G. AND MAYCOCK, R. L. (1953). Studies made by simulating systole at necropsy. II. Experiments on the relation of cardiac and peripheral factors to the genesis of the pulse wave and the ballistocardiogram. *Circulation*, 8, 44–61.

STAUFFER, H. M., OPPENHEIMER, M. J., STEWART, G. H. AND LYNCH, P. R. (1955). Cinefluorography by image amplifier techniques. *J. appl. Physiol.*, 8, 343–6.

STEHBENS, W. E. (1959). Turbulence of blood flow. *Quart. J. exp. Physiol.*, 44, 110–117.

TAYLOR, M. G. (1955). The flow of blood in narrow tubes. II. The axial stream and its formation, as determined by changes in optical density. *Aust. J. exp. Biol. med. Sci.*, 33, 1–16.

— (1956). The mathematical analysis of the pulse wave. *C.R. II Congr. Angiol. Fribourg*, 1955, pp. 412–15.

— (1957a). An approach to an analysis of the arterial pulse-wave. I. Oscillations in an attenuating line. *Phys. Med. Biol.*, 1, 258–69.

— (1957b). An approach to an analysis of the arterial pulse wave. II. Fluid oscillations in an elastic pipe. *Phys. Med. Biol.*, 1, 321–9.

— (1958a). A simple electrical computer for Fourier analysis and synthesis. *J. Physiol.*, 141, 23–25P.

— (1958b). The discrepancy between steady- and oscillatory-flow calibration of flowmeters of the "bristle" and "pendulum" types: a theoretical study. *Phys. Med. Biol.*, 2, 324–37.

— (1959a). The influence of the anomalous viscosity of blood upon its oscillatory flow. *Phys. Med. Biol.*, 3, 273–90.

— (1959b). An experimental determination of the propagation of fluid oscillations in a tube with a visco-elastic wall; together with an analysis of the characteristics required in an electrical analogue. *Phys. Med. Biol.*, 4, 63–82.

TIMM, C. (1942). Der Strömungsverlauf in einem Modell der menschlichen Aorta. *Z. Biol.*, 101, 79–99.

WARBURG, E. (1950). A method of determining the undamped natural frequency and the damping in over-damped and slightly underdamped systems of one degree of freedom by means of a square-wave impact. *Acta physiol. scand.*, 19, 344–9.

WARNER, H. R., SWAN, H. J. C., CONNOLLY, D. C., TOMPKINS, R. G. AND WOOD, E. H. (1953). Quantitation of beat-to-beat changes in stroke volume from the aortic pulse contour in man. *J. appl. Physiol.*, 5, 495–507.

WARREN, J. V. (1948). Determination of cardiac output in man by right heart catheterization. In *Methods in medical research*, vol. 1, ed. Potter, V. R. pp. 224–50. Chicago: Year Book Publishers.

WEBER, E. H. (1850). *Ber. der Sächs. Ges. der Wiss.*, 1850, 166. (Cited by Lambossy, P., 1950.)

WEHN, P. S. (1957). Pulsatory activity of peripheral arteries. *Suppl. Scand. J. clin. lab. invest.*, 9, pp. 106. Thesis: Oslo.

WETTERER, E. (1944). Eine neue manometrische Sonde mit elektrischer Transmission. *Z. Biol.*, 101, 332–50.

— (1954). Flow and pressure in the arterial system, their hemodynamic relationship, and the principles of their measurement. *Minn. Med.*, 37, 77–86.

— (1956). Die Wirkung der Herztätigkeit auf die Dynamik des Arteriensystems. *Verh. dtsch. Ges. Kreislaufforsch.*, 22 Tagung, 26–60.

WETTERER, E. AND DEPPE, B. (1940). *Z. Biol.*, **100**, 205, also *ibid.*, **99**, 320 (cited by Wetterer, 1954).

WETTERER, E. AND PIEPER, H. (1952). Eine neue manometrische Sonde mit elektrischer Transmission. *Z. Biol.*, **105**, 49–65.

WEVER, R. AND ASCHOFF, J. (1956). Durchflussmessung mit der Diathermie-Thermostromuhr bei pulsierenden Stromung. *Pflüg. Arch. ges. Physiol.*, **262**, 152–68.

WEZLER, K. AND BOGER, A. (1939). Die Dynamik des arteriellen Systems. Der arterielle Blutdruck und seine Komponenten. *Ergebn. Physiol.*, **41**, 292–606.

WEZLER, K. AND SINN, W. (1953). *Das Strömungsgesetz des Kreislaufes.* pp. 126. Aulendorf i. Wurtt. Editio Cantor.

WHITBY, L. E. H. AND BRITTON, C. J. C. (1950). *Disorders of the blood.* pp. 759. London: Churchill.

WHITTAKER, S. R. F. AND WINTON, F. R. (1933). The apparent viscosity of blood flowing in the isolated hindlimb of the dog and its variation with corpuscular concentration. *J. Physiol.*, **78**, 339–69.

WIDMER, L. K. (1957). Zur Strömungsgeschwindigkeit in kleinsten peripheren Arterien. *Arch. Kreislaufforsch.*, **27**, 54–81.

WIEDERHIELM, C. A., BRUCE, R. A. AND JOHN, G. G. (1957). Continuous recording of oxygen saturation during cardiac catheterization. *Amer. J. med. Sci.*, **233**, 542–5.

WIGGERS, C. J. (1928). *The pressure pulses in the cardiovascular system.* pp. xi and 200. London: Longmans.

— (1949). *Physiology in health and disease.* 5th Edn. pp. 1242. London: Kimpton.

WINTON, F. R. (1926). The influence of length on the responses of unstriated muscle to electrical and chemical stimulation, and stretching. *J. Physiol.*, **61**, 368–82.

WISKIND, H. K. (1957). Discussion on mechanisms of cardiovascular sound. *Circulation*, **16**, 283–8.

WINTROBE, M. M. (1942). *Clinical haematology.* pp. 792. London: Kimpton.

WITZIG, K. (1914). *Über erzwungene Wellenbewegungen zäher, inkompressibler Flüssigkeiten in elastischen Röhren. Inaug. Diss. Bern.* Bern: Wyss.

WOMERSLEY, J. R. (1954). Flow in the larger arteries and its relation to the oscillating pressure. *J. Physiol.*, **124**, 31–32P.

— (1955a). Oscillatory flow in arteries: effect of radial variation in viscosity on rate of flow. *J. Physiol.*, **127**, 38–39P.

— (1955b). Method for the calculation of velocity, rate of flow and viscous drag in arteries when the pressure gradient is known. *J. Physiol.*, **127**, 553–63.

— (1955c). Oscillatory motion of a viscous liquid in a thin-walled elastic tube. I. The linear approximation for long waves. *Phil. Mag.*, **46**, 199–221.

— (1957). Oscillatory flow in arteries: the constrained elastic tube as a model of arterial flow and pulse transmission. *Phys. Med. Biol.*, **2**, 178–87.

— (1958a). The mathematical analysis of the arterial circulation in a state of oscillatory motion. *Wright Air Development Center, Technical Report WADC-TR*56-614.

— (1958b). Oscillatory flow in arteries: the reflection of the pulse wave at junctions and rigid inserts in the arterial system. *Phys. Med. Biol.*, **2**, 313–23.

WOOD, E. H., LENSEN, I. R., WARNER, H. R. AND WRIGHT, J. L. (1954). Measurement of pressures by cardiac catheters in man. *Minn. Med.*, **37**, 57–62.

WOOD, G. C. (1954). Some tensile properties of elastic tissue. *Biochim. biophys. acta*, **15**, 311–31.

YOUNG, T. (1808). Hydraulic investigations, subservient to an intended Croonian lecture on the motion of the blood. *Philos. Trans.*, **98**, 164–86.

— (1809). The Croonian lecture. On the functions of the heart and arteries. *Philos. Trans.*, **99**, 1–31.